HANDBOOK OF HEARING AID AMPLIFICATION, VOLUME II:

CLINICAL CONSIDERATIONS

AND FITTING PRACTICES

HANDBOOK OF HEARING AID AMPLIFICATION, VOLUME II:

CLINICAL CONSIDERATIONS AND

FITTING PRACTICES

EDITED BY ■

ROBERT E. SANDLIN

ADJUNCT PROFESSOR OF AUDIOLOGY

DEPARTMENT OF COMMUNICATIVE DISORDERS

SAN DIEGO STATE UNIVERSITY, SAN DIEGO, CALIFORNIA

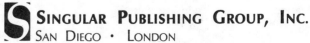
SINGULAR PUBLISHING GROUP, INC.
SAN DIEGO · LONDON

Singular Publishing Group
4284 41st Street
San Diego, California 92105-1197

19 Compton Terrace
London N1 2UN, U.K.

Typeset in 10/12 Times by CFW Graphics
Printed in the United States of America by McNaughton & Gunn

Library of Congress Cataloging-in-Publication Data
  (Revised for volume 2)

Handbook of hearing aid amplification.

   "A College-Hill publication."
   Includes bibliographies and index.
   Contents: v. 1. Theoretical and technical
considerations. — v. 2. Clinical considerations and
fitting practices.
   1. Hearing aids.   I. Sandlin, Robert E.
RF300.H36   1988   617.8′9   88-6832

ISBN 1-56503-399-0 (Volume 1)
ISBN 1-56593-400-8 (Volume 2)

■ CONTENTS

■ PREFACE

Clinical approaches to the selection, fitting, and verification of hearing aid devices used by individuals with acoustic impairments often have appeared contradictory and less than absolute in meeting the needs of persons who use amplification. This text is not intended to offer a resolution to all of the differences existing in decision-making processes regarding hearing aids, but rather to present ideas and clinical experiences of those professionals who deserve to be heard.

In truth, there is no one thought or clinical procedure presented by any one individual or group that has captured the attention of all practitioners involved in fitting hearing aids. However, evident in this textbook is a working premise that there is an *objectivity* that can be brought to bear in determining the most appropriate hearing aid system best meeting the electroacoustic needs of a given hearing loss.

This statement is not to suggest that the "whole person" is ignored in favor of assessing only the electroacoustic needs based on a given formula or clinical procedure, but rather that *objectivity* can add to the success and utility of hearing aid use. To do otherwise is to paint an unrealistic picture of that which can be done and the value to the patient of having done it.

This text represents the collected efforts of a number of well-informed contributors who share their experiences in the various phases of the selection, fitting, and verification of hearing aid instruments, as well as effective patient management strategies. Each is to be congratulated for a difficult task done extremely well.

Ronald Reiter, consistent with his conviction that the dispenser must work with the "whole person," presents an in-depth review of the psychology of the individual with hearing impairment. Based on his experience as an audiologist and clinical psychologist, he presents a unique and sensitive overview of the problems that present themselves. H. Gustav Mueller and David Hawkins skillfully remind us that the hearing health professional must attend to a number of important selection and fitting issues. They discuss the contributions of directional microphones in resolving some of the difficulties associated with hearing aid use, review the role that loudness assessment (loudness discomfort level) plays in the selection and fitting process, and provide a thought-provoking review of binaural amplification and its application to individuals who are bilaterally hearing impaired. David Pascoe offers clinical suggestions in the post-fitting management of the hearing aid patient. His many years of practical experience gained at the Central Institute for the Deaf are evident in his chapter and are of appreciable benefit to the reader. Brad Stach treats with considerable adroitness those problems of hearing aid selection and fitting for individuals with central processing disorders. He stresses the importance of differential diagnosis in determining the presence of central processing dysfunction and the appropriateness of hearing aid use. Jerry Northern, Sandra Abbott Gabbard, and Deborah Kinder combine their years of experience to produce an excellent chapter that defines the important clinical aspects related to fitting hearing aid devices for the young and the care that must be exercised in working with the parents of the children involved. Robert Novak and Aram Glorig perform a most difficult task of bringing into focus the unique problems associated with geriatric populations requiring hearing amplification. Stress is given to the psychosocial behaviors that often may mitigate against hearing aid use. Dan Konkle and Jill Molloy present challenging data questioning continued use of various aspects of speech-based hearing aid evaluation schemes. Although speech-based procedures are not rejected, the authors question the exclusive use of them in the determination of hearing aid need. Dianne Mecklenburg puts into proper perspective the clinical application of cochlear implantation in patients who cannot, or do not, benefit from the conventional hearing aid amplification systems. Michael Seitz and Dennis Kisiel do an outstanding job in presenting data relative to the application of auditory evoked responses in the hearing aid assessment and selection process. Assessment protocols and some of the problems associated with them are emphasized. Support is given to the utility of auditory brainstem response (ABR) measurement when the patient is unable to offer voluntary response to acoustic stimuli. John Tecca does a brilliant job in reviewing the applicability and utility of real-ear probe tube measurements. He emphasizes that recent development of "user friendly" systems have advanced the practice of selection and fitting of hearing aid amplification systems and are of considerable value to the hearing instrument dispenser. Finally, I discuss the application of sound-field audiometry and its clinical utility in hearing aid evaluation practices relative to the selection, fitting, and verification processes.

This book offers the reader information that reflects current practices that have direct clinical value to the practitioner. Acceptance of this book by those involved in the rather wide-ranging field of hearing aid amplification and its application to specific hearing impairments will serve as justification for the considerable effort put forth by those individuals who made it possible.

I am indebted to so many individuals who have served as my mentors over the past several years, that to list them all in a manner consistent with their contribution would be to extend this preface far beyond its normal bounds. Just let me say "thank you" to them all.

Robert E. Sandlin, Editor

■ CONTRIBUTORS

Sandra Abbott Gabbard, M.A.
Clinical Instructor
Department of Otolaryngology
University of Colorado School of Medicine
Clinical Audiologist
Division of Audiology
University of Colorado Health
  Sciences Center
Denver, Colorado

Aram Glorig, M.D.
Senior Advisor
House Ear Institute
Los Angeles, California

David B. Hawkins, Ph.D.
Professor
Department of Communicative Disorders
University of South Carolina
Columbia, South Carolina

Deborah L. Kinder, M.A.
Instructor in Otolaryngology
Division of Audiology
Department of Otolaryngology
University Hospital
University of Colorado Health
  Sciences Center
Denver, Colorado

Dennis L. Kisiel, Ph.D.
Director
Audiology Division
Long Island College Hospital
Brooklyn, New York

Dan F. Konkle, Ph.D.
Director
Department of Communicative Disorders
Children's Seashore House
Associate Professor of Audiology

Department of Otorhinolaryngology and
  Human Communication
University of Pennsylvania School
  of Medicine
Philadelphia, Pennsylvania

Dianne J. Mecklenburg, Ph.D.
Cochlear Implant Specialist
Cavale Consulting
Boulder, Colorado

Jill M. Molloy, M.A.
Senior Audiologist
Communication Disorders Center
Children's Seashore House and
Children's Hospital of Philadelphia
Philadelphia, Pennsylvania

H. Gustav Mueller, Ph.D.
Chief
Division of Audiology and Speech-Language
  Pathology
Letterman Army Medical Center
Presidio of San Francisco
San Francisco, California

Jerry L. Northern, Ph.D.
Professor of Otolaryngology
Associate Professor of Pediatrics
Head
Audiology Division
Department of Otolaryngology
University Hospital
University of Colorado School of Medicine
Denver, Colorado

Robert E. Novak, Ph.D., CCC-A
Associate Professor of Communicative
  Disorders
Department of Communicative Disorders
San Diego State University
San Diego, California

David P. Pascoe, Ph.D.
Associate Professor
Washington University
Clinical Audiologist
Central Institute for the Deaf
St. Louis, Missouri

Ronald S. Reiter, Ph.D.
Director
Counseling Service
Hope for Hearing Foundation
University of California at Los Angeles
Los Angeles, California

Robert E. Sandlin, Ph.D.
Adjunct Professor of Audiology
Department of Communicative Disorders
San Diego State University
San Diego, California

Michael R. Seitz, Ph.D.
Professor of Communicative Disorders
Department of Communicative Disorders
San Diego State University
San Diego, California

Brad A. Stach, Ph.D.
Assistant Professor
Baylor College of Medicine
Director
Audiology and Speech Pathology Service
The Methodist Hospital
Houston, Texas

John E. Tecca, Ph.D.
Partner
Hearing Services and Systems
Portage, Michigan

PSYCHOLOGY OF THE HEARING IMPAIRED AND HEARING AID USE: THE ART OF DISPENSING

RONALD S. REITER ∎

Understanding the *behavior* of people with hearing impairments is of value to professionals who fit and dispense hearing aids. Even to the casual observer, it is apparent that individuals with hearing losses encounter daily experiences that differ from those of persons with normal hearing. This is very evident in the communication process and the problems associated with it. The question is whether persons with hearing impairment differ significantly from persons with normal hearing relative to the stresses and adverse conditions of life and the ways in which they are managed. Is there a unique psychology of the hearing impaired that sets them apart from others who experience different, unwanted life changes that create problems needing resolution? The answer to this question is that hearing-impaired persons do not differ appreciably from normal hearing persons in their reactions to problems or in the way they manage them.

There are a number of possible explanations for the unique behaviors of individuals with hearing impairment, some of which suggest a commonality of reactions and stages through which individuals who lose hearing pass. However, the author feels strongly that there are behaviors that are universal to humans that are independent of hearing impairment or any other disability. If the audiologist or dispenser understands the stages that hearing-impaired individuals pass through in resolving problems, the task of hearing aid selection, fitting, and management becomes much easier. The purpose of this chapter is to review problems encountered by hearing-impaired individuals and to suggest ways in which effective management can be instrumental in gaining acceptance and use of hearing aid devices.

Unless a hearing-impaired individual has accepted the hearing loss and all that it implies relative to emotional, social, and intellectual experiences, the task of management is very difficult. The probability of rejection of amplification remains high among hearing-impaired individuals who are not ready to accept the need for and use of hearing aids.

The human mind is a complex entity, and the resolution of problems that interfere with the enjoyment of life are not simple issues that present themselves in blacks and whites. The hearing health practitioner often deals in shades of gray when attempting to understand the psychology or behavior of hearing-impaired individuals and their utilization of hearing aids. The more one appreciates the complex behaviors of people and learns to deal with them, the more one can appreciate the gray tones. By achieving this understanding, the practitioner can offer better clinical services to individuals with hearing loss who elect to use hearing aid devices. Consider the following personality types and their responses to and need for amplification.

Mrs. G. is an 81-year old widow with a moderately severe bilateral sensorineural hearing loss. Mr. T. is a 57-year-old engineer with one normal ear who is dissatisfied with his bi-cros hearing aid. Ms. L. is a 29-year-old graduate student with a severely fluctuating hearing loss resulting from Meniere's disease. How does the professional hearing aid dispenser get to know these people in order to help them? What will make or break the relationship between the dispenser and these individuals?

This chapter is a segue between the two volumes of this handbook. The reader should understand Volume I, *Theoretical Considerations in Hearing Aid Amplification,* before moving on to Volume II, *Clinical Procedures and Fitting Considerations.* Similarly, the person *between* the ears must be understood, as well as amplification and hearing processes, before dispensing hearing aids. We will refer to understanding individuals with hearing impairments as the psychology of the hearing impaired and to understanding how people (both the client

and the dispenser) behave within the dispensing relationship as the psychology of hearing aid dispensing.

Webster's New World Dictionary (1966) describes human psychology as (1) "the science dealing with the mind and mental processes, as well as feelings, desires, etc.," and (2) "the sum of a person's actions, traits, attitudes, thoughts, etc." What we are talking about is an enormous rubric of what a person, in this case, a person with a hearing loss, is all about. The first task in discussing the psychology of the hearing impaired is a difficult one: reducing hearing-impaired individuals to common personality denominators. Personality factors related to hearing impairment are strongly affected by two variables: age and degree of hearing loss. This discussion, for the most part, will be limited to hard-of-hearing adults who are hearing aid candidates.

The Deaf Population of the United States (Schein & Delk, 1974) is the published report of a national census of the deaf population and also describes the extent and characteristics of the hearing impaired population. Table 1–1 presents the prevalence and prevalence rates for significant bilateral hearing loss by age and sex. Schein and Delk defined significant bilateral hearing impairment as hearing loss that is present in both ears and in which the better ear has difficulty hearing and understanding speech. In a population of 6,549,643 hearing-impaired individuals, only 440,595 developed hearing losses prior to age 17. Those persons born with little or no hearing, whom we usually refer to as deaf, and children with moderately severe losses comprise the populations whose psychology, although of interest, present psychosocial issues that are very different from those that are described in this chapter.

The deaf are a very distinct population. The need for amplification to perceive any type of sound has always been apparent to them. Those persons who use sign language feel that they belong in their own unique world and, therefore, do not need to

TABLE 1-1. Prevalence and prevalence rates for significant bilateral hearing impairment by age and sex in the United States in 1971.

Sex/Age	Number	Rate per 100,000
Both sexes	6,549,643	3,237
Under 6	56,038	262
6 to 16	384,557	852
17 to 24	235,121	862
25 to 44	642,988	1,356
45 to 64	1,870,356	4,478
65 and over	3,360,583	17,368
Females	2,706,124	2,583
Under 6	23,771	227
6 to 16	155,738	701
17 to 24	81,923	568
25 to 44	243,403	990
45 to 64	610,741	2,783
65 and over	1,590,818	14,257
Males	3,843,519	3,938
Under 6	32,267	295
6 to 16	228,819	997
17 to 24	153,198	1,191
25 to 44	399,585	1,749
45 to 64	1,259,885	6,535
65 and over	1,769,765	21,606

Reprinted with permission from Schein, J. D., & Delk, M. T., Jr. (1974). *The deaf populaton of the United States* (p. 29). Silver Spring, MD: National Association of the Deaf.

hide their condition from the normal hearing world. This population does not concern itself with vanity. On the whole it represents a very stable group, especially when deafness is diagnosed and habilitation begins in early childhood.

Children with partial hearing losses grow up feeling somewhat isolated. They rarely meet others with similar problems, and they frequently are the only hearing-impaired children in their elementary schools. Some normal hearing people may treat them as if they are deaf since a hearing aid is often mistakenly seen as a sign of total hearing loss. These children also suffer from stereotypes associated with hearing impairment. Hard-of-hearing children do not feel part

of the deaf community, but they do not fully participate in the normal hearing community either. Hearing aids are seen as necessities, but also as devices that may cause them to be seen as different. The younger an individual is at the time of diagnosis and fitting, the easier the adjustment.

The focus of this chapter is on individuals who develop hearing loss in adulthood. They are the majority of hearing aid clients. What can be said about this population of hearing-impaired adults? How do they act and how do they think? What are their fears and whom do they fear? How do they feel about hearing aids and how do they feel about professionals who advise them about and fit them with these instruments? What makes them good hearing aid candidates and what will likely result in their becoming successful hearing aid users? The following pages provide answers to some of these questions.

The first part of this chapter briefly discusses some of the research about the psychology of the hearing-impaired adult. Theories that are helpful in understanding the adjustment processes clients may experience are presented next, along with the various types of anxieties that can affect clients' responses to amplification. This is followed by a discussion of how anxiety can affect hearing itself. The final and major section suggests the approaches the dispenser should take to address these anxieties and thereby help the client toward successful amplification.

PSYCHOLOGY OF THE HARD-OF-HEARING ADULT

According to Pappas, Graham, and Rolfe (1982), in-depth psychiatric and psychological studies over the last 20 years, although hampered by inadequate measuring tools, have demonstrated that hearing loss has some deleterious effects on personal and social adjustment. Despite the conflicting results from various studies, the authors found considerable evidence showing "increased incidence of emotional problems in the hearing-impaired population." Later studies attempted to enumerate these emotional problems.

In a review article, Barker, Wright, Meyerson, and Gonick (1953) pointed out the great divergence in views regarding the psychological adjustment of hard-of-hearing and deafened adults. Opinions ranged from authors who regarded the hearing-impaired adult as different in personality from normal hearing adults to those who claimed that this population does not differ from the normal hearing population. Goetzinger (1978) pointed out that personality characteristics attributed to hard-of-hearing and deaf adults include "despondency, sense of inferiority, introversion, hopelessness, fear, supersensitivity, bitterness, cruelty, egocentrism, selfishness and lack of sympathy." From reviewing the findings of Barker and colleagues (1953), Goetzinger concluded that several factors in particular contribute to the adjustment problems of hard-of-hearing and deaf individuals, including, "the extra effort they must exert to meet the demands of the environment, head noises, the lack of sound itself, the threat of limited opportunities and second citizenship." Of course, in 1989 it is easy to see that loud sounds, especially noise pollution, have a deleterious emotional effect on individuals with sensorineural hearing impairment who have recruitment.

Jackson (1982) also compiled information about psychological profiles of the "more severely hearing impaired adult." She arrived at the following conclusions based on the work of Schlesinger and Meadow (1972), Levine (1976), Bolton (1976), Schein (1977), and Schein (1978):

1. They tend to be immature
2. They tend to withdraw, especially from communication situations
3. They tend to be less flexible than a normal hearing adult
4. They tend to adhere rigidly to a set routine

5. They tend to demonstrate a negative self-image; this is due in part to a general lack of information concerning the nature of hearing impairment
6. They tend to have a narrow range of interests
7. They tend to show a lack of social judgment
8. They tend to exhibit a lack of regard for the feelings of others
9. They tend to be more naive than the hearing adult
10. They tend to be more dependent than the hearing adult
11. They tend to be irresponsible
12. They tend to be impulsive
13. They tend to be passive and overaccepting, especially if the loss occurred early
14. They tend to be depressed, but generally in cases where the hearing impairment occurred later in life. (p. 29)

Myklebust (1960) conducted the most well known and extensive investigation into the psychology of hard-of-hearing and deaf adults. He found that stresses in the daily lives of his subjects resulted from the following:

■ Considerable patience required at the family level to assist the hearing impaired individual with messages, in seeking employment, and in maintaining friendship
■ Social isolation, loss of friends, and despondency
■ The need to develop identification with other hard-of-hearing individuals

He also found the following:

■ Hard-of-hearing males manifested poorer emotional adjustment than did the comparable female group.
■ The use of a hearing aid was associated with better adjustment for all subjects.
■ No unusual incidence of psychotic responses.
■ Hard-of-hearing subjects estimated their hearing impairment to be a greater

handicap and manifested more depression than did the deaf group. Hard-of-hearing subjects related feelings of depression to their hearing losses.

Myklebust believed that the latter results were related to the deaf groups' "naivete with regard to their handicap" and "could not be regarded as an index of better adjustment." Deaf subjects who claimed that their inability to hear was not a handicap were also found to exhibit the greatest emotional disturbance.

Mykelbust argued that the primary conclusion to be drawn from his study was "that deafness, particularly when profound and from early life, imposes a characteristic restriction on personality, but does not cause mental illness" (p. 158).

Rocky Stone is the founder and director of the International SHHH Organization (Self Help for Hard of Hearing Persons), the largest support organization for both partially hearing-impaired and deaf people. He acquired a profound bilateral hearing loss in adulthood. His writings stem from personal experiences as a hearing-impaired person and as the leader of an organization that fosters his ongoing interactions with thousands of hard-of-hearing and deaf people. The following is Stone's (1986) summary statement regarding the significant differences between people who are born deaf and those who lose their hearing:

> These differences are caused by having lost a precious something once possessed; the ambiguity of a progressive hearing loss; the fear of worse things happening if hearing diminishes; the prejudices of being part of a hearing culture which associates deafness with stigma; the complexities of hearing loss with its many apparent contradictions; the need to adjust to amplification if usable; inadequate alternatives for action; misunderstandings caused by thinking a communication was received accurately when it was not; the humiliation of being no longer able to function adequately on the telephone — the world's most common means of communication; the constant fatigue from straining to hear and to lip read; the embarrassment of being unable to maintain a communicative relationship with one's peers; a feeling of dependence; gradual withdrawal resulting in poor self esteem and low level of life satisfaction.

The list of investigators and studies is growing. I hope that it is apparent to the reader that restricting the personalities or the psychology of hearing impairment to common denominators limits and constricts the relationship between the hearing aid dispenser and clients. The professional who dispenses the hearing aid and searches for common properties by which to characterize all clients faces an impossible task. Sandlin (1974) pointed out that by accepting a single definition of psychology of hearing impairment professionals run the risk of fitting the hearing-impaired person into a particular personality subgroup and reacting accordingly to that individual. He suggested that hearing-impaired individuals need to be classified according to the "properties of the psychological situations in which they live and behave." Each hearing aid candidate needs to be seen as a mini-study regarding the effects of hearing loss on his or her personality and psychological adjustment to hearing loss.

The following sections deal with the practical application of personality factors to the issue of dispensing hearing aids.

Mourning Hearing Loss

Psychological Theories Related to Loss

Understanding certain psychological theories and facts can help hearing aid dispensers understand the needs, feelings, problems, and views of the individuals they are trying to help. Dr. John Bowlby (1969) of the Tavistock Institute of London, England suggested that we must look at the quality of attachments, especially early life attachments, in order to better appreciate how people face separations (losses, for our purposes) later in life.

Attachment-Separation-Loss theory maintains that children who grow up with secure, reliable bases of support usually grow up feeling safe in their environments. They feel free to explore their worlds, knowing their actions will not result in abandonment; they grow up feeling protected. When losses do occur later in life, people who feel secure and worthwhile are able to act with realistic guidelines. On the other hand, children who grow up fearing that their actions will result in separation from their parents often approach adult losses with trepidation and feelings of vulnerability.

The key words to remember are *protection* and *vulnerability*. Both relate to the degree of safety one feels in the face of possible attack, threats to one's being, or threats to one's self-esteem. Individuals differ in the degree of security they feel when revealing their hearing problems to others. Some people will not tell others about their hearing problem because they fear they will be taken advantage of or ridiculed. Others feel that letting people know about the problem will gain their support and cooperation.

Rousey (1971) based his psychology of the reaction to hearing loss on observation of patients at the Menninger Foundation. He claimed that the major effects most often manifested by hearing-impaired individuals are "mourning, pain, and mortification, or some variant of these." He discussed mourning in a sexual context, as the hearing loss on an unconscious level coming to represent a loss of sexual adequacy or potency, including more than just the physical act of sex. Rousey predicted that the effects of a hearing loss would be more severe for a person "who has vacillating or ambivalent feelings about his interaction with the rest of the world." Such a person could also be said to have made poor attachments with important others in the environment. According to Rousey, individuals with long-standing, warm relationships will not resort to pathological mourning.

Parkes (1971), a major proponent of attachment theory, combined stress research with loss research, calling the combined study the field of psychosocial transitions. It is a field that relates directly to an appreciation of the effects of hearing loss. The following transitional events can precipitate severe stress:

- Bereavement, loss due to death, especially a spouse
- Major changes in career, especially being fired
- Calamitous disasters (floods, fires, earthquakes)
- Retirement
- Major illness and disability
- Loss of a body part or function
- Loss of a home due to insufficient funds or disaster
- Migration, especially when under duress

Hearing loss acquired later in life falls into two of the above categories directly (major illness and disability and loss of a body part or function), and may additionally precipitate bereavement over the "lost function," and can provide an impetus to occupational change or even retirement.

For psychologic purposes, the onset of hearing loss is the moment the physician tells the patient, "You will not get better, but can get worse. You have an irreversible hearing impairment." This point is also the moment of transition. Up to this time some people may have been able to fool themselves into believing that their hearing problem was temporary. Now their worst fears about their hearing have been confirmed. Some people hear the word "deafness" instead of hearing loss (i.e., they see the loss in an all-or-nothing fashion). For most people the transition does not begin easily. They have been hit over the head with a glass hammer and are attending to their pain while at the same time trying to pick up the pieces resulting from the blow. The physician may see a quiet, pensive response, while in reality the patient is experiencing an emotional storm.

Stages of Mourning

The patient is left to grieve the lost hearing. Psychological theory dealing with bereavement can help hearing aid dispensers to be cognizant of the patient's emotional state of acceptance. Bowlby and Parkes (1970) identified four phases involved in the grief and mourning process that can be applied to the hearing aid candidate (and to parents who have been told that their child is hearing impaired):

- Numbness that usually lasts a few hours to one week
- Yearning and search for the lost figure or object
- Disorganization and despair
- Greater or lesser degree of reorganization

NUMBNESS. Unwanted and sometimes shocking news makes us feel jarred out of what we think of as a normal or typically reactive state of mind. This state of mind is a kind of pinch-me-and-see-if-I'm-awake state. At this point the disappointed and somewhat dumbfounded patient and the family need precise direct advice as to how the problem should be handled.

The physician is also disappointed by the news. Otolaryngologists would like to cure the problem, and many physicians do not want to give the patient any more bad news than is necessary. Therefore, when the patient asks the question: I do not need a hearing aid, do I? the answer is frequently a tentative and negative, "Not yet." These physicians do not want to disturb the patient further with such terrible news as having to wear hearing aids. Of course, much of the problem lies in the poor question: Do I *need* a hearing aid? A person does not need hearing aids. The word "need" refers to something mandatory for sustaining life. Many otolaryngologists, however, do recognize the importance of proper encouragement regarding amplification and respond appropriately.

The physician's positive attitude toward amplification could shorten the duration of the mourning stage of numbness. Hearing aids do not really make you live longer, but they certainly can lead to a happier life. The better question is: Will hearing aids improve the quality of my life? Physicians can, in most cases, give a more complete and most likely affirmative response to such a question. Their answers would thus shift the focus to hope instead of fear. Nevertheless, not all patients are responsive to physician's hearing aid recommendations and they go from feeling numb to experiencing denial.

At this point it should be mentioned that sometimes the audiologist or hearing aid specialist is the first to confirm the findings of sensorineural hearing impairment. Some people avoid physicians; others feel that being evaluated by someone other than a physician means that the situation is less critical. Therefore, the hearing aid specialist must be aware of the numbness which occurs following a description of the condition.

Some patients leave the ear specialist's office without really understanding that they have a confirmed irreversible hearing loss. They do not know why they have a prescription blank with a hearing aid dispenser's telephone number on it. Here again, the dispenser may be the first person to drive home the numbing information.

YEARNING AND SEARCH FOR THE LOST OBJECT. In the second stage of mourning, disbelief sets in and the patient sets out to prove the physician, the hearing aid dispenser, and the family are wrong. Family members sometimes collude by saying: See, you can hear when you really want to! This statement is said at times when there is an absence of competing signals and when concentrated lip reading is utilized. Such family members do not want to accept the hearing loss as real, fearing it could mean that the person is deteriorating or that they will have to "eventually learn sign language" to communicate with their loved one. Nonsensical myths about hearing impairment exist, and many newly diagnosed hearing-impaired persons, as well as family members, accept these myths as real.

This period can also be described as the *time of strain,* because the patient strains to hear and blames others when messages are misunderstood. "I could hear you if you would not mumble!" is a common complaint. Some people attempt to deny the loss altogether. They attend movies, plays, and lectures to prove that they really can hear. When they fail in their attempts, they blame the acoustics of the theater or auditorium, the strange speaking habits of those speaking, and background noise. These factors do make it much more difficult for the damaged cochlea to interpret the signal. *The strain to hear produces anxiety and fatigue, which further inhibit hearing,* and the person must look for other ways to deny the hearing loss.

The same phenomenon is frequently manifested in hearing testing. Fearing a diagnosis of hearing loss, many clients strain to hear during the audiometric evaluation. Jaws and fists are clenched in a strange attempt to block out all possible head noises so the pure tones will be easier to identify. Of course, this increases the chances of tinnitus due to stress.

Amplification should not be suggested during the second stage of mourning. The clients' search is not for anything other than proof that their own hearing is normal. Hearing aid suggestions are usually rebuked. This strong state of fear must be respected. In this stage, pressuring the person about amplification could result in a deeper state of denial which would make the eventual acceptance of hearing aids a good *im*possibility.

Yes, some hearing aid dispensers are able to talk such denying people into buying hearing aids. However, do not assume that the aids are used.

DISORGANIZATION AND DESPAIR. In the third stage of mourning, disorganization and despair, typical thoughts include: I get a startling pain when people talk louder and I still do not understand them! and What is the use? I might as well stay home and read a book or watch television, but these newscasters talk lousy too!

Anger and depression act together to bring about a greater withdrawal from society and even from the family. The hearing loss is finally accepted as valid, but the individual's mental attention is given to the loss instead of the desire to overcome the difficulties precipitated by the loss. "Leave me alone about a hearing aid!" greets family members who attempt to intrude on the individual's desire to be left alone to deal with the sadness over the loss. Heavy-handed suggestions do not help in this stage because clients are not ready to hear anything they interpret as a demand. Overcoming a loss usually requires a period of calmness to get used to the idea of change and to act on it. When depression goes on for too long, it is advisable to seek professional help to overcome the grief.

Emergence from this stage usually requires considerable understanding and patience from family and friends. Positive, nonforceful comments regarding amplification by the physician could help get the person over the hump, but a return visit to the medical ear specialist rarely occurs once the diagnosis has been established. This situation is unfortunate because during a second visit the person is likely to be more accepting of the hearing loss and in a better position to let rehabilitation information penetrate the depression.

Aural rehabilitation programs related to adjustment to hearing loss provide a setting in which hearing-impaired individuals and family members can help one another to get through the sense of disorganization that plagues them. Experiencing the commonality of the problem makes people with newly diagnosed hearing impairments feel less alone and more willing to move toward amplification. Many people who enter such rehabilitation programs are in the process of emerging from this stage and are beginning to want answers, but are not fully ready to accept amplification as the only answer. A good aural rehabilitation program teaches realistic attitudes about hearing loss and hearing aids, which results in a desire to get back to what one has been missing. Despair fades and the shattered pieces begin to come together again. This point is the beginning of the fourth stage.

REORGANIZATION. The final stage of mourning deals with reorganization. At this point, patients are willing to try anything that will put their lives back on a growth-oriented course. Denial and withdrawal have resulted only in mental pain for all those involved (i.e., family, co-workers, and friends). Finally, the person is capable of seeing the hearing aid as a friend and not the enemy that could defeat him or her in the quest to deny the loss. Now the hearing aid . specialist can be viewed as a helpful professional instead of an opportunist who takes advantage of people who really do not need those unnecessary devices.

This final stage can be very tricky. Poor results with hearing aids can throw a person back into depression and withdrawal. The need for careful advice regarding expectations about amplification along with helpful instruction and counseling on good lip reading and listening habits cannot be stressed enough. In the period of reorganization clients desire to once again learn skills for a healthy manipulation of the environment. Understanding the need to pay attention, the need to speak in the same room, and awareness of situations that reduce hearing ability are just a few of the counseling tips that make for better hearing aid wearers. This type of instruction helps hearing-impaired individuals to accept the loss and amplification because now there are things they *can do* to get back a part of the world they have been missing. The greater the reorganization, the sooner the mourning will give way to a healthy *acceptance* of the hearing problem and a healthy *control* of the problem.

The stages of mourning have been presented to give readers an idea of some of the mental processes that could affect their clients when they are confronted with their hearing losses. Each person passes through these stages in different ways. Some take years to get to the point of reorganization. Some never make it. Others take a day. Nevertheless, do not be fooled by this last group. Most likely, they had been thinking about the hearing problem for quite a while and had accepted the possibility of hearing aids long before consulting the physician.

The next section addresses the effects of anxiety on the dispensing of hearing aids, on adaptation to hearing aids, and on the hearing aid itself.

Anxiety and the Hearing Aid Candidate

Anxiety is an emotional mixture of apprehension, uncertainty, and fear. To understand the overall anxiety of a person who is in the process of being fitted with hearing aids, the following component categories will be discussed: consumer anxieties, attention anxieties, mechanical anxieties, and separation-rejection anxieties. Chances are very high that hearing aid candidates fit into one or a combination of these anxiety categories.

Consumer Anxieties

Democratic countries offer people the chance to purchase items from people in private businesses who have much to gain from these purchases. Such entrepreneurship has given rise to apprehension by the consumer toward the private practitioner. It is only normal that there is some degree of suspicion on the part of the clients, especially when they are spending many hundreds of dollars. Car dealers and other commissioned salespeople, such as insurance agents, as well as physicians in private practice and even hearing aid specialists themselves are thought to have the same question in mind: What's in it for me? Consumer anxiety affects everyone and leads to a certain amount of inner dialogue before going out and purchasing something at face value. Typical worries about purchasing hearing aids include:

- How do I know I am being sold the proper hearing aid?
- Why is the person down the street cheaper?
- Why are hearing aids so expensive?
- Do I really need two hearing aids?
- How do I know this dispenser is really any good?
- How can I really know this is the best brand when I have never heard of it?
- How do I know I am not being ripped off?
- Why should I buy hearing aids when they really are not any good because my friend does not wear his any place but the chest of drawers?

The list is extensive. Readers can come up with their own lists of such questions regarding many things they are about to purchase.

The main component of consumer anxiety is the *fear that someone will take advantage of us because of what we do not know.* Clients feel that they are at the mercy of someone else's judgment and intentions. They place themselves in the position of being a child in that they must rely on someone else to give them what they need. It is the hearing aid specialist's responsibility to help turn these fears, more reminiscent of childhood, into trust, more typical of adulthood, by serving as a listening and caring guide. Trust comes from the good recommendation of other users and through a positive direct relationship. The keys to a good relationship between practitioner and client are *mutual respect* and *mutual goals.* The dispenser who takes great pleasure in the client's success communicates this pleasure during the interactions. Of course, the sale and the income derived from the sale are important, but the client becomes leery when these appear to be the hearing aid specialist's sole motivation. Empathic physicians who are able to listen are a prototype for other health professionals who want to succeed in helping people achieve healthier lives.

Attention Anxiety

This type of anxiety is a very difficult concept, and it affects only a small number of clients. Some people live in constant fear of being noticed for anything at all. Unable to tolerate attention, they shy away from any comments concerning them, whether positive, negative, or even neutral in nature. They fear attention. Therefore, they especially fear being noticed because of the hearing aid or the hearing loss. These individuals have difficulty with communication in general, and this difficulty becomes worse when they must ask someone to do anything to help them hear better. A person who has difficulty asking for water in a restaurant would certainly cringe at asking someone to face him or her when speaking.

The psychological roots of this problem extend back to childhood. People afflicted with attention anxiety feel they do not have a right to attention from others. They view acceptance of another's attention as a major transgression. Others who have never received any positive attention fear that attention, in general, may bring them great hurt and pain. Their only security is in not being noticed at all. The client who never complains may suffer from attention anxiety.

People with attention anxiety are the most difficult group to help, and most of these people will never show up for a fitting. However, their anxieties can often be reduced by a genuine display of *positive* attention on the part of the professional. Persons with attention anxiety need many visits to understand that the hearing aid dispenser is on the same team and that they are not alone regarding their hearing problem. These people need contact with a consistently approving adult figure who will work with them at their own pace.

Mechanical Anxiety

People have varying capacities for operating mechanical equipment. Some people feel that they never could learn to operate a television, use a food processor, preset a video recorder, ride a bicycle, drive a car, play a musical instrument, operate a computer, fly a plane, or manipulate a hearing aid. Others fear that they do not have the potential to remember what the dispenser has taught them and are embarrassed to admit that they forget. Some fear that they will never understand how to place the earmold in the canal and concha. Others worry that they will not be able to operate the volume and on-off switch while the instrument is being worn. Persons who fear rejection worry that they will not be able to operate the equipment and that others will notice them trying to fiddle around with it. These clients spend considerable time in bathrooms to make sure others do not see them fidget with the aid. They also fear the terrible feedback noise which definitely calls attention directly to them. This fear results in a constant inconspicuous removal of the aid from the ear to adjust the volume.

The skilled hearing aid specialist can go far to alleviate mechanical anxiety. It requires additional time during the initial visit, but in the long run, clients will make fewer visits due to mechanical anxiety. People who understand how to use the hearing aid because of the specialist's care and attention are usually pleased with their aids. Good, careful instruction is also quite useful in decreasing consumer anxiety while giving the client tools for improving hearing ability. Recognition that they are able to operate the hearing aid should re-

sult in clients feeling in good control of their communication. Insecurities about not being able to hear should decrease when insecurities regarding the operation of mechanical devices decrease. When people feel secure in the operation of hearing aids, they feel more independent and in control of their hearing. More information on this important aspect of dispensing is presented later in this chapter.

Separation (Rejection) Anxiety

This psychological term usually connotes a *normal* reaction to an unwilling separation; the reaction is greater when the separation could lead to possible danger. The concept is extensive. Only features that relate separation anxiety specifically to fears involved with wearing hearing aids are considered here. (The term "rejection" is included when talking about separation to elaborate on this concept, which is new to most hearing professionals.) The ways in which wearing hearing aids can bring up fears regarding how an individual feels about him- or herself are addressed first. Then situations that bring up fears individuals have regarding the ways others will feel about them are discussed.

HOW DO HEARING AIDS MAKE ME FEEL ABOUT ME? Acceptance of amplification is the cementing action in accepting the hearing *loss.* Wearing hearing aids can bring up anxieties related to what it means to separate from one's hearing. This concept was discussed in the section on mourning, but it can also be applied in relation to anxieties regarding self-concept. Some individuals feel that by accepting the use of hearing aids they are betraying their lost hearing or rejecting their remedial hearing. Typifying statements are: I cannot wear a hearing aid because it is a crutch that keeps me from using my real hearing. If I wore a hearing aid, I would become dependent on it and that would mean giving up my independence.

These attitudes arise from misunderstanding the function of hearing aids. Clients must be taught that amplification works to assist residual hearing instead of working to make up for lost hearing. In the author's opinion, the word "crutch" is also inappropriate. In ambulatory problems, a crutch is something that affords the ability to do things that could not be done without it; a crutch is very useful. Unfortunately, the word has received a bad press and is often used to connote taking advantage of something one really does not need. Used in this way, another person can be a crutch for the hearing-impaired person who rejects amplification. An example of a negative crutch is a person who hears and interprets for a person who will not consider hearing aids. Normal hearing spouses act like negative crutches when they:

■ Answer for the client
■ Encourage the client to stay at home due to the hearing loss
■ Gesture to others that the client cannot hear instead of encouraging the client to ask others for assistance to hear better
■ Make all verbal plans for the spouse who has sufficient hearing ability to make plans on his or her own

These spouses need assistance in understanding the problem and should be instructed directly in ways they can best assist their hearing-impaired husband or wife to hear better (e.g., helping the hearing-impaired spouse to become more assertive in telling others about the problem).

To some people, the acceptance of hearing aids represents a concrete example of a separation from their youth. The hearing aid may be seen as a sign that the body is deteriorating, and clients are reminded of this every time they go to put that "damn gizmo" in their ear. For these people, amplification signifies a separation from the feeling that they have young, indestructible bodies. People experiencing separation anxiety regarding their youth see the hearing aid as symbolic of the body's vulnerability to attack.

The hearing aid should be a source of feeling more complete. Hearing aid specialists need to emphasize that hearing aids are meant to enrich life, regardless of age. Hearing aids should be regarded as partners in reducing stress. (Actually, stress is more likely to bring on physical deterioration.)

HOW DO HEARING AIDS CAUSE OTHERS TO FEEL ABOUT ME? Feeling vulnerable to attack forms the basis for separation anxiety experienced by hearing aid candidates, and some hearing aid users as well. Separation anxiety also can be regarded as rejection anxiety because vulnerability to rejection is the primary fear. The fear of being alone is directly related to the feeling of being unprotected in the world.

Ramsdell (1964) described three functions of hearing: communication of ideas, thoughts, and feelings through the verbal exchange of language, known as the *symbolic function* of hearing; the signal or *warning function,* which allows us to be aware of approaching danger; and the use of one's auditory sense *to feel a part of the world,* providing the world with an "affective tone." It seems obvious that hearing loss results in massive insecurity in regard to all three of these functions. When the ability to understand speech is impaired, communication with others is also impaired. Not hearing a prowler or an approaching ambulance makes one vulnerable to physical danger. Missing the friendly at-home sounds of a populated world gives way to a sense of isolation.

Logically, a person who is missing these things would run out and obtain hearing aids to overcome all of these deficits and thus feel more protected and a part of the world. Nevertheless, many people approach amplification with trepidation and have preconceived ideas that predispose them to reject the instruments. Many of these people fear that others will see the hearing aids and label them as less than fully functioning people.

The fear of being devalued by others is a pivotal motivating factor in many hearing aid rejections. Do we devalue people with handicaps? Do we devalue people with prostheses? Do we devalue people who wear things in their ears? Do we devalue people who look aged? The answer to these questions lies in looking different. We live in a society that has trouble handling differences. In our educational system, although children are taught about people who are different, they are not taught how to act toward people who are different. Many people who are hearing impaired fear the hearing aid acts as a beacon that announces "Look at me!" Unfortunately, it does sometimes result in others looking away out of ignorance.

The Western world is smothered in its aesthetic trappings. We fear that looking different will result in rejection. The media upholds beauty and appearance as the standards for acceptance. People fear that hearing aids will detract from their attractiveness and will make them undesirable to others, who will not want to be seen in public with an individual who is wearing hearing aids. In reality, most people respect those who are tolerant of individual differences. It should not take bravery to associate with hearing aid users.

Another fear is that hearing aids will make them look old. They worry: It is a sign to *others* that my body is deteriorating and that I am no longer useful to society. And they ask the question: How can a hearing aid add to my life? It can only take away. Our society certainly needs to change its attitudes toward the aging process and the aged to reach, support, and rehabilitate those persons who are affected by such fears.

Hearing-impaired individuals may fear that the hearing aid will be a symbol to others that they are not perfect or that they are not whole. People with such fears should be reminded that perfection or wholeness of human beings depends on their actions and treatment of others, and not on whether they have perfect hearing. Epitaphs do not contain engravings of audiograms but the essence of one's character.

A common fear is that people who see the hearing aids will treat the user as a child. People spend a lifetime trying to achieve and maintain the feeling of being an adult. They do not want a hearing aid to threaten this perception.

Miniaturization has become a main activity of the hearing aid industry in an attempt to help people allay their fears of looking different and being rejected. The author is not against miniaturization, but the industry also needs a public relations campaign to notify an ignorant hearing public that the hearing impaired are not different. The public also must be instructed on how it can help.

Hearing aids need to be regarded as devices that will increase the chance of public acceptance and not as equipment to be feared as the source of ridicule. Amplification should result in a greater sense of security. Fear of rejection should be superseded by fears of vulnerability over being unable to hear. Desire for the best possible hearing, instead of desire to conceal the instrument, should be stressed. Better hearing through appropriate amplification is the best possible sales pitch to change attitudes of rejection into a healthy desire to again communicate with the world.

This extended discussion of separation anxiety with its many component tensions has been presented because anyone who dispenses hearing aids needs to understand the feelings behind fears of rejection. Many hearing-impaired individuals feel that their very being is at stake when it comes to disclosing their hearing problem through the use of amplification. Fears involving possible abandonment bring up childhood anxieties that cause people to reject amplification or to conceal the instruments in a desperate manner. One role of the hearing aid specialist is to provide a healthy support base from which the hearing-impaired individual can learn to explore accepting relationships and receive encouragement regarding realistic interactions with the normal hearing and, unfortunately, ignorant world. It would be helpful for those who read this book to consider themselves as dispensers of *hearing*.

RASH

Whether in response to amplification, to others, or to themselves, it is quite obvious that the lives of hearing-impaired adults are full of anxiety. At the UCLA Hope for Hearing Community Outreach Program over 3000 hearing-impaired adults and their family members were interviewed. Through these interviews, phenomena that produced potentially crippling anxiety in the daily lives of these people were observed. It takes the form of a vicious cycle, or syndrome, and can best be explained by an example.

Mr. Z., age 56, is an aerospace engineer with a moderately severe hearing loss. He holds a high-ranking managerial position at work, and at the time of this example, he was about to lead a major meeting regarding a new aerospace design which he had helped to develop. Events occur in the following order:

Mr. Z. leaves home in the morning wearing his binaural hearing aids. While in the car driving to the meeting, Mr. Z. has the following thoughts:

Should I wear my hearing aids? Most of the people there do not know I have a hearing problem. The hearing aids will call attention away from the project, or maybe they will think less of me if they know I have this problem. They might even reject the project.

I will wear the aids. But what happens if I do not understand their ques-

tions? Do I tell them I have a hearing problem? They might laugh; they might not take me seriously. How often can I ask them to repeat without getting them ticked off? I know I will make a fool of myself and wreck this project.

Of course, these thoughts lead to considerable anxiety (stress, tension, fear). Most readers probably remember the Alfred Hitchcock films. A good director of mystery adventure films can keep an audience on the edge of its seats for the majority of the film, particularly the last 20 minutes. My favorite example is "North by Northwest." Such a film usually has the audience taking a huge breath and feeling somewhat exhausted.

With anxiety comes fatigue. The anxiety provoking scripts going on in Mr. Z's head result in his feeling quite fatigued, even before he gets to work. *Fatigue has a negative effect on hearing;* consequently, Mr. Z. arrives at work with poorer hearing than when he left home.

Mr. Z. enters the meeting room wearing his hearing aids and has them turned on. However, he notices that he is not hearing as well as usual even during conversational speech. He starts playing with the hearing aids, hoping that will make a difference. He starts to *strain* to hear. In other words, he begins to do some maneuvers like eye squints, jaw exercises, and swallowing.* These exercises are to no avail, they are rarely helpful. *Straining to hear results in fatigue.*

The sense of decreased hearing also causes additional anxiety which will affect Mr. Z.'s general presentation. Mr. Z. gets up to give his presen-

---

* This may also remind readers of some of the maneuvers people perform during hearing tests to give the very best hearing test results, which were briefly discussed in the previous section on mourning, including attempts to block out tinnitus and other extraneous noises. However, straining to hear results only in fatigue and may result in poorer thresholds than if the person was relaxed during the session.

tation and is overcome by his sense of reduced hearing, increased fatigue, and overwhelming anxiety. An extreme response, which occurs with very few people, would be for Mr. Z. to develop a conversion hysteria such as sudden temporary hemiplegic paralysis or sudden temporary blindness in one eye. (There have been undocumented reports of such occurrences with people in this stage.) A more typical response is considerable jitteriness, blinking, and heavy breathing.

The meeting begins with Mr. Z. in a terribly anxious and fatigued state and with a hearing level reduced by stress and anxiety. The vicious cycle will continue as long as Mr. Z. continues to anxiously strain and fatigue himself while paying more attention to what he is missing and worrying about the missed information than attending to what he is actually able to hear.

The only way to break this cycle is to be aware of it. Mr. Z. needs to see a red light go off in his head and have it register *stop!* This awareness should be followed by a relaxing deep breath of relief and a sense of once again being in control of the situation, including his level of tension, fatigue, and fluctuating hearing.

The author terms this phenomenon Reiter's Anxiety Syndrome re-Hearing (RASH), because it is like a rash, which worsens the more it is irritated.* Improvement comes when an individual learns to stop concentrating on the rash, and instead pay attention to the world outside of it.

Other examples of RASH are the middle-aged woman at a church social who entertains mind scripts about revealing her hearing loss and the college student who does not want to be seen as different. The RASH phenomenon becomes a direct adversary to good self-esteem. It also relates directly to the dispenser–client relationship. The client may be concentrating on residual fears about hearing aids and experiencing anxiety, fatigue, and reduced hearing while in the dispenser's office. These clients may be so preoccupied with their anxiety that they really cannot listen to what the dispenser is trying to teach them and thus are not in the right state of mind for judging the usefulness of amplification.

The next section on the psychology of dispensing addresses these issues. It discusses how to minimize the client's stress and achieve a more open state of mind so that the hearing aid fitting process can shift from a source of anxiety to a successful adaptation to life.

THE PSYCHOLOGY OF THE PROFESSIONAL DISPENSER

Excellent dispensing of hearing aids is both an art and a science. Physiology and anatomy are the scientific disciplines of dispensing. Psychology, understanding human beings, is also a prerequisite to working in the area of human rehabilitation. The art of successful dispensing results in a satisfied user.

The foregoing section was intended to provide a psychological background for deeper understanding of the hearing aid candidate. Awareness of these mental processes will prove helpful in choosing the questions to ask clients. "I wish he would listen to me instead of his machine!" is a frequent complaint made by clients regarding hearing health professionals. The successful fitting of hearing aids requires 40 percent understanding of the audiogram and 60 percent understanding of the particular person and his or her life-style, which includes understanding how the client interprets his or her hearing problem. All in

---

* This term is a fancy way of including myself in the theory's name. It is not to be confused with Reiter's syndrome, a venereal disease that Columbus and his group brought to the natives of the New World.

all, this is the psychology of approaching individuals who must be seen as unique regarding hearing and their individual lives.

When lecturing on the professional role of the dispenser in treating the hearing impaired, the author uses the acronym PEOPLE (proper fit, expectations, openness, personality, listening, education) as a guide and checklist for working with and dispensing hearing aids to that *special* individual between the ears. The components of PEOPLE are not mutually exclusive, and no single component is more important than another. These components or elements should be viewed as fitting together in order for the dispenser to understand the client and the client to understand the dispenser. This checklist is of considerable value in determining the origin of problems that need to be solved before, during, and after the dispensing process.

Proper Fit

The first element of PEOPLE is proper fit. Much of this book is devoted to teaching excellent hearing aid *fitting*. The best possible acoustical fitting of hearing aids is only one aspect of dispensing amplification, but it is the lead aspect. Understanding the person will not go far if the client feels that sound-wise the hearing aid is wrong. The dispenser must be certain that the acoustic fit is proper before searching for emotional reasons to explain the client's dissatisfaction.

The dispenser should be reminded that going for the best fit will usually result in satisfaction for both client and dispenser. Doing the best job possible is a psychological reward in itself, which is felt by all parties involved. The sense of offering the client the best possible fit gives the dispenser a more meaningful role in the healing partnership between dispenser and client.

The best possible fit is not based on the audiogram alone. The right questions need to be asked throughout the fitting period to arrive at this desired result. Two elements of

PEOPLE, expectations and personality, help to answer some of these questions.

Expectations

Mr. X., Countess Y., and Ms. Z. are in the office waiting room. What do they expect from the hearing aid dispenser? Understanding clients' expectations is a major way to understand the dispenser-client relationship. Again, an organized approach to asking questions can help to reduce anxiety about obtaining answers. This includes questions that deal directly with hearing and amplification. To get the best understanding and appreciation of clients' attitudes toward the hearing problem, it is best to use open-ended questions. These questions require explanations as opposed to yes or no responses. The following questions are recommended:

Describe your hearing loss in your own words. Clients usually will repeat phrases and descriptions regarding their hearing problems that they picked up from other professionals, particularly the physician who diagnosed the hearing loss, for example: I have nerve deafness. I am slightly deaf. I really do not need a hearing aid yet. My hearing loss is not bad enough for two hearing aids, or I have a 60 percent loss in one ear and a 20 percent loss in the other. What do clients mean by these phrases? How do they know that their hearing is going to deteriorate? It is very important to know who told them these facts. Using universal, understandable terminology helps clients feel more grounded and sets the basis for understanding the language being used to help them. In other words, the hearing aid specialist should talk in terms of degrees of severity and should try to eliminate the words "deaf" or "deafness" from the description of hearing losses by persons with partial hearing impairments.

How has the hearing loss affected your life? The least invasive questions usually deal with work. Therefore, it is a good idea to begin with questions regarding how the loss has affected a change in occupation, layoffs, choice of occupation, anxiety over the feared loss of work, and relationships with coworkers. Do the people at work, including employers and employees, know about the hearing loss? How is the problem interfering with the best possible job performance? Is occupational noise a problem? Has it contributed to the degree of impairment?

The next area of inquiry should be the relationship between hearing loss and education, including leisure activity classes. Have instructors been helpful and understanding? How has the hearing problem changed the client's social life, hobbies, and favorite entertainment? These questions help the client to voice frustrations related to persons outside the family. Questions about family are frequently more touchy and may involve accusations directed toward an accompanying spouse, child, or parent. It is best to ease into discussions of family issues by first addressing frustrations that occur outside the home. Once work, educational, and leisure frustrations about hearing loss have been voiced, it is easier to introduce problems concerning communication breakdown due to hearing loss within the family.

How has your hearing loss affected your relationship with your spouse? What are your chief complaints and your spouse's chief complaints? The client should be asked to assess the level of cooperation regarding hearing in the home. *Do family members treat you differently because of the hearing problem?* Of course, any family relationship can be substituted or added.

Sometimes it is necessary for the dispensing professional to bring up issues of loneliness and isolation. Anxious clients may forget to bring up these issues or feel that they are too painful to bring up on their own. Others may feel that the dispensing professional is not capable of hearing emotional information. Emotional issues have a strong effect on expectations regarding amplification; therefore, understanding

these issues is an integral part of the fitting procedure.

It is also important to separate issues regarding hearing loss from those regarding hearing aids. Information about the hearing loss is gathered to keep the client's attitudes regarding hearing impairment separate from attitudes regarding amplification. Both clients and family members frequently confuse hearing loss and hearing aids as is evident in the following self disclosures: "I have hearing aids" versus the more definitive and personal "I have a hearing loss" or "I am worried someone will see my hearing aids" instead of "I am worried someone will learn that I am hard of hearing." These statements indicate the need for clients to detach the hearing loss from themselves by referring instead to hearing aids.

After obtaining a good hearing loss history, the professional dispenser can begin to question the client regarding hearing aid history and, of course, expectations regarding *amplification.* Much of this chapter is geared toward working with first-time hearing aid users, but an understanding of the psychology of dispensing also involves understanding experienced users' attitudes and anxieties regarding amplification. This information must be acknowledged and understood to have a successful subsequent fitting. Dispensing professionals may have to work hard to establish a trusting relationship due to a client's negative experience with another dispenser. At all times, it is in the new dispenser's interest to treat comments about previous fittings with respect. The experiences and the way the client perceives them should be acknowledged without criticizing the efforts of a colleague. The focus should always be on the client's present needs and the current fitting.

To understand the client's expectations about amplification, the hearing aid specialist should have a working knowledge of the client's attitude toward hearing aids in general. Many clients are overwhelmed by negative stereotypes about hearing aids. These myths need to be addressed and dispelled before progressing to the client's expectations. Some general questions to ask include: What do you think of people who wear hearing aids? and How would you describe hearing aids, and what exactly do they do? Initially, it is important to ask these questions in the third person so that clients are allowed some distance from the problem before directly relating it to themselves. It is sometimes easier to get clients to talk about the world in general before mentioning their own fears. Clients are thus encouraged to talk about hearing aid issues that they might not introduce on their own.

Some people are frightened of hearing aids. Many people are overwhelmed by mechanisms they do not understand, and especially by uncommon objects that fit into orifices of the human body. The thought of earmolds filled with cerumen makes some people cringe, for others any thought of closing off the ear canal with a foreign object is seen as damaging or painfully unnatural for the body. These are further examples of the need to dispel myths before dealing with expectations.

Finally, the issue of expectations regarding amplifications must be confronted. *Why, really, are Mr. X., Countess Y., and Ms. Z. at the dispenser's office?* Are they visiting the dispenser to appease their spouse, a relative, their doctor, or friends, or are they there to improve communication?

What do they think the hearing aid will do for them? This issue is crucial regarding expectations about hearing aid use, and the dispenser must be able to pinpoint it. Some clients expect complete cures (e.g., "I will hear everything perfectly with hearing aids." "I will be able to keep my hearing loss a secret because no one will know that I have trouble hearing as long as the aids are hidden!" or "Now only the sounds I have diffculty hearing will be made louder while the sounds I can hear well and noise will not be made louder"). Unrealistic expectations result in strong disappointments,

which are difficult to remedy. Good attitudes toward amplification change into poor attitudes when initial hopes fade into disappointment. To avoid these pitfalls, the dispenser should deal with specific situations regarding the client's life-style, work, family, and social relationships.

What are the client's expectations regarding the hearing aids and work? How will hearing aids enhance job performance? How will hearing aids threaten job performance? Improved hearing should be regarded as a means toward improvement of the work situation. However, many clients fear that advertising their hearing problems by using hearing aids will cause them to lose the respect and confidence of coworkers, employers, and employees. They fear that wearing hearing aids may even cause them to be terminated from their jobs. This fear is a good example of separation anxiety in regard to fears surrounding amplification. These people expect perfect hearing but also expect perfect concealment to keep their jobs.

Unfortunately, the pronouncement of a hearing problem may actually endanger the employment of some clients. This problem needs to be evaluated, through careful questioning. Clients whose livelihood is threatened are good candidates for aural rehabilitation programs where they can receive career advice, career counseling, and suggestions for introducing realistic aspects of their hearing problems to their employers, coworkers, and employees.

What are the clients' expectations regarding hearing aids and their spouse or other family members? These expectations include clients' expectations of how things will or will not be different as well as the expectations of spouses or other family members. Clients may complain that the family has unrealistic expectations because "what they really want is for me to be cured." Or they may think things such as: "I understand the extent of help the hearing aid can give, but my family will not. They will still get upset when I miss one word or ask them to repeat things, thinking that I should be hearing perfectly with the hearing aids." "My family believes that now my problem is going to go away." The hearing aid specialist will be assisted in understanding these comments regarding family expectations through direct questioning of family members. Family members, as well as clients, need to be counseled regarding good communication with hearing aids (i.e., maintaining good eye contact, speaking from the same room, getting the person's attention before speaking). More of this is addressed in the section on education.

What are the client's expectations regarding hearing aids and social relationships? It must be determined whether clients look forward to the use of hearing aids as a means of enhancing their life-styles, or whether they fear that using hearing aids will be a source of ridicule that will lead to embarrassment and their withdrawal from social events. Of course, even for those who anticipate an enhancement of their social lives through hearing aid use, there must be proper instruction as to where and how to maximize the benefits of amplification. For most hearing aid users, groups of people all talking at once will present a problem, just as it usually does for normal hearing people. Clients must be warned against using such situations as the primary test of success with the instruments.

Clients who expect social ridicule and rejection suffer from anxiety about being left out. They need to provide specific examples of these situations for the dispenser to understand and to help them overcome their fears. Focusing on hiding the instrument, as opposed to its communication enhancing qualities, causes anxiety that will result in the expected negative result. As with normal hearing people, expecting to be rejected frequently leads to rejection. The psychology of dispensing involves the client's and the dispenser's awareness of these negative expectations so that they can change them.

The issue of expectations applies not only to clients and their families but also to hearing aid specialists' expectations for their clients and of themselves. Determination to handle difficult challenges results in specialists having higher expectations of themselves. Expecting to be more thorough is more likely to lead to careful and satisfying work. Part of this thoroughness is making sure that clients understand the specialist's expectations for the client regarding amplification. Addressing this important and often neglected issue of expectations helps bring a greater measure of reality to the dispensing situation for both the client and the specialist.

For more information on initial client interviewing, the reader is referred to Reiter (1985).

Openness

Americans born prior to 1950 grew up in a society in which it was very unusual to discuss private matters outside of the family. It was not normal for people to discuss their handicaps or human differences with strangers. Discussing emotional issues regarding disabilities was highly unlikely in the years prior to the humanistic 1960s. Sure, Jim Anderson on "Father Knows Best" was always around to help the family with whatever emotional needs required discussion, and the Cleavers were always helping Beaver with everyday life, but were these scenes typical of family life? Hardly. Most people who will be fitted with hearing aids prior to the twenty-first century grew up prior to the 1960s. In other words, the majority of people fitted for hearing aids for the next 10 years will be people who are used to communication patterns of emotional secrecy instead of openness.

Clients may be fully aware of their emotional feelings toward their hearing losses and toward amplification, but in most cases, these thoughts and feelings have never been shared with others. They may fear that sharing emotional issues will leave them open to negative criticism and eventual rejection. Their fears stimulate or exacerbate separation anxieties. Anxieties, in turn, can result in rejection of amplification.

To help clients with difficulties in being open to discuss the emotional problems with the hearing loss and amplification, hearing health professionals need to bring up two essential issues. The first is confidentiality. One would not ordinarily think that information regarding hearing loss or hearing aids needs to be kept confidential, but to the hearing-impaired person, keeping such information "under wraps" may be as essential as keeping the aids hidden. Letting clients know that any information they impart will not be shared with any other person, including family members, unless their consent is given, helps to reassure them that their feelings are respected and will remain in the office.

To ease open communication, the dispenser also needs to directly address emotional issues. The professional should describe and explain that discussion of the emotional side of the problem in the dispenser's office may be thought of as unusual by the client, but that it is indeed normal and can help obtain the best possible hearing aid fitting. Dispensers may also want to say that they know that discussion of emotional issues may be difficult, regardless of the subject, but regarding hearing loss and amplification the hearing aid specialist represents an open and interested party whose job it is to help through understanding.

During the interview process, certain areas of discussion can be used to guide the client toward a greater degree of openness. Many of these topic points are covered in the sections on personality and expectations. The issue of openness addresses the need for the dispenser to take the discussion onto a different plane of greater insight and understanding. Family issues are the most likely example. What are the bruises

hurts, and entanglements that affect the client's relationship with his or her family? Does Mr. Jones or Mrs. Smith feel isolated in his or her own home? Has the hearing loss resulted in feelings of being rejected by loved ones? These issues are tricky and involve difficult questions. However, being asked the right in-depth questions is frequently what the client needs to address the *need for* as well as the *fear of* hearing aids.

This discussion is not to suggest that the hearing aid specialist fulfill the role of a psychotherapist. Clearly, hearing aid professionals are not trained to engage clients in this capacity. The hearing aid specialist's reason for asking these questions is to learn what it feels like to be Mr. Jones or Mrs. Smith.

It behooves the specialist to behave in a professional manner, which will assist the client toward giving important information that will assist the dispensing process. For example, dispensers should appreciate clients' fears of being rejected due to hearing impairment, and dispensers should understand what hearing aid-related issues result in clients' feelings of embarrassment, incompetency, and sadness.

The hearing health professional must provide an open atmosphere in which it is all right to talk about fears of rejection or embarrassment. A conscious attempt must be made not to ridicule clients because of these voiced anxieties. Expressions such as "Do not be silly, people will not reject you!" do not foster trust from the client and will certainly make the dispensing local appear to be everything but an open, understanding environment.

The atmosphere must also be open for the family members to engage in dialogue with the client and the dispenser. What are the spouse's chief complaints regarding having a hearing loss in the family? Stone (1986) claimed misunderstanding develops easily in such families. According to Stone, "the hearing impaired person feels the family does not understand the problem and the family feels the person is not 'accepting' the hearing loss; is not adjusting properly." Both parties should be encouraged to describe the mutual frustrations of having a hearing problem in the family. Frequently, it is appropriate for the dispenser to arbitrate by asking each to listen to what the other is saying before defending or accusing. The dispenser should not play family counselor but should afford clients and family members the opportunity to voice their frustrations so that the dispenser can eventually describe how amplification, along with good listening, will make things better. However, the dispenser, the client, and family members must first develop, through an open dialogue, an understanding of what the problems are.

Is the client *open* to change? Many hearing-impaired people are quite used to a life-style that places them apart from society at large. The sense of feeling withdrawn is normal and, in some instances, is a very safe feeling. The dispenser, the source of amplification, and the prospect of a new life-style may be viewed by such clients with fear and negativity. The hearing health professional may be seen as forcing them into a world where they will be expected to perform and where they may fail. They fear that change will not be for the good. The hearing health professional is the key person in helping the client understand that changes resulting from amplification are for the good of the client and that amplification is consistent with human growth. However, this process takes time and patience on the part of the dispenser.

How open is the dispenser to change? This point is the flip side of the openness issue, involving openness on the part of dispensers toward how they view clients, themselves, and the roles dispensers play in the client–dispenser relationship.

The issue of proper fit has already been discussed. Is the hearing aid professional open to the idea that there may be a substantially better set of hearing instruments for the client than the ones chosen? Is the hearing aid professional open to say-

ing that maybe he or she has made an error in judgment and is willing to try something else? Is the hearing aid professional open, in general, toward admitting to clients and/ or colleagues that he or she made such an error? Is he or she open toward learning new information about the client, the instruments, and him- or herself? People who are willing to address these issues and deal with changes are professionals who want to continue to grow and mature in their work. Such professionals need to present the facts with confidence and understanding. In this way clients understand that the professional is competent, forthright, and human. The result is a greater degree of confidence in the professional and, thus, a very likely successful fitting.

Openness also refers to the hearing health professional's willingness to seek outside consultation to provide the very best hearing health care. Classes in aural rehabilitation aid the fitting process and enhance the credibility of the dispenser. Yet, many dispensers are hesitant to refer their clients to aural rehabilitation because they fear that the client will be referred to another dispenser or that those teaching the class will take issue with the hearing aid fitting. Attitudes like these leave little room for a positive team approach toward the best possible treatment of the client. The dispenser who holds such attitudes must look deep into his or her fears of being found out for not being perfect. This professional suffers from the fear of rejection and separation anxiety. Openness toward referral of clients for consultation or aural rehabilitation will be appreciated by clients and is another way in which the dispenser can be recognized for providing help instead of "just a hearing aid."

There is yet one more type of openness regarding the dispenser. Openness toward seeing oneself as more than the person who fits hearing aids is an attitude that gives audiologists who dispense hearing aids an expanded role and image over dispensers without graduate degree credentials. A creative approach to rehabilitation, especially with atypical populations, gives audiologists who dispense this expanded image. A good example can be illustrated with teenage clients with partial hearing losses who are mainstreamed into normal classrooms. At Hope for Hearing UCLA, there is an ongoing support group for this population. However, most hearing aid offices do not provide aural rehabilitation for adults or support groups for teenagers. The audiologist who sees his or her role as providing more than just a hearing aid fitting offers special programs for his or her clients. Bringing teenagers who have no way of meeting others with their unique problems together is such a program. Dispensers who are open to creative programming will find their work more fulfilling. Openness refers to a professional climate in which the professional is open to recognizing that creative programming is necessary for work fulfillment.

Personality

Hilgard, Atkinson, and Atkinson (1979) described personality as "the individual characteristics and ways of behaving that, in their organization of patterning, account for an individual's unique adjustments to his or her total environment (syn. Individuality)." In lay terms, personality is thought of as the way a person comes across or how the way they behave is described. Opinions of clients are frequently shaped by what the specialist thinks of the client's personality. This assessment can affect the specialist's dispensing behavior.

Just as attachment-separation-loss theory formed a good basis for understanding the mourning process surrounding hearing loss, the phenomenological approach to the study of personality forms a good basis for understanding the information that clients present about their lives and behavior. The phenomenological approach includes a number of theories that, although different in some areas, share a common emphasis on the individual's *private view of the world*. In other words, the reporting of subjective experience highlights the phenomenological approach. It concentrates on the whole person, seen as basically healthy, and emphasizes a positive, optimistic view of human nature.

Rather than looking for unconscious impulses, phenomenologists focus on the individual's subjective view of what is taking place in the *present*. They are concerned with how the individual perceives and interprets events. The hearing aid candidate who says that a hearing aid is unnecessary because there is nothing worthwhile to hear may be seen by the specialist as a resistant client when, in actuality, the client could very well be speaking about how he or she views the world. The woman who claims that all she needs is for people to speak louder could be experiencing the reality of improved hearing every time people do speak louder. In other words, we cannot form opinions about people until we really understand how they perceive themselves, the world, and their relationship to that perception. Amplification needs to be based on how the hearing aid candidate sees this relationship and not on how the hearing aid specialist sees it. The specialist's understanding of clients' personalities helps to bridge the gaps between possible differences in the experienced realities of the specialist and the client.

Questions asked should provide answers about how clients live their lives, as well as what they see as missing in their lives. Obtaining a *medical history* is a good, nonthreatening means of beginning the questioning and dialogue with clients. The information is usually viewed as objective by clients, and it is reassuring to them that the specialist is interested in their overall health. Get them to describe any severe illnesses and chronic problems that interfere with daily living. Talk with them about any medication they are taking. Counseling regarding possible toxicity of certain drugs and the need to consult a physician, when warranted, helps clients understand that the hearing aid specialist is interested in their overall well being.

An appropriate manner of asking questions about *work history* is also not obtrusive. Is the client presently working? Retired? Laid off? Was it forced or voluntary? Why? What jobs would the client like to hold? (Perhaps women who answer with "just a housewife" in answer to "present career" should be corrected. This occupation is demanding work that requires good on-the-job hearing.) Get clients to talk about the work they do or did; a simple job classification, such as engineer or teacher, is not sufficient. If clients understand that their work is important to the hearing health professional, they will provide details without coaxing. They will also be offering a subjective description of how environmental noises have and do interfere with work. The specialist should have clients describe their education.

Once medical and work information have been obtained, it is easier to address more personal family, marital, and social questions. Understanding a client's marital history helps the specialist learn about the client's close relationships, which require good ongoing communication, as well as understand losses which the person may have experienced. If a person is widowed or divorced, it is important to know how recently the loss took place. The specialist needs to know if clients are in a new marriage or relationship or if they have developed years of communication patterns with their partners.

The recent loss of a spouse due to death or divorce may affect a new candidate's adjustment to amplification. It is difficult to cope with acceptance of a hearing loss at the same time one is trying to get used to the loss of a loved one. Compassion and patience help the bereaved. They need time to cope with the many changes in their lives. The recently widowed often

feel rejected and that they are a burden to their family, friends, and society. They fear that their hearing problems make them an even greater source of irritation. Therefore, they are in a position to change their subjective experience of amplification. They can be taught that hearing aids can be "friends," which will bring them into a greater connection with others and away from isolation. These issues relate directly to the earlier discussion on separation anxiety. To be accepted, the hearing aid must be perceived as a source of connection to others and not as a source of further rejection.

Does the person live alone or with whom does he or she live? Frequently, hearing-impaired persons complain of a very uncooperative world in which others really do not care if they hear or not. They may answer that they do not associate with people and therefore do not actually need hearing aids. This is the experiential reality of the person making the statement. The hearing aid specialist may not view this statement as a healthy or positive perception regarding good social interaction, but the professional should try to avoid reinforcing it. Treat the person as if his or her opinion matters.

Get an appreciation for the client's general family history. Does the client have children? Do they live nearby? How often does the client see them? Are parents living? How many siblings does the client have and where do they fit in the birth order (oldest to youngest)? These questions help the hearing aid specialist understand the client's perception of past and present family support systems. Are these supports available or are they the source of much frustration and disappointment?

Sometimes the hearing specialist learns that the client has survived a child. This situation is one of the greatest burdens for an adult. Such a tragedy could result in a depressed personality and feelings that improved hearing is of no avail as life is perceived as empty.

Hearing-impaired adolescents may view the family as the sole element of an accepting world. The hearing aid dispenser may be the first opportunity for a young person to discuss problems with someone outside the family. Encouragement of social participation will help broaden a very constricted world. Families, as well as depressed clients, can often benefit from professional psychological counseling.

Finally, the specialist will find descriptions of the clients' leisure time valuable in understanding clients' social sense of themselves. Do they participate in organizations? Religious activities? Social get-togethers? Entertainment? What are their hobbies? With whom do they share these things?

All of this information helps the hearing specialist know who these people are and the direction in which they see their lives moving. Carl Rogers and Abraham Maslow are two phenomenologists who have delved deeply into the area of self-actualization. Rogers (1951) stated that, "The organism has one basic tendency and striving to actualize, maintain and enhance the experiencing organism" (p. 457). Maslow was an emphatic advocate of a person's tremendous positive potential for growth and fulfillment. He saw striving toward actualization of this potential as a basic quality of being human. This information is introduced here because it is important to regard clients as having this potential for continued growth and to convey this to clients so that they feel the dispenser can be of benefit in making positive changes in their communication and communication modes.

The flip side of the issue of personality is the personality of the dispenser. How hearing aid specialists act, the emotions they display, and their sense of self affect the dispensing process and is a focal point in the psychology of dispensing. Hilgard and colleagues (1979) paraphrased Maslow regarding characteristics of self-actualizers and behaviors that lead to self-actualiza-

tion. Their list, which was modified by Maslow, appears in Table 1–2.

Alfred Adler (1956), one of Sigmund Freud's most well know disciples, coined the term "social interest" to refer to the successful fulfillment of life's three most important tasks: love, friendship, and work. Dispensers who follow Maslow's list are certainly succeeding in social interest. The approach to work colors the personality of the dispenser and has an ongoing effect on the client–dispenser relationship which, in turn, makes for more successful dispensing and more enjoyment at work. This concept is elucidated further by other elements of the PEOPLE acronym.

Listening

Is the client taking in what is being said or is he or she distracted? The hearing aid specialist must constantly check to see if the client is "tuned in." The smiling elderly lady who shakes her head as if to indicate perfect agreement with what is being said may be thinking, "I wish this person would be quiet already because I cannot understand a word being said" or "I have only 10 minutes until the bus comes."

The dispenser should make clear distinctions between the words "hearing" and "listening" to the client. *Hearing* should be used to indicate sufficient loudness and clarity to *understand* what is being said. The word *listening* should indicate that one is paying sufficient *attention* to understand what is being said. Hearing is not always under one's control due to noise, health, and acoustical factors. Listening, or paying attention, is almost always under the individual's control. Another interesting point about the word listening is that it frequently connotes obeying orders or following through with an action. A parent frequently asks a child, "Were you listening to me?" or "Did you listen?" The dispenser must be certain to use listening in a way that indicates that the client needs to pay attention

TABLE 1–2. Maslow's characteristics of self-actualizers and behaviors leading to self-actualization.

CHARACTERISTICS OF SELF-ACTUALIZERS

Perceive reality efficiently and are able to tolerate uncertainty

Accept themselves and others for what they are

Spontaneous in thought and behavior

Problem-centered rather than self-centered

Have a good sense of humor

Highly creative

Resistant to enculturation, although not purposely unconventional

Concerned for the welfare of humanity

Capable of deep appreciation for the basic experiences of life

Establish deep, satisfying interpersonal relationships with a few, rather than many, people

Able to look at life from an objective viewpoint

BEHAVIORS LEADING TO SELF-ACTUALIZATION

Experience life as a child does, with full absorption and concentration

Try something new rather than sticking to secure and safe ways

Listen to your own feelings in evaluating experiences rather than to the voice of tradition or authority or the majority.

Be honest; avoid pretenses or "game playing"

Be prepared to be unpopular if your views don't coincide with those of most people

Assume responsibility

Work hard at whatever you decide to do

Try to identify your defenses and have the courage to give them up

From Hilgard, Atkinson, and Atkinson (1979), paraphrased with modifications from Maslow (1954, 1967). Reprinted with permission.

and never to obey, which could result in the client feeling like a child.

Unless the client is actively listening to the dispenser, the dispenser is not being heard and therefore is not being understood. The needed connection for transmitting information that ends in successful aiding of the individual never materializes.

Why is the client not listening? When does he or she stop listening? What turns the client off? The issue of preoccupation was addressed in the section on anxiety. Many people with hearing impairments are so preoccupied with worrying about what they are going to miss that they do not pay attention to what they do hear. They are preoccupied with not hearing. Others are preoccupied with questions such as: Will the dispenser like me if I ask questions? I am worried I cannot tell the difference between wearing and not wearing the hearing aids. Will it show? or Will I be able to hear once I get out of this office? Much needed information is lost when the mind is filled with other thoughts and questions. The dispenser may as well be speaking to the hearing aids and not to the person wearing them. The client must be brought back from preoccupation or distraction in a gentle way. It is always good to have the client repeat some of the dispenser's comments and explain certain facts. This reassures the dispenser that the information is being received.

During our hearing loss workshops at the UCLA Hope for Hearing Foundation, participants are asked to list their responses to the statement: I stop listening when . . . . This technique, adopted from Margaret Fleming Haspiel of the San Francisco Veterans Hospital, helps participants recognize that their lack of listening, which they can control, rather than their hearing loss is frequently responsible for problems in communication. The same technique can be applied in the dispenser's office. Major distractions that interfere with listening include the emotions of anger, fear, joy, and sadness along with the emotional feelings and thoughts that the listeners have about the persons speaking to them.

Many people who have hearing impairments learn to tune out when they no longer feel a part of the communication world. Poor listening behavior becomes a major component of their communication style. Clients who have tuned out may smile and shake their heads but they do not attempt to tell the speaker that they do not understand. Some may not attempt to understand what is being said. They tune out in a way that they believe is polite. However, speakers feel annoyed and, without really understanding the problem, begin to distance themselves from the seemingly "air-head" head nodder.

In the dispenser's office, clients frequently tune out because they are bored or because the information is too far above their understanding. If they miss one piece of critical information, they assume that they will not understand the next piece of information. At this point, they are tuned in to being lost and fear that the dispenser is just one more person who represents the unavailable status quo.

This scenario brings up the role of the hearing health professional as a listener. How good a listener is the dispenser? When clients are speaking is the dispenser thinking about the next client, why the session is taking so long, or what will be said to the next client if this session runs late? It is very normal to be distracted by thoughts while a person is speaking. However, the dispenser must be willing to say, "Excuse me, I missed that point" or "Pardon me, I was distracted and did not get what you just said." In this way, the hearing health professional also becomes a good role model in that listening, not hearing, is put forward as the reason something is missed. Of course, the healthy assertiveness with which such a statement is made also demonstrates good modeling: It is okay to say that you were not listening. It is not okay to fool someone into thinking that information, which is probably important for them to impart, was received and understood when it was not.

Dispensers need to be aware of what causes them to tune out. Listing exercises are good tests for hearing aid specialists to give themselves, especially responding to the statement, "I stop listening when . . . ." Dispensers will probably be surprised to see the myriad ways in which they tune out. These range from fatigue to just finding a client's speaking pattern irritating. However, good hearing health care requires good listening, and dispensers must also find ways to alert themselves to their own tuning-out behavior.

The dispenser has an even more important task to perform regarding the issue of listening. As mentioned earlier, many hearing-impaired people feel quite isolated. Clients' feelings of isolation include a general sense that no one is really interested in them or in what they have to say. Their physician, who could not help them via medicine or surgery, has sent them to someone else, whom clients may feel will also give them the "brush off." Their families seem too absorbed in daily living to take the time to listen. Their friends do not understand the situation any better than family members. Subjects that hearing-impaired clients want so badly to address with others include the issue of faulty hearing and their tremendous desire to once again engage the world as before.

The hearing health professional cannot take the place of former friends or family members who do not understand. The hearing health professional can, however, be a person who demonstrates that people do listen and that there are others who are willing to listen to hearing-impaired persons discuss the issues that most concern them.

Clients' statements about their hearing losses and their negative feelings regarding amplification have often fallen on deaf ears. "Go get a hearing aid!" may seem to be the only thing family and friends understand. The dispenser can be a person who demonstrates that there are people who are willing to listen to reasons why amplification may be difficult and frightening. The dispenser, through listening, can verify or disagree with what is being said, but what clients say should be examined and discussed further. In the dispenser's office hearing-impaired clients can feel like they are an active part of the conversation and not an extra party to it. Challenging the client can be done in a genuine way when the dispenser is really listening to what is being said.

The hearing health professional has the opportunity to bring dialogue back into clients' lives. By being listened to, hearing-impaired people begin to regain former good feelings of self-esteem and self-acknowledgment. Of course, the reverse is also true. The dispenser who appears too busy to listen or too disinterested to pay attention to what clients have to say communicates to clients that they are really unimportant and just a means of commercial gain for the dispenser. This type of communication increases the likelihood that the aids will not be purchased or that the chest of drawers will have a full-time occupant.

Empathic listening is really quite easy. Being heard and understood is a normal human desire. Adult clients wish to be treated as adults and not dismissed as children. Empathic listening means that agreement or disagreement is not routine but comes as an honest response to what the dispenser feels about what the client has said. This response is not a critical or judgmental one, but one that is used to guide clients toward accepting the most realistic and healthiest (both physical and mental) approach in dealing with hearing problems. Paying attention to what is being said makes work more fulfilling because dispensers will experience themselves as more active participants in the dispensing process and clients will receive more positive feelings from the on-target exchange.

Education

Education is the final element in the PEOPLE acronym. It calls for the most active participation by the hearing aid specialist. Frequently, proper fitting, which appears to be the most central issue in hearing aid fitting, is out of the hands of the dispensing agent and under the domain of the referral source. The dispenser's role as an instructor and guide will be the long-lasting, pivotal ingredient in the client–dispenser relationship. Good educators help their students reduce tensions through careful instruction, consistent checking or feedback, and long range planning. The issue of education is discussed at the end of the PEOPLE section because it influences and is influenced by all of the other elements as Figure 1–1 illustrates.

In the recent pop psychology literature, considerable attention has been given to the negative characteristics of parent-child-type relationships when both parties are adults. The dispenser–client relationship can be viewed as a parent–child relationship that has some very healthy aspects. Most new hearing aid candidates are fledglings who, if left on their own, will find very little security in the noise bombarding world. They need to be guided through all of the stages that will make them satisfied and successful hearing aid users. A good

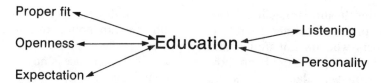

FIGURE 1-1. Diagram of the PEOPLE acronym describing the role of the hearing aid dispenser in treating the hearing impaired.

parent cares for his or her offspring through good instruction, watchful eyes and ears, and realistic communication of what can be expected in the world, and continues to support them through gentle and productive criticism. The educational role of the hearing aid professional, it is hoped, will be as constructive and effective as that of the positive parent prototype.

From their first interaction with a client, professional hearing aid specialists should act as guides who will see the client through the amplification process. Careful explanation of the fitting procedure reassures the client that he or she will not be alone, that the fitting of hearing aids is neither too simple nor too complex, and that the fitting process requires planning and checking. Clients can begin to arrange their schedules based on the timing of appointments with the understanding that several appointments will likely be required. It is understood from the beginning that there will be no *instant* cures.

Explanations of what hearing aids are and how they work help to reduce consumer and mechanical anxieties. When clients understand the apparatus, they begin to trust the person who did the fitting and also to trust their own manipulation of the apparatus. This process results in increased self-confidence. Fears such as "What will I do if the aid whistles?" are eliminated because the client has information about what can be done. In this way the dispenser not only teaches the client how to operate the hearing aid but also increases the client's self-confidence as well.

With increased self-confidence comes a reduction in attention anxiety. As people

are taught more and more about how to control and manipulate hearing aids, they begin to perceive hearing aids as a part of themselves. Therefore, they begin to feel less self-conscious and do not worry as much about being noticed because of the hearing aids. In this way, the hearing aid specialist can also be regarded as an instructor in self acceptance. People tolerate themselves better when they stop perceiving themselves as irritating light beacons drawing negative attention.

A dispensing audiologist who educates his or her clients also reduces separation anxiety. Part of the dispensing process is teaching the client to understand and operate the hearing aid. Another part is teaching the client how to explain the nature of the hearing loss and amplification to normal hearing people. Knowing how to put the instrument in the ear and how to operate it does not mean the clients are any less fearful of being rejected by someone who recognizes that they have a hearing loss or that they wear hearing aids. Instructing the client to tell others that hearing aids are limited in what they can do and how others can help serves two functions. First, the client is told how to explain the aids to others, and second, the client receives the same message. The client must be educated regarding amplification expectations and how to clearly explain such expectations to others. The client must also be given distinct guidance on how to instruct others to help: to speak at understandable rates, to keep the mouth visible, to face the hearing-impaired person, to get the person's attention before speaking, to make sure that the sun and other bright light is not hampering lip reading visibility, and that loud voices and noises are painful.

One form of anxiety has not yet been discussed: competency anxiety. The general population fears disabled, handicapped, or just plainly different people because the general population does not know what to do about such people when the occasion arises. Therefore, they try to avoid or ignore people who are different.

Hearing-impaired persons recognize the tremendous stress they feel when trying to communicate with normal hearing people. What a hearing-impaired person does not realize is that the same interchange is filled with tension for the normal hearing person as well. Normal hearing people often feel that their judgment, their ability to make themselves understood, and their speech characteristics are being scrutinized and judged by hard-of-hearing people. These normal hearing people feel that their competency as communicating human beings is being questioned, and they feel insecure and inadequate because they really do not know what to do.

The aged hearing-impaired person fears being thought of as too old because of the loss of hearing, while the aged normal hearing person who is talking to a hearing-impaired person also feels too old because of his or her inability to get the message across to the hearing-impaired person. For both the result is a sense of inadequacy and frustration. Teaching clients how to explain the hearing loss to others also leads to a reduction in competency anxieties in the normal hearing.

A suggested teaching technique is to relate the training of the normal hearing world by hearing-impaired persons to the guidance of first-time tourists in a foreign country. Tourists are usually ignorant of the customs, language, and nuances of the native population. They must be educated in these important facts to be understood, for their needs to be met, and for an enjoyable interchange to occur between hosts and visitors. The same is true for the normal hearing person who feels as though he or she has landed on foreign turf when encountering a hearing-impaired person.

In the author's research (Reiter, 1985) on adjustment to hearing aids and its relationship to the dispenser's role as a teacher, excellent adjustment to hearing aids was found to be positively correlated with the degree to which subjects valued the dispenser's instructions. These results were statistically significant at the 0.001 level, meaning that these results were likely to have occurred by chance only one time per thousand cases. These findings, which support the claim that the dispenser–client relationship is as important, if not more important, than the apparatus–client relationship, should not be underestimated.

Continuing education also has a psychological effect on the professional. Constant awareness and retraining in new instruments and procedures brings continued self-confidence and self-satisfaction to the hearing aid specialist. In the psychological literature, learning is synonymous with growth and change. Such powerful change will have a comforting and reassuring effect on the client–dispenser relationship as well as an effect on the actual dispensing.

This chapter presented a particular way of looking at clients and the dispensing process from a psychological perspective. It also presented a way of looking at the dispensing audiologist from a psychological perspective. Satisfaction with amplification and growth in communication are facilitated through the dispensing audiologist's awareness of the client's personality dynamics, listening skills, anxieties, and expectations. The professional dispenser guides clients via careful listening, providing an open atmosphere, awareness of his or her own behaviors, a presentation of realistic expectations, and careful instruction and follow-up on the operation and maintenance of hearing aids as well as understanding of the hearing loss. The projected results are new hearing and improved communication through amplification and awareness.

REFERENCES

Barker, R. G., Wright, B. A., Meyerson, L., & Gonick, M. (1953). *Adjustment to physical handicap and illness: A survey of the social psychology physique and disability* (Bull. No. 55). New York: Social Science Research Council.

Bolton, B. (1976). Introduction and overview. In B. Bolton (Ed.), *Psychology of deafness for rehabilitation counselors* (pp. 1–18). Baltimore: University Park Press.

Bowlby, J. (1969). *Attachment and loss: I. Attachment.* New York: Basic Books.

Goetzinger, C. (1972). *The psychology of hearing impairment.* In J. Katz (Ed.), *Handbook of clinical audiology.* Baltimore: Williams & Wilkins.

Hilgard, E. R., Atkinson, A., & Atkinson, A. (1979). *An introduction to psychology.* New York: Harcourt, Brace, Jovanovich.

Jackson, P. (1982). A psychological and economic profile of the hearing impaired adult. In R. Hull (Ed.), *Rehabilitational audiology* (pp. 27–33). New York: Grune & Stratton.

Levine, E. S. (1976). Psycho-cultural determinants in personality development. *Volta Review, 78,* 258–267.

Myklebust, H. (1960). *The psychology of deafness: Sensory deprivation, learning, and adjustment.* New York: Grune & Stratton.

Pappas, J., Graham, S., & Rolfe, R. (1982). Psychological problems associated with hearing impairment. *Hearing Instruments, 32*(10), 54–55.

Parkes, C. M. (1971). Psycho-social transitions: A field for study. *Social Science and Medicine, 5,* 101–115.

Ramsdell, D. A. (1964). The psychology of the hard of hearing and deafened adult. In H. Davis & S. R. Silverman (Eds.), *Hearing and deafness* (pp. 459–473). Holt, Rinehart & Winston.

Reiter, R. S. (1985). Patient information and history. In R. Sandlin (Ed.), *Hearing instrument science and fitting practices.* Livonia, MI: National Institute of Hearing Instrument Studies.

Rousey, C. (1971). Psychological reactions to hearing loss. *Journal of Speech and Hearing Disorders, 36*(3), 382–389.

Sandlin, R. (1974). The psychology of the hearing impaired. *Hearing Instruments, 25*(11), 22–23.

Schein, J. D. (1977). Psychology of the hearing impaired consumer. *Audiology and Hearing Education, 3,* 12–14, 44.

Schein, J. D. (1978). The deaf community. In H. Davis & S. R. Silverman, *Hearing and deafness* (4th ed., pp. 511–524). New York: Holt, Rinehart, & Winston.

Schein, J., and Delk, M., Jr. (1974). *The deaf population of the United States.* Silver Spring, MD: National Association of the Deaf.

Schlesinger, H. S., & Meadow, K. P. (1972). *Sound and sign: Childhood deafness and mental health.* Berkeley: University of California Press.

Stone, H. (1986). Psychology of people who are hard of hearing. *Encyclopedia on deafness.* New York: McGraw-Hill.

Webster's New World Dictionary of the American Language (College Ed.). (1966). Cleveland: World Publishing.

2

■ THREE IMPORTANT CONSIDERATIONS IN HEARING AID SELECTION

H. GUSTAV MUELLER ■

DAVID B. HAWKINS ■

*T*he obvious goal of the hearing aid selection process is to determine the best amplification system for a given patient. Traditionally, audiologists have devoted the greatest amount of time and effort to the selection of the hearing aid's frequency response curve. In the past, this often was measured indirectly through repeated speech testing with different hearing aid models. In recent years, because of the popularity of prescriptive fitting approaches, functional gain, and probe tube microphone measures, greater attention has been given to the direct assessment of gain at specific frequencies. While the importance of appropriate gain across frequencies is obvious, other selection options also play a critical role in the overall success or failure of the hearing aid fitting. Many of these factors, however, are given little attention, and are sometimes overlooked, in the hearing aid selection process. In this chapter the discussion focuses on three such factors that are useful in improving speech intelligibility and enhanc-ing user satisfaction. They are directional microphones, binaural amplification, and loudness discomfort level (LDL) testing.

DIRECTIONAL MICROPHONE HEARING AIDS

The foremost goal in the majority of hearing aid fittings is to improve speech intelligibility when background noise is present. Many of the hearing impaired, especially those with only high-frequency impairment, express little communication difficulty in quiet non-reverberant listening environments. It is the difficult listening situations involving background noise that prompt many of these people to try hearing aid use. For example, Bender and Mueller (1984) surveyed 300 people who were obtaining hearing aids for the first time and asked them to rate their reasons for seeking amplification. Of the seventeen different factors mentioned, the most common rea-

son given was communication difficulty in
noise; 82 percent of those surveyed stated
that this was a significant factor.

To understand the communication difficulties experienced by people with hearing impairments, it is important to consider that background noise affects these
individuals to a greater extent than it does
normal-hearing individuals. This point is
illustrated in Figure 2–1, taken from the
work of Hawkins and Yacullo (1984). In
this experiment, the authors measured the
50 percent speech recognition level for NU-
6 monosyllabic words presented with a
multitalker speech babble for normals and
a group of hearing-impaired subjects. To
obtain the 50 percent correct recognition
point, the level of the background noise was
varied using an adaptive procedure. The resulting mean signal-to-noise (S/N) ratios
for three different reverberation times (0.3,
0.6 and 1.2 s) for the two groups are shown

in Figure 2–1. Observe that across reverberant conditions, the scores of the hearing-
impaired groups are separated by approximately 10 to 13 dB from those of the normal-hearing group. Stated differently, to attain the same performance as the normal-
hearing group, the hearing-impaired group
required a listening situation with 10 to 13
dB less noise. Although performance for
both groups predictably becomes poorer as
reverberation time increases, it appears
that increasing the reverberation also wid-
ens the gap between the two groups. These
findings of Hawkins and Yacullo serve to
illustrate the difficulties faced by individuals who are hearing-impaired and the importance of providing them the most favorable S/N ratio possible. Until the time that
digital processing hearing aids with effective noise reduction circuitry become the
routine fitting, the directional microphone
hearing aid (DMHA) remains one of the

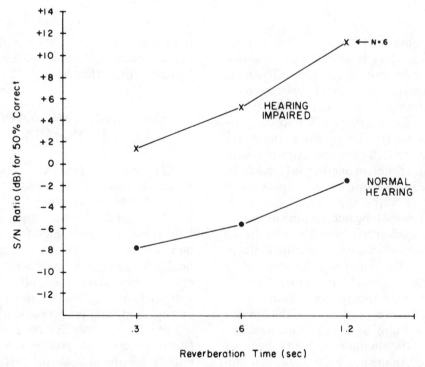

FIGURE 2–1. Illustration of the effect of different mean S/N ratios for hearing-impaired and normal hearing groups. Results shown for the S/N ratios yielding 50 percent correct performance at three reverberation times. From Hawkins and Yacullo, 1984. Reprinted with permission.

most effective methods of improving the S/N ratio at the ear of the listener.

Design of the DMHA

In May of 1971, a new type of hearing aid was introduced to the American market that contained a Linear Array Dephasing microphone, commonly referred to as a directional microphone. This style of hearing aid originally was developed by the Wilco firm of Hamburg, Germany in the late 1960s. Directional microphones themselves, however, had been used in the recording industry since the early 1940s (Bauer, 1942). The only previously reported attempt of "directional amplification," was by Lybarger (1947), who designed a hearing aid that provided some cancellation of sounds arriving from other than a 0-degree azimuth. Research with this early version of a directional hearing aid apparently was not successful, and it received little attention in the commercial market.

The DMHAs of today do not differ substantially from the models introduced in the early 1970s. Summary articles are available that describe the design of the directional microphone used for DMHAs (e.g., Knowles Electronics, 1980; Hillman, 1981). Shown in Figures 2-2 and 2-3 are cross-sectional drawings of an omnidirectional pressure type microphone (Figure 2-2) and a directional microphone (Figure 2-3). Briefly, as shown in Figure 2-3, the directional microphone has two inlets that allow sound to enter both the front and rear acoustical cavities and impinge on either side of the microphone diaphragm. Pressure differences exerted on the diaphragm cause it to move and are converted to an electrical output signal. If the air pressure in both cavities is the same phase and magnitude, cancellation occurs. The time delay acoustic network (shown in the rear microphone inlet) is selected so that if a sound strikes the rear inlet first, the arrival time of this sound will be reduced so that it reaches the diaphragm of the microphone at the same time as the sound entering the front inlet, causing cancellation. Of course, the time delay required for maximum cancellation varies for different frequencies. DMHAs, therefore, tend to have varying amounts of directional effect across frequencies. Be-

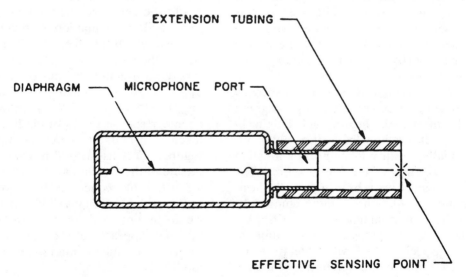

FIGURE 2-2. Diagramatic cross-sectional view of an omnidirectional pressure type microphone. From Hillman, 1981. Reprinted with permission.

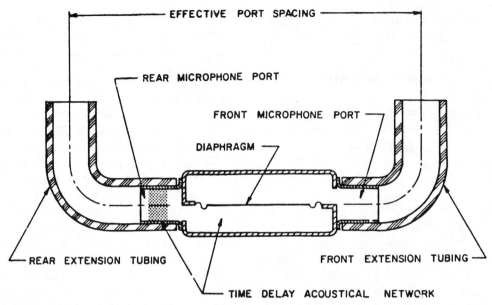

FIGURE 2-3. Diagramatic cross-sectional view of a directional microphone. From Hillman, 1981. Reprinted with permission.

cause background noise is primarily low frequency, the DMHA usually is designed to provide maximum attenuation for this frequency range.

Due to the nature of the design of the DMHA, traditional electroacoustic measures (e.g., frequency response, gain, SSPL90) provide little information regarding the hearing aid's directional effectiveness. It is necessary, therefore, to conduct additional measurements that reveal the ability of the DMHA to attenuate sound from specified directions or azimuths. The measurement customarily is accomplished by conducting a receptor intensity polar graph (polar plot) of the hearing aid. This technique indicates how the hearing aid is differentially sensitive to sound as a function of the azimuth of the sound source. The plotting can be made by using only the hearing aid in isolation or, more commonly, with the hearing aid mounted on a KEMAR. Polar directivity patterns have become familiar aspects of the DMHA literature and often are shown for different frequencies of interest (e.g., 500 Hz, 1000 Hz, 2000 Hz). A sample polar plot is shown in Figure 2-4.

This example is from Preves (1976), and is obtained from an in-the-ear (ITE) DMHA mounted in the right ear of a KEMAR. The difference between the dotted response (directional) and the solid line (non-directional) ITE hearing aid reveals the amount and azimuth of the attenuation provided by the directional microphone. This response would indicate a good DMHA design, as 15 to 25 dB of attenuation is provided from the rear quadrants (i.e., 90–270°), yet, as shown, the aids perform essentially equally for sound originating from the front (e.g., 315–45°). Another method of illustrating the DMHA characteristics is through frequency response curves of the hearing aid taken at 0 and 180-degree azimuths (see Figure 2-5). This method provides a clear picture of the directional characteristics as a function of frequency. The curve shown in Figure 2-5 is perhaps slightly better than would be obtained from all DMHAs, as this aid appears to provide substantial front-to-back attenuation ranging from 250 to 4000 Hz.

The variability of the directional effectiveness of DMHAs from different manufac-

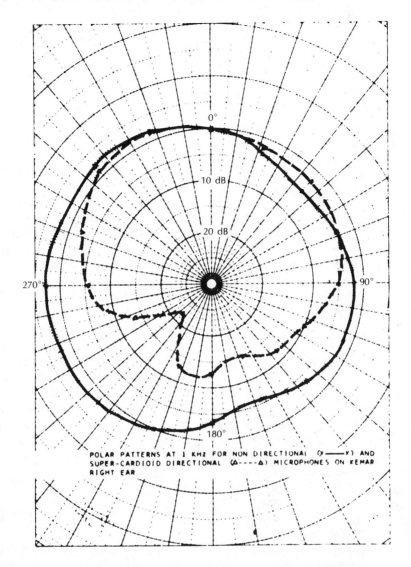

FIGURE 2-4. Polar plotting at 1000 Hz for an omnidirectional (solid line) and a directional (dotted line) in-the-ear hearing aid mounted in the right ear of a KEMAR. From Preves, 1976. Reprinted with permission.

turers was illustrated in an electroacoustic comparative study by Beck (1983). In this study, DMHAs and omnidirectional microphone hearing aids (OMHAs) were rated on three electroacoustic indices: directional efficiency, equivalent acoustic distance, and directivity index. These indices, discussed in detail by Preves (1976), are described briefly here as follows: (1) directional efficiency: The ratio of microphone output from a 0-degree incident sound to the microphone output resulting from random sounds incident all around an imaginary sphere (a microphone that is perfectly omnidirectional would have a ratio of 1.00); (2) equivalent acoustic distance: This measure relates how far the microphone may be from the signal source, in the presence of noise, to produce a given signal-to-noise ratio (in the 1983 Beck study, improvement

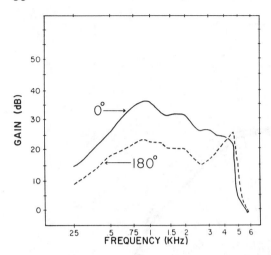

FIGURE 2–5. Insertion gain frequency response curves for a behind-the-ear directional microphone hearing aid. The curves were obtained with the hearing aid mounted on a KEMAR in an anechoic chamber with speakers at 0 and 180 degree azimuths. From Hawkins and Yacullo, 1984. Reprinted with permission.

is expressed by a shorter equivalent distance, using 10 feet as a reference); (3) directional index: This measure represents the ratio of the microphone output from sounds originating in an imaginary front hemisphere to the microphone output for sounds originating in an imaginary rear hemisphere.

Beck (1983) reports on these three measures in comparing 10 behind-the-ear (BTE) DMHAs and 4 BTE OMHAs using a speech spectrum noise. The hearing aids were mounted on a KEMAR in an anechoic chamber. As shown in Table 2–1, Beck's results illustrate that the directivity of DMHAs varies substantially across manufacturers and that some poorly designed DMHAs offer little, or no more, directionality than some OMHAs. In general, however, it appears that most DMHAs provide a 2 to 3 dB improvement in the S/N ratio over similarly designed OMHA instruments. The significance of this improvement for speech intelligibility is discussed in a later section of this chapter.

Although the polar plots, the 0- to 180-degree frequency response curves, or other electroacoustic comparisons serve as useful tools in designing DMHAs, comparing one DMHA with another, or estimating directional efficiency, they often present somewhat misleading information concerning the performance of the DMHA in everyday listening situations. These electroacoustic measurements usually are obtained in anechoic chambers. It is known, however, that the DMHAs directional characteristics are considerably reduced in reverberant listening environments. The degree to which reverberation affects the performance of DMHAs was studied systematically by Studebaker, Cox, and Formby (1980). These authors conducted 0- to 180-degree frequency response curves for DMHAs mounted on a KEMAR when the manikin was placed in rooms of varying reverberation times. Their findings showed that when the reverberation time reached 0.8 s or greater, little directionality remained. This raises on obvious and important question: Does the remaining directionality observed for the DMHA in reverberant listening conditions result in improved speech intelligibility in noise for the hearing-impaired listener? Considerable research has addressed this question.

Behavioral Studies of DMHA Use

Shortly after the DHMA was introduced, several studies emerged comparing this hearing aid with the more traditional omnidirectional microphone models. These studies typically based the comparison on the results of monosyllabic speech recognition testing in noise for subjects using the two instruments in an audiometric test booth (an experimental paradigm consistent with the method of evaluating hearing aids that was used in the early 1970s). As pointed out by Mueller and Grimes (1977), the results of these studies were largely dictated by the azimuths that the researchers chose for presenting the speech or noise signals, for example, if speech was presented

TABLE 2-1. Results of the analysis of ten directional and four omnidirectional hearing aids, rank ordered according to degree of directionality from greatest to least based on three measures of directional characteristics.

Hearing Aids	Directional Efficiency	Equivalent Acoustical Distance (re: 10 ft.)	Directivity Index (in dB)
DIRECTIONAL			
A	0.64	8.02	1.92
B	0.65	8.06	1.87
C	0.71	8.41	1.50
D	0.76	8.72	1.19
E	0.80	8.98	0.93
F	0.81	9.03	0.89
G	0.85	9.25	0.68
H	1.02	10.09	−0.08
I	1.06	10.30	−0.26
J	1.09	10.45	−0.38
OMNIDIRECTIONAL			
A	1.03	10.17	−0.15
B	1.44	12.02	−1.60
C	1.46	12.07	−1.63
D	1.55	12.45	−1.90

From Beck, 1983. Reprinted with permission.

from the front and noise from behind, the DMHA had a distinct advantage. In summarizing many of these articles, Mueller (1981) concluded that in almost all instances the DMHA was found to be superior. He further stated that in the few studies that did not favor DMHAs (e.g., similar results were obtained for the two microphone types) it was only because adequate background noise was not utilized, the azimuth(s) of the speech or noise signal(s) was in opposition to the design of the DMHA, or the DMHA used in the experiment was poorly designed and actually functioning as an OMHA. In an attempt to develop a method of evaluating DMHAs in the clinic setting without establishing a bias for the DMHA, Mueller and Sweetow (1978) suggested presenting the competing signal from an overhead location. The authors reported that this location had the desired effect of surrounding the listener with noise, yet did not require the use of several loudspeakers. In an experimental application of this presentation method, Mueller and Johnson (1979) evaluated the effects of varying the front-to-back ratio of a DMHA on speech understanding for a group of hearing-impaired listeners. Using the synthetic sentence identification (SSI) test, Figure 2–6 illustrates the improvement observed in speech understanding for three levels of background competition (0 dB, -10 dB, and -20 dB) as directivity increased (aids A to D, respectively). A systematic improvement of 8 to 12 percent occurs for all three listening conditions as the directional efficiency of the hearing aid is increased. (Front-to-back ratios at 1000 Hz ranged from 6 dB for aid A to 20 dB for aid D.)

Although the results of Mueller and Johnson (1979) showed a significant ad-

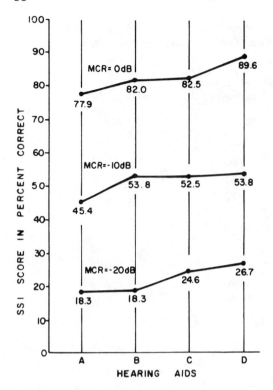

Synthetic sentence identification (SSI) scores at three different message-to-competition ratios (MCRs) for four hearing aids differing in degree of directionality. From Mueller and Johnson, 1979. Reprinted with permission.

vantage for DMHAs, it must be pointed out that this testing was conducted in a relatively non-reverberant audiometric test booth. Recall that Studebaker and colleagues (1980) reported that at least some DMHAs lose their directivity in more reverberant listening environments. In recent years, Hawkins and colleagues have studied the important effects of the interaction of speech recognition in noise, DMHAs, and reverberation.

In the first of these studies, Madison and Hawkins (1983) conducted speech recognition testing using NU-6 monosyllabic words in both an anechoic chamber and a reverberant room (0.6 s) with a hearing aid that could be switched between omnidirectional and directional reception. In both listening environments, the background noise was altered to obtain a 50 percent speech recognition score. The results for 12 subjects are shown in Table 2-2. Observe that for the anechoic environment a mean improvement in S/N ratio of 10.7 dB was found for the directional setting. While this mean advantage decreased in the reverberant room, a significant 3.4 dB improvement remained, and 11 of the 12 subjects contin-

TABLE 2-2. S/N ratios for 50 percent correct performance for the omnidirectional and directional microphone in an anechoic and reverberant room.

Subject	Anechoic Room			Reverberant Room		
	Omni	Direct.	Difference	Omni	Direct.	Difference
1	−5.4	−16.1	10.7	−2.7	−5.0	2.3
2	−5.9	−14.8	8.9	−2.3	−7.3	5.0
3	−3.4	−14.1	10.7	−1.1	−5.4	4.3
4	−3.6	−13.4	9.8	−2.3	−5.4	3.1
5	−3.9	−14.8	10.9	−1.8	−3.4	1.6
6	−5.9	−14.8	8.9	−2.5	−2.1	−0.4
7	−6.6	−18.2	11.6	−2.3	−9.6	7.3
8	−3.6	−16.4	12.8	−0.2	−6.8	6.6
9	−4.3	−17.5	13.2	−3.2	−5.2	2.0
10	−3.6	−14.1	10.5	2.9	0.7	2.2
11	−4.3	−14.5	10.2	2.3	0.7	1.6
12	−5.4	−15.0	9.6	−1.1	−6.6	5.5
Mean	−4.7	−15.3	10.7	−1.2	−4.6	3.4
S.D.	1.2	1.5	1.4	1.9	3.1	2.3

From Madison and Hawkins, 1983. Reprinted with permission.

ued to show improvement for the directional setting. These results clearly demonstrate that if a well-designed DMHA is chosen, directional advantages remain even in a moderately reverberant listening condition.

The performance of DMHAs in reverberation was explored further in a study reported by Hawkins and Yacullo (1984). In this experiment, 50 percent speech recognition scores in noise were established for both normal-hearing and hearing-impaired individuals in three levels of reverberation. As shown in Figure 2–7, an advantage for the DMHA of 4 to 6 dB emerged for reverberation times of 0.3 and 0.6 s. The advantage was similar for both groups and was not dependent on whether the listening condition was monaural or binaural. (At the 1.2 s reverberation time, the DMHA advantage was not significant

for the normal-hearing group; and many of the hearing-impaired subjects could not attain a 50 percent score; therefore, mean scores could not be calculated.) Again, these findings of Hawkins and Yacullo (1984) demonstrate the potential advantage of a DMHA over an OMHA for typical listening environments.

In a third investigation related to the effectiveness of DMHAs in everyday listening conditions, Hawkins (1984) included directional microphones as a variable in the study of speech recognition in noise for hearing-impaired children using hearing aids and FM systems. Directional microphones were shown to be superior for two separate conditions. First, when the hearing aid was used alone, without the FM system activated, the directional microphone showed a 2.6 to 2.8 dB S/N advantage. Sec-

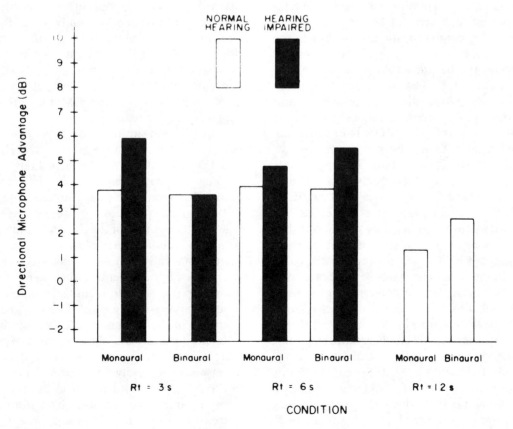

FIGURE 2–7. Directional microphone advantage in dB for monaural and binaural hearing aids at three reverberation (Rt) conditions. From Hawkins and Yacullo, 1984. Reprinted with permission.

ond, when the FM system was utilized, a directional teacher's microphone was found to provide a significant improvement in S/N ratio (3.3 dB) over the omnidirectional microphone.

The results of these three studies by Hawkins and colleagues clearly illustrate the advantages available from directional microphones. A S/N improvement of 3 to 6 dB was consistently present for the majority of test conditions and reverberation levels. One method of determining the significance of this improvement in S/N ratio is to survey hearing aid users after they have compared an OMHA to a DMHA.

Survey Reports of DMHA Users

It is well recognized that the results of speech intelligibility testing in the clinical hearing aid evaluation may bear little relationship to successful hearing aid use in everyday communication. In regard to the DMHA, this gap has been bridged to some degree by the previously reported work of Hawkins and colleagues, as these researchers created "real-life" experimental conditions. An important additional measure of the benefits of the DMHA is to solicit the opinions of users who have compared an OMHA to a DMHA. Early research of this type was reported by Nielsen (1973) and Nielsen and Ludvigsen (1978). In both of these studies, preferences emerged for DMHAs in some listening conditions, but not in others. One limitation of these early studies was that two different hearing aids were used for comparative purposes, one featuring a directional microphone and the other an omnidirectional microphone. While the electroacoustic characteristics of the two hearing aids in the studies were similar, the possible influence of other uncontrolled variables existed. Recent studies of subjective ratings of DMHAs have used a hearing aid that allows the user to switch between omnidirectional and directional microphones. Very little change other than

directivity occurs when the hearing aid is changed from one microphone type to the other.

Mueller, Grimes, and Erdman (1983) reported two experiments of user ratings of hearing aids that could be switched between omnidirectional and directional microphones. In the first of these studies, the authors discuss 30 subjects who used the hearing aid in a variety of listening situations for a 6-week period. The results showed that for listening situations in quiet, the majority of responses (42%) were in the no-preference category, and no significant preference for microphone type emerged. For the situations when background noise was present, 31 percent of the responses remained in the no-preference category. However, when preferences were present, the DMHA outweighed the OMHA by a 2 : 1 margin (47 vs. 22%). This ratio remained constant across other variables such as age of respondent, daily use of the hearing aid, and amount of communication with others. For individuals who reported that 50 percent or more of their daily communication was in a noisy environment, preferences for the OMHA setting dropped to 12 percent.

In a second similar study, Mueller and colleagues (1983) compared the OMHA and DMHA settings for 30 individuals attending a 10-day aural rehabilitation program. This group differed from the group in the first study in that they were younger (age 21–49), eighteen of the thirty were fitted with non-occluding earmolds, and all were fitted binaurally. The subjects were instructed to alternate between the two microphone types in four different listening conditions varying in degree of difficulty. For example, in the optimum listening condition, the listener was close to the talker, there was no background noise, and the room was only mildly reverberant. In each of the three more difficult listening conditions, distance from the talker, background noise, and room reverberation were increased. The results of the user ratings are shown in Figure 2–8. Preferences for the DMHA were observed for all listening conditions, although these preferences increased as the listening situations became more difficult. Preferences for the DMHA were also greater for individuals fitted with occluding molds, presumably because there was more low-frequency amplification, which potentially could be attenuated. When the listening situation was moderately adverse, preferences for the OMHA were only 5 percent.

Importantly, and consistent with previously mentioned research, these results illustrate that, while it is possible that little or no difference exists between OMHAs and DMHAs for some listening conditions, whenever a preference does exist, it favors the DMHA. When these subjective reports are considered in conjunction with the behavioral studies (e.g., Hawkins & Yacullo, 1984), there appears to be no compelling reason to fit omnidirectional microphone hearing aids.

Clinical Implications

As discussed in a review article by Mueller, Hawkins, and Sedge (1984), there appears to be a sizable gap between the proven advantages of the DMHA and its share of overall hearing aid sales. For example, although research shows that DMHAs are beneficial for almost all hearing aid users, Mueller (1981) reported that audiologists recommend DMHAs for only 20 percent of their patients. This low rate of use in 1981 probably could be attributed in part to the manner in which candidacy for DMHAs was determined. For example, rather than simply considering everyone a candidate for a DMHA, many clinicians or dispensers viewed this as a "special fitting" and reserved this microphone type for individuals who had exceptional complaints involving communication in noise or someone who had experienced repeated failure with OMHAs. A separate group of dispens-

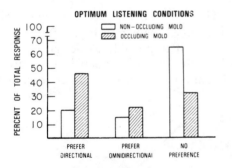

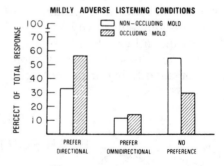

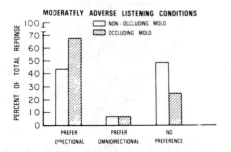

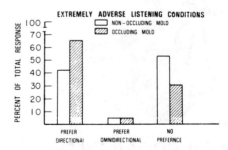

FIGURE 2-8. Patient preference for directional versus omnidirectional microphone types in four different listening environments. From Mueller, Grimes, and Erdman, 1983. Reprinted with permission.

ing audiologists did not even consider whether a hearing aid had a directional microphone, and selected the hearing aid based on other electroacoustical features, behavioral test results, or cosmetic appeal. Both of these approaches would result in few DMHA fittings. Over the years clinicians have maintained a remarkably indifferent attitude regarding directional amplification.

Nearly 10 years have passed since the Mueller (1981) survey, and DMHA use is now estimated at below 5 percent. An issue that weighs heavily on the present low use of DMHAs is the popularity of the ITE hearing aid. This hearing aid style currently represents nearly 80 percent of hearing aid sales (Mahon, 1988), and few if any manufacturers offer a directional microphone as an option for their ITE models. This is somewhat surprising, as limited research has shown that directional microphones work as well in an ITE (full-concha) as in a conventional behind-the-ear (BTE) model (Griffing & Preves, 1976; Preves, 1976; Rumoshosky, 1977). Recall that the polar plot shown earlier in this chapter representing substantial directivity was that of an ITE hearing aid (see Figure 2–1).

The reason commonly given by manufacturers for not offering or promoting di-rectional ITE aids is the difficulty created by space limitations and with the front and rear port alignment. Although these factors are obvious concerns, they do not seem to prevent successful production of directional ITE aids. For example, Figure 2–9 shows two ITE directional instruments. The aid on the left is a low profile ITE model and the aid on the right is a standard full-concha model. The only noticeable difference between these hearing aids and their omnidirectional counterparts is the presence of two, rather than one, microphone openings on the superior portion of the faceplate. Figure 2–10 shows the real ear aided response (**REAR**) of these two instruments measured at 0- and 180-degree azimuths with a probe tube microphone system in a moderately reverberant room (measurements taken a 1 m). Observe that considerable attenuation is present for both models when the signal originates from behind the user (the directional effect probably would be reduced at distances greater than 1 m).

The 0- to 180-degree frequency response curves, shown in Figure 2–10 illustrate that it is possible to design an ITE DMHA that provides a satisfactory directivity pattern. It is probable, therefore, that

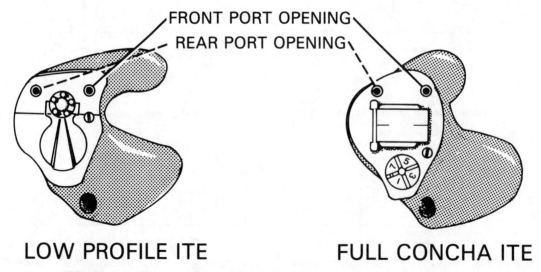

LOW PROFILE ITE   FULL CONCHA ITE

FIGURE 2-9. Illustration of two types of in-the-ear (ITE) directional hearing aids.

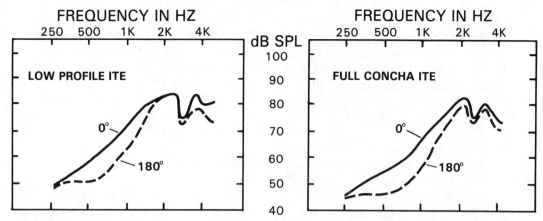

FIGURE 2-10. Real Ear Aided Response (REAR) for two different in-the-ear (ITE) hearing aids measured using a probe tube microphone system. Measurements obtained in a moderately reverberant room with the input presented at 0 and 180 degree azimuths. Hearing aid user was 1 m from input source.

a primary reason for the absence of directional microphones for ITE hearing aids is that this option is not considered, or requested, by many professionals who recommend and dispense hearing aids. The same indifferent attitude that was prevalent for BTE DMHAs 10 years ago also seems to exist for ITE DMHAs today.

In summary, as Mueller and colleagues (1984) pointed out, it is difficult to find reasons not to fit a directional microphone instrument. With the exception of canal aids, space for the two microphone ports should not be a major limitation. While the DMHA advantage sometimes may be small, and may even be absent for some extreme listening conditions, the potential for an improved S/N ratio is present continually. The worst possible outcome is that the DMHA will function as an OMHA.

BINAURAL HEARING AIDS

A second important consideration in the hearing aid selection process is whether to fit an individual with one or two hearing aids. The seemingly simple answer — if both ears are impaired, the individual is fitted with two hearing aids — has been complicated through 50 years of research. While logic would dictate that most indi-

viduals who are hearing impaired are candidates for binaural amplification, two recent surveys have shown that only 40 to 50 percent of hearing-impaired adults are fitted binaurally (Curran, 1985; Cranmer, 1988). It is appropriate, therefore, to review briefly some of the advantages of binaural hearing aids.

Benefits of Binaural Hearing Aids

Many of the reported advantages of binaural hearing aids are similar to the benefits of binaural hearing for normal-hearing individuals. Research has shown that the majority of these advantages also exist for hearing-impaired individuals if the hearing loss is relatively symmetrical. (For review, see articles by Byrne, 1980; Hawkins, 1985; Mueller & Grimes 1987.) Three of these advantages are directly related to the overall improvement of speech recognition: binaural summation, elimination of head shadow, and binaural squelch.

Binaural Summation

When a sound is presented binaurally, it is perceived as louder than if the sound is presented monaurally. For threshold measurements, it has been shown that the binaural threshold is approximately 3 dB better than the threshold of the best ear. This appears to be true for both pure tones and speech (Hirsh, 1948; Licklider, 1948). The binaural summation effect increases at suprathreshold levels and may be as large as 10 dB at levels of 90 dB SPL (Reynolds & Stevens, 1960).

Binaural summation effects also have been demonstrated for the hearing impaired. For example Byrne (1980) reported the results of comparing binaural with monaural thresholds for 265 hearing-impaired children 9 to 11 years of age. The mean binaural improvement in threshold was 3.2 dB at 500 Hz, 2.1 dB at 1000 Hz, and 2.5 dB at 2000 Hz, values that are equivalent to those measured for normal-hearing individuals. Research by Dermody and Byrne (1975) has shown that, as with normals, this summation effect also increases at suprathreshold levels for persons with conductive hearing losses. The recent work of Hawkins, Prosek, Walden, and Montgomery (1987) extended these findings to persons with sensorineural hearing loss. Subjects with a bilateral high-frequency sensorineural hearing loss demonstrated 6 to 10 dB of suprathreshold loudness summation, equivalent to that found for normal-hearing subjects.

These summation effects offer some obvious benefits to the hearing-impaired person using hearing aids. First, for those with severe hearing impairments who use their hearing aids at or near the maximum gain setting, the additional 3 to 5 dB increase in the speech signal may provide a significant improvement in speech detection and intelligibility. For individuals with mild or moderate impairments, the summation effect allows for equivalent loudness at a lower volume control setting, thus reducing feedback problems and prolonging battery life for some hearing aids. The reduction in feedback is especially noticeable when open earmolds or IROS ITE hearing aids are utilized for high-pass fittings. A third possible advantage, recently reported by Hawkins (1986), relates to the

individual's binaural LDL. Hawkins' research showed that while a binaural summation of 6 to 10 dB occurred for a group of hearing-impaired listeners, binaural LDLs were not reduced from monaural LDLs. This would allow the binaural hearing aid user to enjoy a wider perceived-loudness dynamic range of hearing.

Elimination of Head Shadow

An individual with a bilaterally symmetrical hearing impairment who is aided monaurally is at a distinct disadvantage when speech is presented from the nonaided side. This is especially noticeable when the hearing aid users are placed in a listening situation where repositioning themselves or the speaker is difficult (e.g., seated at a table, travelling in an automobile).

Recently, Feston and Plomp (1986) reported on the acoustic head shadow (mean of 8 subjects) measured for 1/3 octave bands from 80 to 8000 Hz. As shown in Figure 2–11, little or no attenuation from the head occurs at 1000 Hz and below. Observe, however, that for frequencies above 1500 Hz, attenuation of 10 to 16 dB is present at the ear canal entrance. The solid line shown in Figure 2–11 represents measurements taken at the approximate location of the microphone of a BTE hearing aid. These values are not as reduced as those measured at the ear canal, but attenuation of 6 to 12 dB remains.

Clearly, the acoustic head shadow can have a significant effect on speech intelligibility for someone who is aided monaurally. In a worst case situation, the monaural hearing aid user may receive 10 to 18 dB less high-frequency gain than the binaural user (see Figure 2–11 for differences of baffle side/shadow side for each frequency).

Binaural Squelch

Binaural squelch refers to the reported ability of the auditory system to "squelch" noise or reverberation more efficiently when

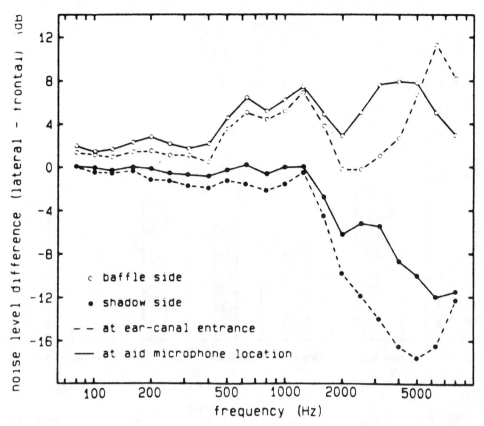

FIGURE 2-11. Average level difference between noise from the front (baffle side) and from lateral positions (shadow side) measured for eight subjects in one-third octave bands at the ear canal entrance and at the hearing aid microphone location. From Feston and Plomp, 1986. Reprinted with permission.

input is received from two ears rather than one. The expected outcome for the binaural hearing aid user is improved speech intelligibility, especially for noisy listening conditions. Traditionally, audiologists frequently have based their decision to fit an individual monaurally or binaurally on this one potential advantage. Considerable research has been conducted on this topic and review articles have been written by Ross (1980), Byrne (1980), and Nabalek (1980). As summarized in these articles, the majority of research has shown that speech intelligibility in noise improved with binaural amplification, although this advantage may not be apparent in relatively easy listening conditions.

One area of interest regarding binaural squelch concerns the effects of different levels of reverberation. Recently, Hawkins and Yacullo (1984) studied the effects of monaural versus binaural amplification for three reverberation times (0.3, 0.6, and 1.2 s). As described previously in this chapter, the authors measured the S/N ratio necessary for a 50 percent correct score for NU-6 monosyllabic words. The binaural advantage observed for normal-hearing and hearing-impaired listeners is shown in Figure 2-12. (Aided testing was conducted with both an omnidirectional and directional microphone hearing aid.) Observe that a binaural advantage to 2 to 3 dB is present for both the normal-hearing and hearing-

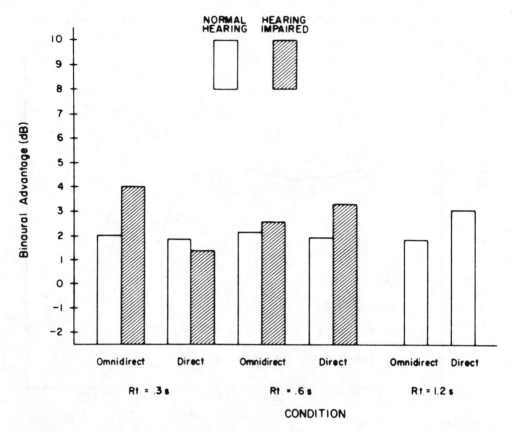

FIGURE 2-12. Binaural advantage in dB for omnidirectional and directional microphones at three different reverberation (Rt) conditions. From Hawkins and Yacullo, 1984. Reprinted with permission.

impaired groups across all three reverberation times. The binaural advantage, therefore, does not appear to be unique to a particular level of reverberation or to a particular microphone type.

The findings of Hawkins and Yacullo illustrate the potential advantages of binaural hearing aids for improving speech recognition. While a 2 to 3 dB improvement in the S/N ratio may not be significant when the listening task is either very easy or very difficult, this improvement can have a substantial effect in some common listening situations. For example, Walker and Byrne (1985) showed that intelligibility ratings for continuous discourse in speech spectrum noise improved from 25 to 75 percent with only a 3-dB reduction in the noise signal.

In addition to binaural summation, elimination of head shadow, and binaural squelch, other commonly reported advantages of binaural hearing aids include improved localization, spatial balance, relaxed listening, and relief from tinnitus. These factors may not be readily apparent in a 1- or 2-hour clinical hearing aid evaluation. It has been customary, therefore, for many professionals to rely on patient report following a trial period with binaural hearing aids.

Surveys of Binaural Hearing Aid Users

In general, most studies that have relied on patient reports of binaural versus monaural hearing aid use have shown a significant preference for binaural aids. Several surveys have revealed such pronounced advantages for binaural amplification that these findings seem to overshadow the small binaural–monaural differences measured in the clinical setting. For example, Erdman and Sedge (1986), summarizing their cumulative findings from three separate surveys, reported that 84 of 89 subjects preferred binaural over monaural amplification.

The results of two other surveys, Schreurs and Olsen (1985) and Chung and Stephens (1986), are displayed in Tables 2–3 and 2–4, respectively. Although similar, some interesting contrasts exist in these two surveys. The results of both studies demonstrated that preferences for binaural amplification are greater when the listening situation is quiet than when background noise is present. A similar finding also was reported by Byrne (1980). The subjects of Chung and Stephens (1986), however, showed a significantly greater overall preference for binaural amplification than

did the subjects of Schreurs and Olsen (1985). These preferences were also reflected in the subjects' reported use of binaural rather than monaural hearing aids, or not using hearing aids at all. Chung and Stephens reported that only 19 percent of their subjects selected monaural over binaural aids, and that 7 percent were not using hearing aids. In contrast, Schreurs and Olsen reported that 57 percent of their subjects selected monaural over binaural hearing aids, and that 17 percent of the subjects chose not to use hearing aids. Two factors that may partially explain the greater preferences for binaural amplification observed by Chung and Stephens are (1) their respondents had used hearing aids for at least 6 months as compared to 1 month in the Schreurs and Olsen study and (2) their subjects were provided hearing aids free of charge. Additionally, Schreurs and Olsen stated that they did not promote the advantages of binaural amplification to their patients, an important variable not discussed by Chung and Stephens.

TABLE 2–3. Number of better responses when comparing monaural and binaural hearing aid use in various listening situations for 30 subjects.

Listening Situation	Better		No Difference	No Response
	Monaural	Binaural		
Conversation in quiet room	7	16	6	1
Conversation while others are talking nearby	18	11	1	0
Quiet restaurant	5	19	5	1
Noisy restaurant	20	8	1	1
Listening to radio or TV in quiet	5	16	9	0
Listening to radio or TV while others are talking nearby	14	11	4	1
When listening in church, theater, or other large room	10	15	3	2
When driving or riding in a car	14	11	5	0
When listening via telephone	17	1	11	1
When trying to locate source of sound	5	14	11	0

From Schreurs and Olsen, 1985. Reprinted with permission.

TABLE 2–4. Summary of preferred mode of amplification for subjects categorized as full-time hearing aid users.

Listening Situations	Preferred Mode of Amplification		
	2 Hearing Aids	1 Hearing Aid	No Difference
Listening to speech in quiet situations involving 1 or 2 persons	92%	0%	8%
Listening to speech in noisy situations	56	21	23
Listening to TV, radio, or records	92	0	8
Listening to conversation from the front at close range (20' or less)	92	4	4
Listening to conversation from behind	71	4	25
Listening to conversation from a distance (over 20')	69	2	29
Locate sounds, e.g., car horn	76	8	16
Recognize sounds, e.g., dripping tap	72	2	26
Listening to group conversation (3 or more persons)	69	10	21
More comfortable listening	94	4	2
Ease of listening at meeting, church, picture or theatres	85	4	11

From Chung and Stephens, 1986. Reprinted with permission.

Schreurs and Olsen's (1985) study represents one of the few user survey studies in which binaural amplification was not reported as the fitting of choice. It is tempting to attribute this negative finding to the additional cost of the second hearing aid, since many other studies of this type have utilized subjects who were provided the hearing aids at little or no cost (e.g., Markides, 1977; Byrne, 1980; Erdman & Sedge, 1981). The 1984 Hearing Industries Association (HIA) survey, however, suggests that the cost of hearing aids may be less of a deterrent to the potential user than normally is believed. In their survey of 1050 hearing-impaired adults who did not own hearing aids, only 0.8 percent cited cost as the reason they had not purchased hearing aids. The leading reason given for not using a hearing aid was that a professional had advised against hearing aid use. (*The Marketing Edge*, 1986, 1987). While the HIA survey was directed at hearing aid use in general, it is reasonable to believe that the same factors may relate to the acceptance and use of binaural amplification.

Contraindications for Binaural Hearing Aids

Given the research favoring binaural hearing aids, it seems appropriate to consider this arrangement the standard fitting. An important question then becomes: Who is *not* a candidate for binaural hearing aid use? Two non-auditory factors that are often cited are financial constraints and cosmetic concerns. The significance of the additional expense for a second hearing aid was discussed briefly in the preceding section. While the majority of patients are willing to spend the extra money for two hearing aids if they have been convinced this fitting arrangement is the best for them, some individuals simply cannot afford the second hearing aid. Some reports suggest that many of the elderly may fall in this category (Davies & Mueller, 1987). Obviously, a monaural fitting is superior to no hearing aid at all for these individuals.

Cosmetic concerns do not appear to be a strong deterrent to binaural hearing aid use. It is likely that this factor will be even less of a concern as the popularity of ITE and in-the-canal (ITC) hearing aids increases. Table 2–5, taken from the previously mentioned survey of Chung and Stephens (1986), displays the frequency of problems with binaural aids reported by 53 full-time users and 39 non-users. Observe that cosmetic problems were not cited by any of the full-time users and only 5 (13%) of the non-users. A similar finding was reported by Mueller (1986a) on 134 patients who preferred to be fitted monaurally rather than binaurally. Only 16 percent cited cosmetic factors as a significant influence in their choice of a monaural fitting.

Two auditory factors that have been reported to contraindicate binaural hearing aids are the presence of an asymmetrical hearing loss and a central auditory deficit. Of these two, asymmetry in pure-tone thresholds is the easiest to quantify and also has been studied the most frequently. While most researchers agree that some asymmetry is acceptable, the degree of asymmetry that prevents reasonable benefit from a second hearing aid is not clearly understood. Perhaps the best clinical guidelines have been provided by the work of Davis and Haggard (1982) and Gatehouse and Haggard (1986). These authors suggest that an asymmetry of 12 to 15 dB or less should have a minimal effect on the success of the binaural fitting. They caution, however, that when asymmetry exceeds 30 dB, the benefits of binaural amplification may be marginal. These recommendations are based primarily on psychoacoustic laboratory testing and have not been studied systematically through user ratings in everyday listening situations.

A final possible contraindication to the use of binaural amplification is the

TABLE 2–5. Summary of problems reported by full-time users and non-users of binaural hearing aids.

Problems Stated	Full-time Users N	Non-users N
Background noise	2	8
Difficulty with clarity for speech	3	—
Acoustic discomfort	4	2
Physical discomfort	4	7
Difficulty in use	9	6
Telephone	2	2
Whistling	3	—
Wind noise	3	—
Too deaf/not deaf enough	1	2
Cosmetic	—	5
Change of life-style	—	2
Headache	—	2
No advantage	—	3

From Chung and Stephens, 1986. Reprinted with permission.

presence of a central auditory processing disorder (Corso, 1977; Del Polito, Smith & Dempsey, 1980). This is most commonly noted in the elderly individual. Presumably, the central processing disorder prevents the benefit of binaural squelch, an advantage of binaural amplification that was discussed earlier in this section. Unfortunately, there is not an accepted clinical method of identifying these individuals prior to the fitting of hearing aids, nor is there conclusive research showing that these patients actually will not benefit from binaural hearing aid use. Arnst (1986), for example, has suggested that patients with generalized central auditory processing problems may need to rely *more* heavily on the additional auditory cues provided by binaural stimulation. Mueller and Calkins (1988) reported that individuals with central processing dysfunction (as measured by a dichotic speech test) favor binaural over monaural amplification to the same degree as patients with only peripheral disorders. Patients' overall satisfaction with hearing aids in general, however, was reduced. Clearly, several issues involving central auditory processing and binaural amplification are unresolved. Further discussion of this topic can be found in Chapter 4.

Clinical Implications

The preceding review of research clearly indicates that the majority of hearing-impaired individuals should be fitted binaurally. While contraindications sometimes exist, these factors apply to only a small percentage of potential binaural hearing aids users. Given the overwhelming evidence in support of binaural amplification, the results of surveys showing monaural amplification as the customary fitting are somewhat puzzling (e.g., Curran, 1985; Cramer, 1988). There appears to be a discrepancy between professionals' acceptance of the theoretical advantages of binaural fitting and their application of this belief to

clinical practice. As discussed by Hawkins (1985) and Mueller (1986a, 1986b), in recent years there does seem to be a gradual shift in favor of binaural fitting among audiologists. In addition to the already mentioned accumulating research in favor of binaural amplification, this shift may also be due to alterations in hearing aid selection methods (audiologists are no longer trying to prove binaural is better through word recognition testing) and the changing occupational setting of the audiologists. Approximately 30 percent of all audiologists are now in private practice, and nearly 40 percent dispense hearing aids (Cherow, 1986).

Assuming that the professional hearing aid dispenser is convinced that binaural fittings are superior, it is necessary to consider the views of the prospective binaural hearing aid user. Mueller (1986a) surveyed 282 individuals prior to their hearing aid fitting. Subjects were asked to state their preference for using binaural or monaural amplification and to rate the influence that several factors had on their decision. Because all of the subjects were retired military, the hearing aids were provided at no cost to the patient.

Mueller reported that despite the fact that these patients knew that they could receive two hearing aids free of charge, only 43 percent of the respondents stated a preference for binaural amplification. The reasons for preferring binaural amplification are shown in rank order in Table 2–6. Persons disposed to wearing binaural amplification reported that they are significantly influenced by several factors (see Table 2–6). The overall high ratings seem to indicate a high level of enthusiasm for hearing aids in general for this group of respondents.

Results for the 57 percent who preferred monaural amplification are shown in Table 2–7. The most noticeable aspect of these results is that the mean influence ratings for monaural preferences are considerably lower than those shown in Table 2–6 for binaural. This could be interpreted to mean that these patients are considering

TABLE 2–6. Influence ratings on seven factors for persons (*n* = 91) stating binaural amplification as their preference. (Mean rating obtained by assigning 3.0 = strong influence, 2.0 = moderate influence, 1.0 = mild influence, and 0.0 = no influence.)

Reasons for Preferring Binaural Amplification	Distribution (%)			
	Mean Influence Rating	Strong Influence	Mild or Moderate Influence	No Influence
Hear (understand) better	2.74	83	15	2
Most natural/balanced	2.48	70	23	7
Severity of loss	2.41	63	31	6
Two-sided hearing	2.31	58	34	8
Advice from medical professional	1.73	50	15	35
Observation/advice from other users	1.34	30	27	43
Spare aid/always have one working aid	1.14	19	38	43

From Mueller, 1986a. Reprinted with permission.

TABLE 2–7. Influence ratings on seven factors for persons (*n* = 134) stating monaural amplification as their preference. (Mean rating obtained by assigning 3.0 = strong influence, 2.0 = moderate influence, 1.0 = mild influence, and 0.0 = no influence.)

Reasons for Preferring Monaural Amplification	Distribution (%)			
	Mean Influence Rating	Strong Influence	Mild or Moderate Influence	No Influence
Hearing loss not severe enough to use two aids	1.86	38	44	18
No expected improvement in hearing (understanding) with second aid	1.45	27	41	32
Observation/advice from other users	1.29	31	20	49
Advice from medical professional	1.19	26	23	51
Convenience/second aid too much bother	1.10	23	27	50
Cosmetic aspects	0.81	16	25	59
Appear less handicapped with one aid	0.58	11	22	67

From Mueller, 1986a. Reprinted with permission.

binaural amplification and therefore do not have strong reasons for choosing a monaural fitting. A more likely explanation, however, is that respondents in this group simply are less enthusiastic about amplification in general and are considering not a binaural fitting, but rather no hearing aid at all.

If Mueller's findings are typical, the obvious question facing clinicians is: What is the appropriate fitting approach for the large percentage of binaural candidates who prefer a monaural fitting? Audiologists typically have favored a conservative approach, either to fit the patient monaurally or to recommend a binaural-versus-monaural trial period. An approach that may be more appropriate, however, is to inform the patient that the hearing loss dictates the use of two hearing aids and to proceed with a binaural fitting unless the patient objects strongly. Evidence supporting this approach is shown in Table 2–6, where 50 percent of the respondents preferring a binaural fitting cite advice from a medical professional as a strong influence in making this decision. At least one study has shown that the use of and satisfaction with binaural hearing aids is influenced by the type of counseling provided at the time of the hearing aid fitting (Mueller & Reeder, 1987).

In summary, the practicing clinician must assume that (1) most bilaterally hearing-impaired persons will benefit from binaural amplification, and (2) most patients are willing to purchase two hearing aids if they are convinced that the second aid will be beneficial. With these assumptions in mind, a clinical protocol for providing the optimum hearing aid arrangement can be developed.

LOUDNESS DISCOMFORT LEVELS (LDLs) AND SSPL90

A third important preselection consideration is the determination of the maximum output, or SSPL90, of the hearing aid.

Walker, Dillon, Byrne, and Christen (1984) stated that "of the parameters of hearing aids which are selected for the client, maximum power output (MPO) (saturation sound pressure level SSPL90) has received the least attention yet it may be the parameter most closely related to user acceptance of the aid" (p. 23).

The importance of an appropriate SSPL90 may be inferred from the data of Franks and Beckmann (1985), who studied several groups of geriatric hearing aid users. In a group of 25 subjects who had worn a hearing aid but rejected it, 88 percent indicated that hearing aids "make sounds too loud." In a second group of 25 subjects who were still wearing hearing aids, 32 percent indicated that sounds were too loud. If the hearing aids had been set such that the SSPL90 was just below the LDL, theoretically, these percentages should have been zero.

For a successful hearing aid fitting, the SSPL90 should be set just below the LDL. If the SSPL90 exceeds the LDL, a number of unfortunate consequences can occur. The worst, mentioned above, is ultimate rejection of the hearing aid due to loudness discomfort. Other consequences outlined by Hawkins (1984b) include (1) reduction of the volume control wheel to a less than optimum position in order to minimize the number of times the LDL is exceeded; (2) constant volume control wheel manipulation, especially when louder sounds occur or are anticipated; and (3) restriction of hearing aid use to quieter environments to avoid high level inputs in a noisy situation that might cause LDL to be exceeded. In the reverse situation, if the SSPL90 is set too low, the dynamic range of the instrument will be unnecessarily restricted.

Given the consequences of an inappropriate SSPL90, care should be taken in deciding where to set this electroacoustic parameter. Three approaches to determining where to set the SSPL90 have been described: (1) estimating the LDL based on pure-tone thresholds and setting the SSPL-90 based on the LDL, (2) setting the SSPL90 based on a suprathreshold measure other than the LDL, and (3) measuring the LDL and setting the SSPL90 just below this value.

Estimating the LDL from Pure-Tone Thresholds

Basing the SSPL90 on a predicted LDL obtained from pure-tone thresholds is an attractive alternative for a number of reasons. First, it saves time since LDLs do not have to be obtained. Data from a routine hearing assessment are sufficient. Second, the method is particularly useful for patients who are incapable of performing suprathreshold loudness judgment tasks such as LDLs. If such a procedure is to be defensible, however, the errors associated with making individual predictions based on group data must be acceptable. Two major sets of data that show LDLs as a function of degree of hearing loss are available (Kamm, Dirks, & Mickey, 1976; Dillon, Chew, & Deans, 1984). An example of these data is shown in Figure 2–13. Notice the range of LDLs that can be obtained for a given degree of hearing loss. It is clear from these data that under- and overprediction of an individual's LDL can easily occur based on degree of hearing loss.

Cox (1985) calculated regression equations to determine the best prediction of LDL from pure-tone thresholds. She concluded that the equation

$$LDL = 100 + 1/4 \text{ Hearing Loss}$$

provided an acceptable fit to the data for clinical purposes. For example, if an individual had a hearing loss of 80 dB HL, then the predicted LDL would be 100 + 20, or 120 dB SPL, and the SSPL90 would be set to 120 dB SPL. If the approach chosen is to use a prediction scheme, this equation would seem defensible. However, one must be concerned with the high probability of over- and underfitting on an individual case basis.

Determining SSPL90 from Suprathreshold Loudness Measures

A second approach to selecting SSPL-90 has been to base the SSPL90 on a suprathreshold loudness measure, but not the LDL. Two examples of this approach are the suggestions by Cox (1983) and Skinner and colleagues (1982). In both of these, the purpose is not strictly to prevent loudness discomfort, but also to avoid having the peaks of speech saturate the hearing aid and thus create excessive distortion. Cox suggested that an appropriate place to limit is the Upper Limit of Comfortable Loudness (ULCL) plus 12 dB. This assumes that the average amplified levels of speech would, at their maximum, be placed at the ULCL, with the peaks extending 12 dB above the average. An SSPL90 set at this level would not produce excessive distortion. Cox cautioned that in some cases such a setting might exceed the LDL, so the patient should be questioned about any loudness discomfort after the initial fitting of the hearing aid. More recently, Cox (1988) has modified the ULCL plus 12 dB formula so that different constants are added at different frequencies. The new values range from 0.2 dB at 250 Hz to 17.6 dB at 2500 Hz.

A similar idea was expressed by Skinner and colleagues (1982). These authors suggested that the SSPL90 be set to the lower of two values: the LDL or the MCL plus 15 dB. The idea is that the user will set the volume control wheel such that the average speech levels will be at MCL. If the peaks exceed this level by 15 dB, then an SSPL90 setting of MCL plus 15 dB should prevent the peaks from saturating the hearing aid. It is reasoned that, even if the LDL is greater than MCL plus 15 dB, there is no reason to set it any higher, because one risks potential overamplification for no obvious benefit. If the LDL is less than the MCL plus 15 dB, then the SSPL90 should be set equal to the LDL in order to prevent loudness discomfort. Perhaps the only disadvantage of this approach is that it as-

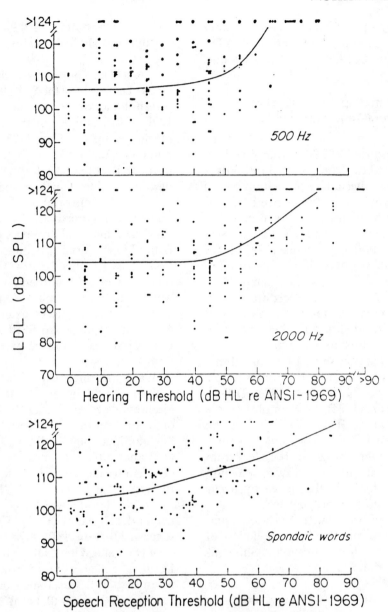

FIGURE 2-13. Loudness discomfort levels (LDLs) as a function of hearing loss for 500 and 2000 Hz pure tones and spondaic words. Each dot represents an individual subject and the solid lines are best fit curves. From Kamm, Dirks, and Mickey, 1978. Reprinted with permission.

sumes that the MCL is (a) a reliable measure, and (b) static and does not change over time or as a function of listening environment. Several studies have questioned the first assumption, and there are no data concerning the second.

Setting SSPL90 Based on Measured LDLs

The final possibility in determining the SSPL90 is to base it on measured LDLs. While this approach has obvious face validity, there are numerous problems and issues that must be dealt with in implementing this apparently straightforward strategy. The major variables that affect the LDL, and thus the SSPL90 setting, are the instructions to the patient, type of stimulus, and stimulus delivery system.

Instructions

The instructions that are given to the patient probably constitute the largest source of potential variability in measurements of the LDL. Over the years instructions to the user have ranged from "tell me when it hurts your ears" to "tell me when sound first becomes annoying." The same user might well give values of 130 dB SPL and 95 dB SPL for these two sets of instructions. Hawkins (1980) characterized the above two instructions as representing "extreme discomfort" and "initial discomfort." The majority of other recommended instructions fall in between these two, a category described as "definite discomfort," for example, "tell me when the sound becomes uncomfortably loud." Hawkins, Walden, Montgomery, and Prosek (1987) recently recommended a different approach to LDL measurement, wherein the client labels each presented sound with a loudness category judgment. The client is given a sheet of paper with nine vertically arranged loudness categories. The loudness category sheet is shown in Table 2–8. The following instructions are then given:

> We need to do a test that will help me decide where to set the amplifier on the hearing aid. We want to set it so that sounds to not get so loud that they are uncomfortable. If we set it too high, sounds could get too loud for you, and you may no want to wear the hearing aid.
> You will hear some tones, and after each one I want you to tell me which of the loudness categories on this sheet best describes the sound to you. So after each tone, tell me if it was "Comfortable," or "Com-

fortable, But Slightly Loud," or "Loud, But O.K.," or "Uncomfortably Loud."

> I will be zeroing in on this "Uncomfortably Loud" category, because that's where we want the hearing aid to stop. We want to keep the sound down in this region [point to the three comfortable categories] and not let the sound get up into here [point to the top three categories]. So for each tone, tell me which category it falls into. Understand? (p. 163)

This instructional set has been shown by Hawkins and colleagues (1987) to produce stable LDLs over time, whereas a more typical set of instructions resulted in rather large variations in the LDL over a 1-week period. Since the LDL instructions can play such an important part in the final value, each clinician should pay close attention to this part of the LDL procedure, striving for instructions that are clear to the layman, provide anchors for loudness judgments, zero in on a reasonable level of loudness discomfort, and produce stable measurements.

LDL Stimuli

The second major variable in LDL measurements is the type of stimulus that is employed. The stimulus most often used is

TABLE 2–8. Loudness category sheet used in LDL measurement.

Levels of Loudness
Painfully Loud
Extremely Uncomfortable
Uncomfortably Loud
Loud, But O.K.
Comfortable, But Slightly Loud
Comfortable
Comfortable, But Slightly Soft
Soft
Very Soft

From Hawkins, Walden, Montgomery, and Prosek, 1987. Reprinted with permission.

speech, probably because of its face validity. There are, however, good reasons for using more frequency-specific signals, such as pure tones or narrow bands of noise. First, SSPL90 curves can vary significantly as a function of frequency. Even with relatively smooth curves, the SSPL90 can be quite different across frequency. This fact, combined with the finding that LDL curves vary across frequency when expressed in 2 cc coupler values (Dillon, Chews, & Deans, 1984; Hawkins et al., 1987), suggest that, if the goal is to maximize the dynamic range across frequency, it is necessary to determine the LDL at several places and then attempt to best match the SSPL90 curve to the LDL curve. If a broad-band signal is used, the LDL may be based on the area of greatest energy, the area of the lowest LDL, or both. For these reasons, it would appear best to obtain measures of the LDL in several frequency regions for the purpose of accurately and specifically defining SSPL90 characteristics. Pulsed pure tones, warble tones, or narrow bands of noise are all adequate stimulus choices.

LDL Stimulus Delivery

The last major variable that affects the LDL is how the stimulus is delivered to the ear and how the delivery system is calibrated. The most common delivery method is the standard audiometric earphone, which is calibrated in a NBS-9A 6 cc coupler. Using this delivery system, an LDL is obtained in dB HL for pure tones, narrow bands of noise, or speech. These values are then converted to dB SPL using the appropriate conversion values. For instance, if an LDL of 100 dB HL is obtained at 1000 Hz, this value is then converted to 107 dB SPL. If an LDL for speech is obtained at 90 dB HL, then the value is 110 dB SPL, adding the 20 dB conversion factor. The typical procedure is to then take these values, which are SPL developed in a 6 cc coupler with a TDH-39, 40, or 50 earphone, and select a hearing aid whose SSPL90 (which is de-

fined as output in a 2 cc coupler) is just less than the LDL. There are problems with this approach. First, values from the 6 cc coupler are being compared to the 2 cc coupler. There are differences between what is developed in a 6 cc coupler and in the real ear (Cox, 1986), as well as between the 2 cc coupler and the real ear (Sachs & Burkhard, 1972). Further, the magnitude of the 2 cc–real ear difference will depend on the earmold configuration used and how it differs from the earmold simulator in the coupler, as well as the hearing aid microphone location. Direct comparison of an earphone-based LDL to hearing aid specifications is a tenuous procedure.

In an effort to overcome some of the above problems with earphones, Hawkins (1980), Cox (1981), and Dillon, Chew, and Deans (1984) have recommended delivering stimuli for LDLs through a hearing aid receiver, the output of which has been calibrated in a 2 cc coupler. In this approach, an electrical signal is fed to the hearing aid receiver, which is attached to the client's personal earmold. In this way, the signal is modified by the appropriate earmold acoustic alterations, the residual volume of air in the ear canal, and the user's middle ear impedance. Finally, the LDL is measured in dB SPL referenced to a 2 cc coupler so that the value can be taken directly to the hearing aid specification sheet for SSPL90 selection.

A recent modification of the above hearing aid receiver presentation method has been described by Hawkins and colleagues (1987). In their procedure, the patient wears a high-output hearing aid coupled to a personal or stock earmold. Stimuli are presented via a loudspeaker in sound field and the LDL is defined as the SPL entering the hearing aid microphone at the point of loudness discomfort plus the 2 cc gain of the hearing aid. In other words, the input to the hearing aid microphone at loudness discomfort plus the 2 cc gain yields a value of the SPL developed in a 2 cc coupler that is uncomfortable to the user. This approach incorporates the advantages of the earlier procedures plus the inclusion of head and body diffraction effects. Data reported on the stability and validity of the procedure are encouraging, suggesting that the LDL instructions employed (the ones given earlier in this section) yielded stable LDLs and the signal delivery system produced LDLs, and thus SSPL90 values, that were valid. Figure 2–14 shows data obtained with the Hawkins and colleagues (1987) procedure and how the results compared to those obtained using the same instructions, but standard earphones.

Another alternative in stimulus delivery, which allows direct specification of the LDL in 2 cc coupler values, is to utilize an earphone that has been calibrated in a 2 cc coupler. An example of this is the Etymotic ER series earphones. Libby (1985) has ex-

plained how the LDL can be obtained with an ER-3A earphone. Because the earphone can be calibrated in a 2 cc coupler, the LDL values can be directly compared to hearing aid specifications sheets.

In summary, the selection of SSPL90 is an important preselection decision, and must be followed up by questioning the new hearing aid user to determine if an appropriate setting, which prevents loudness discomfort, has been chosen. The goal should be to maximize the user's residual dynamic range, yet avoid uncomfortable loudness. Less accurate ways of doing this are to predict LDLs, and thus SSPL90, by using pure-tone thresholds. A potentially more accurate method is to measure LDLs, but problems in measuring LDLs, such as the best instructional set to utilize, the most

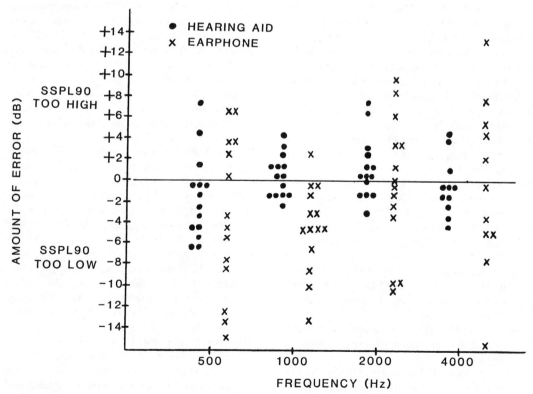

FIGURE 2–14. The amount of error in the recommended SSPL90 setting for 14 hearing-impaired subjects using a hearing aid presentation method where the output was calibrated in a 2 cc coupler and a typical earphone delivery system. From Hawkins, Walden, Montgomery, and Prosek, 1987. Reprinted with permission.

valid stimuli, and the best delivery system, still exist. Regardless of which approach is used, SSPL90 selection should receive careful attention from the hearing aid dispenser if the goal is a satisfied hearing aid user.

REFERENCES

Arnst, D. (1986). Binaural amplification in cases with central auditory deficits. *The Hearing Journal, 39*(11), 27–29.

Bauer, B. (1942). Supra-cardioid directional microphone. *Electronics, 1,* 31–33.

Beck, L. (1983). Assessment of directional hearing aid characteristics. *Audiological Acoustics, 22,* 178–191.

Bender, D., & Mueller, H. (1984). Factors influencing the decision to obtain amplification. *ASHA, 26*(10), 120.

Byrne, D. (1980). Binaural hearing aid fitting: Research findings and clinical application. In E. Libby (Ed.), *Binaural hearing and amplification,* Chicago, IL: Zenetron, Inc.

Cherow, E. (1986). The practice of audiology — a national perspective. *ASHA, 28*(9), 31–38.

Chung, S., & Stephens, S. (1986). Factors influencing binaural hearing aid use. *British Journal of Audiology, 20,* 129–140.

Corso, J. (1977). Presbycusis, hearing aids and aging. *Audiology, 16,* 146–163.

Cox, R. M. (1981). Using LDLs to establish hearing aid limiting levels. *Hearing Instruments, 32,* 16–20.

Cox, R. M. (1983). Using ULCL measures to find frequency/gain and SSPL90. *Hearing Instruments, 34,* 17–21, 39.

Cox, R. M. (1985). A structured approach to hearing aid selection. *Ear and Hearing, 6,* 226–239.

Cox, R. M. (1986). NBS-9A coupler-to-eardrum transformation: TDH-39 and TDH-49 earphones. *Journal of the Acoustical Society of America, 79,* 120–123.

Cox, R. M. (1988). The MSU hearing instrument prescription procedure. *Hearing Instruments, 39*(1), 6–10.

Curran, J. (1985). ITE aids for children: Survey of attitudes and practices of audiologists. *Hearing Instruments, 36*(4), 20–23.

Cranmer, K. (1988). Hearing aid dispensing. *Hearing Instruments, 37*(5), 6–12.

Davies, J., & Mueller, H. (1987). Hearing aid selection. In H. Mueller & V. Geoffrey, (Eds.),

Communication disorders in aging: Advances in assessment and management. Washington, DC: Gallaudet University Press.

Davis, A., & Haggard, M. (1982). Some implications of audiological measures in the population for binaural aiding strategies. In O. Pederson & T. Paulson (Eds.), Binaural effects in normal and impaired hearing. *Scandinavian Audiology,* (Suppl. 15), 167–179.

Del Polito, G., Smith, D., & Dempsey, C. (1980). Central auditory testing: Implications for hearing aid candidacy. In E. Libby (Ed.), *Binaural hearing and amplification,* (pp. 201–216). Chicago: Zenetron, Inc.

Dermody, P., & Byrne, D. (1975). Loudness summation with binaural hearing aids. *Scandinavian Audiology, 4,* 23–28.

Dillon, H., Chew, R., & Deans, M. (1984). Loudness discomfort level measurements and their implications for the design and fitting of hearing aids. *Australian Journal of Audiology, 6,* 73–79.

Erdman, S., & Sedge, R. (1981). Subjective comparisons of binaural vs. monaural amplification. *Ear and Hearing, 2*(5), 225–229.

Erdman, S., & Sedge, R. (1986). Preferences for binaural amplification. *The Hearing Journal, 39*(11), 33–36.

Feston, J., & Plomp, R. (1986). Speech reception threshold in noise with one and two hearing aids. *Journal of the Acoustical Society of America, 79,* 465–471.

Franks, J. R., & Beckmann, N. J. (1985). Rejection of hearing aids: Attitudes of a geriatric sample. *Ear and Hearing, 6,* 161–166.

Gatehouse, S., & Haggard, M. (1986). The influence of hearing asymmetries on benefits from binaural amplification. *The Hearing Journal, 39*(11), 15–20.

Griffing, T., & Preves, D. (1976). In-the-ear aids: Part II. *Hearing Instruments, 27*(5), 12–14.

Hawkins, D. B. (1980). Loudness discomfort levels: A suggested procedure for hearing aid evaluations. *Journal of Speech and Hearing Disorders, 45,* 3–15.

Hawkins, D. B. (1984a). Comparisons of speech recognition in noise by mildly-to-moderately hearing-impaired children using hearing aids and FM systems. *Journal of Speech and Hearing Disorders, 49,* 409–418.

Hawkins, D. B. (1984b). Selection of a critical electroacoustic characteristic: SSPL90. *Hearing Instruments, 35,* 28–32.

Hawkins, D. B. (1985). Selection of hearing aid

characteristics. In W. Hodgson (Ed.), *Hearing aid assessment and use in audiologic habilitation* (3rd ed.). Baltimore: Williams & Wilkins.

Hawkins, D. B. (1986). Selection of SSPL90 for binaural hearing aid fittings. *The Hearing Journal, 39*(11), 23–24.

Hawkins, D. B., Prosek, R., Walden, B., & Montgomery, A. (1987). Binaural loudness summation in the hearing impaired. *Journal of Speech and Hearing Research, 30,* 37–43.

Hawkins, D. B., Walden, B. E., Montgomery, A. A., & Prosek, R. A. (1987). Description and validation of an LDL procedure designed to select SSPL90. *Ear and Hearing, 8,* 162–169.

Hawkins, D. B., & Yacullo, W. (1984). Signal-to-noise ratio advantage of binaural hearing aids and directional microphones under different levels of reverberation. *Journal of Speech and Hearing Disorders, 49,* 278–286.

Hearing Industries Association. (1984). A market research study of the U.S. hearing impaired population. Washington, DC: Author.

Hillman, N. (1981). Directional hearing aid capabilities. *Hearing Instruments, 32*(7), 7–11.

Hirsh, I. (1948). The influence of interaural phase on interaural summation and inhibition. *Journal of the Acoustical Society of America, 20,* 544–557.

Kamm, C., Dirks, D., & Mickey, M. (1978). Effect of sensorineural hearing loss on loudness discomfort levels and most comfortable loudness judgments. *Journal of Speech and Hearing Research, 21,* 668–681.

Knowles Electronics, Inc. (1980). Directional hearing aid microphone application notes. *Technical Bulletin 21B.* Franklin Park, IL: Author.

Libby, E. R. (1985). The LDL to SSPL90 conversion dilemma. *Hearing Instruments, 36,* 15–16.

Licklider, J. (1948). The influence of interaural phase relations upon the masking of speech by white noise. *Journal of the Acoustical Society of America, 20,* 150–159.

Lybarger, S. (1947, November). Development of a new hearing aid with magnetic microphone. *Electrical Manufacturing,* 19–29.

Madison, R., & Hawkins, D. (1983). The signal-to-noise ratio advantage of directional microphones. *Hearing Instruments, 34*(2), 18, 49.

Mahon, W. (1988). 1988 U.S. hearing aid sales summary. *The Hearing Journal, 41*(12), 9–13.

Markides, A. (1977). *Binaural hearing aids.* London: Academic Press.

Mueller, H. (1981). Directional microphone hear-

ing aids: A 10 year report. *Hearing Instruments, 32*(11), 18–20.

Mueller, H. (1986a). Binaural amplification: Attitudinal factors. *The Hearing Journal, 39*(11), 7–10.

Mueller, H. (1986b). Binaural: The remaining questions. *The Hearing Journal, 39*(11), 4.

Mueller, H., & Calkins, A. (1988). Dichotic speech measures for predicting hearing aid benefit. *ASHA, 30*(10), 104 (Abstract).

Mueller, H., & Grimes, A. (1977). A review of experimental results with directional hearing aids: The relationship to the testing paradigm. *Audiology and Hearing Education, 10*(11), 26–28.

Mueller, H., & Grimes, A. (1987). Amplification systems for the hearing impaired. In J. Alpiner & P. McCarthy (Eds.), *Rehabilitative audiology: Children and adults* (pp. 115–160). Baltimore: Williams & Wilkins.

Mueller, H., Grimes, A., & Erdman, S. (1983). Subjective ratings of directional amplification. *Hearing Instruments, 34*(2), 14–16.

Mueller, H., Hawkins, D., & Sedge, R. (1984). Three important options in hearing aid selection. *Hearing Instruments, 35*(11), 14–17.

Mueller, H., & Johnson, R. (1979). The effects of various front-to-back ratios on the performance of directional microphone hearing aids. *Journal of the American Audiological Society, 5,* 30–34.

Mueller, H., & Reeder, P. (1987). Success with binaural amplification: Two important contributing factors. *ASHA, 29*(10), 161 (Abstract).

Mueller, H., & Sweetow, R. (1978). Clinical rationale for using an overhead speaker in the evaluation of hearing aids. *Archives of Otolaryngology, 104,* 417–418.

Nabalek, A. (1980). Effects of room acoustics on speech perception through hearing aids by normal-hearing and hearing-impaired listeners. In G. Studebaker & I. Hochberg (Eds.), *Acoustical factors affecting hearing aid performance* (pp. 25–46). Baltimore: University Park Press.

Nielson, H. (1973). A comparison between hearing aids with directional microphone and hearing aids with conventional microphone. *Scandinavian Audiology, 2,* 173–176.

Nielson, H., & Ludvigsen, C. (1978). Effect of hearing aids with directional microphones in different acoustic environments. *Scandinavian Audiology, 7,* 217–224.

Preves, D. (1976). Directivity of in-the-ear aids

with non-directional and directional micro-phones. *Hearing Aid Journal, 29*(6), 9–12.

Reynolds, G., & Stevens, S. (1960). Binaural sum-mation of loudness. *Journal of the Acoustical Society of America, 32,* 1337–1344.

Ross, M. (1980). Binaural versus monaural hear-ing aid amplification for hearing-impaired individuals. In E. Libby (Ed.), *Binaural hear-ing and amplification* (pp. 1–21). Chicago: Zenetron Inc.

Rumoshosky, J. (1977). Directional microphone in ITE aids. *Hearing Aid Journal, 30*(11), 48–50.

Sachs, R., & Burkhard, M. (1972). Earphone pres-sure response in ears and couplers. Paper presented at the 83rd Meeting of the Acousti-cal Society of America.

Schreurs, K., & Olsen, W. (1985). Comparison of monaural and binaural hearing aid use on a trial period basis. *Ear and Hearing, 6,* 198–202.

Skinner, M. W., Pascoe, D. P., Miller, J. D., & Popelka, G. R. (1982). Measurements to de-termine the optimal placement of speech en-ergy within the listener's auditory area: A basis for selecting amplification characteris-tics. In G. A. Studebaker & F. H. Bess (Eds.), *The Vanderbilt Hearing Aid Report.* Mono-graphs in Contemporary Audiology. Upper Darby, PA: Associated Hearing Instru-ments.

Studebaker, G., Cox, R., & Formby, C. (1980). The effect of environment on the directional per-formance of headworn hearing aids. In G. Studebaker & I. Hochberg (Eds.), *Acousti-cal factors affecting hearing aid performance.* Baltimore: University Park Press.

The Marketing Edge. (1986). Hearing Industries Association, 1(2) 2–3.

The Marketing Edge. (1987). Hearing Industries Association 2(1) 2–3.

Walker, G., & Byrne D. (1985). Reliability of speech intelligibility estimation for measur-ing speech reception thresholds in quiet and noise. *Australian Journal of Audiology, 7,* 23–31.

Walker, G., Dillon, H., Byrne, D., & Christen, R. (1984). The use of loudness discomfort levels for selecting the maximum output of hear-ing aids. *Australian Journal of Audiology, 6,* 23-32.

3

POST-FITTING AND REHABILITATIVE MANAGEMENT OF THE ADULT HEARING AID USER

DAVID P. PASCOE ■

*T*his chapter is intended to be an overview of rehabilitative management practices that have proven beneficial in working with individuals who are experiencing hearing aid amplification for the first time. As such, it represents fundamental approaches to patient management that have provided effective procedures designed to encourage hearing aid acceptance and use.

The contents of this chapter have value for the neophyte audiologist or the dispenser and also for the experienced practitioners who want to review their established practices in rehabilitative management of the adult hearing aid user.

There is no general consensus regarding how the problems faced by adults who use hearing aids should be managed or what sequence of events should be followed by any individual practitioner. For most, the rationale adopted to guide fitting practices has been developed through trial and error. This chapter serves as a reference for those who seek alternative approaches to

an augmented management strategy. To that end, the information presented is basic, unadorned with supposition and not burdened by theoretical dogma. The procedures recommended have been arrived at empirically and found to be effective in achieving desired goals.

Most people feel apprehensive when starting something new, but most people have experienced the joy of seeing tasks that once seemed difficult become easy, even natural. Beginning to use hearing aids can be just such an experience for the hearing-impaired listener. This chapter reviews the factors involved in helping the new hearing aid user proceed from fear to satisfaction and gives suggestions for possible action.

FIRST STEPS

Before sending clients home to start using their first hearing aids, the following procedures should be clearly understood, practiced, and learned.

Correct Insertion and Removal of Hearing Aids and Earmolds

This activity must be learned by doing, not by explanation. People differ so much in their dexterity and there are so many shapes of ears that clinicians should avoid teaching a single procedure. Each person must find and learn an efficient way to hold and to insert the earmold or the hearing aid. Suggestions and demonstrations can be given, their fingers can be guided, but hearing aid recipients must learn by trying, by putting the hearing aids in and taking them out several times. A double-mirror can be helpful if it gives a clear impression of how the hearing aid or earmold should fit within the concha or sit behind the ear, but further practice should focus on *feeling* the positions and actions required.

One common error of insertion is to fit the hearing aid or the earmold shaft into the canal and leave the top "hook" or helix outside of the pinna's front folds, just above the tragus. This position can be uncomfortable and usually allows feedback. In this case the user needs to be taught how to twist the aid or the earmold back so that it will slide correctly into the proper place.

Removing the aid from the ear can also be a problem if the thumb is inserted behind the rear edge of the aid's faceplate, forcing the hand to turn forward and pull the rear edge out first. This motion makes the aid's canal shaft hook against the ear canal wall and impedes removal of the hearing aid or earmold. Since most people's ear canals turn toward the rear of the head, unless their shafts are short and straight, hearing aids and earmolds should be extracted by turning them toward the rear of the head. In other words, the front edge of the aid or of the earmold should be pulled out first.

Hearing aid devices should be turned off to avoid feedback when they are being inserted or removed. The battery doors of in-the-ear (ITE) hearing aids and the tubing of behind-the-ear (BTE) hearing aids should not be used as handles for insertion or removal. To help individuals who have poor dexterity, fingernail grooves or removal handles should be specified when ordering the instruments.

When necessary, relatives or caretakers should be shown how the hearing aid looks when it is properly inserted so that they can give appropriate help at home. In most cases, the proof of an efficient insertion is the absence of feedback when the volume of the hearing aid is turned up to a desired loudness level.

Learning to Operate the Hearing Aid

Moving the volume control, whether it rotates on the face of ITE and canal hearing aids or moves up and down as in the BTE hearing aid, is the most frequent action that the listener must learn. It seems simple to say: Raise the volume until it sounds comfortable. The trouble is in defining *what* should be made comfortable. If it is conversation, how is the user to control the level of other people's voices? Relatives often retain the habit of talking louder to hearing aid users, as a residue of the gradual adjustment they have made to a gradual increase in the new hearing aid users' hearing loss. Except for listeners with severe and profound hearing losses, loud voices rarely require amplification.

Another strategy is to adjust the volume so that the user's amplified voice sounds "normal" to the user. The problem in this case is that people usually define "normal" as the way their voices sound without an aid. Should the volume be adjusted when listening in a quiet room? Or should the listener learn to adjust the volume to fit each situation? These questions may not have single answers, and listeners may have to find their own preferred methods. The audiologist or the dispenser must beware of presenting pat, single patterns, no matter how common they may be, as "expert" advice.

Since the level of amplified sound cannot be increased in the same gradual manner that the loss of hearing has usually increased, amplified sound cannot be introduced without some degree of rejection. It is possible, for example, to assume that each listener knows what is best and let it go at that (whatever gain is chosen must be correct). Unfortunately, new users sometimes set their aids at levels that give no gain and may even create some loss. Some users of hearing aid devices may say that their aids sound "wonderful" when they are actually turned off!

For the new user, selecting an acceptable and useful volume is a search into unknown dimensions. It is useful to demonstrate several ways to approach the problem:

1. A simple approach is to ask the listener to raise the volume, as the clinician speaks, to reach a level that sounds louder than desired and then to reduce the volume slowly until the level is acceptable. If clients complain that their own voices are too loud at this level, *they should lower their voices not their hearing aids.*

2. The audiologist or the dispenser can also pre-adjust an aid's volume in a test box by following one of several well-known assumptions, such as the one-half or the one-third rules that predict "use" gain from the listener's average hearing levels (HLs).

3. If one has a reliable estimate of the listener's comfortable loudness range, another way of setting a predetermined gain, is to define *desired gain* as the difference between the mean comfortable level and an estimate of the average speech input levels. This method can be as simple as the formula:

Mean or Average
Comfort Level
(in dB HL) − 55 dB = Desired Gain

The pre-adjusted levels should not be used to show the listeners where the hearing aid's volume must be set but simply to give them an idea of the levels that can be used after amplified sound becomes more acceptable. Often, users like to know the "number," or the relative position of the volume control, so that they can set it at the desired level before insertion. Sometimes marking the correct setting with a dot or a mark made with bright fingernail polish can be helpful.

When two hearing aids are adjusted, the first should be set to a softer level than would be chosen if it was worn as a single aid. Then the volume of the other hearing aid should be raised until sound is perceived in that ear and then lowered so that sound is perceived in the center of the head, or so that sound is not louder in either ear.

A good way to assure a well-adjusted binaural balance is to turn on a radio or television set and, with eyes closed, turn around at least once until the exact location of the sound source can be pinpointed. If the source is not located correctly, one ear is receiving more sound than the other and an adjustment must be made. The final test of a true binaural fitting is an improved ability to detect the direction of audible sounds, as well as the resulting capacity to separate one source from another, which facilitates the reception of speech in noisy surroundings.

If hearing aids include other controls, such as an on-off switch or a "phone" or a "tone" position, these controls should be pointed out and their effects tested. Some ITE aids include an on-off position in the volume control that must be demonstrated by feel or sound. When hearing aids do not turn off, the user must be shown how the battery door should be opened to interrupt function and thus increase battery life. Some BTE instruments use the battery door as a switch, and the direction of their on-off action (in contrast to the normal opening motion), should be shown to new users. Practice in this operation should also be given.

If the hearing aid device includes a phone or tele-coil switch, an actual demonstration of telephone use should be given. If there is more than one telephone line in the clinic or office building, telephone conversations should be carried out for practice. The placement of the telephone handset over the hearing aid, so that the most effective contact can be made with the coil, must be demonstrated. In some cases, after the hearing aid has been set to the "T" position, the volume can be turned up to improve reception since feedback will not occur. Furthermore, when the telephone conversation is over, the user must remember to reset the switch to "M" for normal function. These details may sound overly simple, but their omission or insufficient emphasis on them in training new hearing aid users often causes unnecessary problems.

Since many of the newer telephones are not compatible with hearing aids, other alternatives must be discussed, and the availability of acoustic and electromagnetic couplers should be mentioned.

In some cases, telephone reception can be achieved through the hearing aid's microphone. For this option, it is important to show the listener how the telephone should be kept close to the ear but not touching the hearing aid and also how the fingers can be used to maintain the handset a specific distance from the head. The vent, in fact, can be used as direct path for telephone reception when an individual has sufficient low-frequency hearing.

Sometimes people spend time and effort to come to see the audiologist or the dispenser because they think that their hearing aids are not working, only to discover that the problem is as simple as a switch in the wrong position. These undesirable events can be avoided with proper instruction. When they do occur, they can often be solved over the telephone by asking the caller to move the appropriate switch back and forth, or to take the battery out and put it back in, while the audiologist or the dispenser listens for the onset of feedback.

Understanding Feedback

Even experienced hearing aid users may not understand what feedback is or what causes it. In many cases, that annoying squeal is the guideline people use to set hearing aid volume. People often say, "I raise the volume up until I hear the whistle, and then I set it back a little." This error is common, but misinformation of this sort can reach amazing extremes, for example, the client who was told that feedback is a device used by the hearing aid manufacturer to warn the listener when sound is over-amplified, somewhat in the spirit of an escape valve in a pressure cooker or a whistling teapot. Without any doubt, feedback is a major problem in achieving efficient amplification. It must be avoided, not by turning the aid's volume below a desired level, but by solving the acoustic factors that cause it.

A hearing aid that functions well, that fits into the ear canal and concha and makes an efficient closure or seal, does not cause feedback when it is properly inserted. A hearing aid that fits well, by this definition is one that can be turned up to a desired loudness level without causing feedback. Nevertheless, even with a hearing aid that fits properly, the user should understand that feedback can still occur if the hearing aid is not inserted properly, if a hand is cupped over the microphone, if the ear canal is partially blocked with ear wax, or if the instrument has developed internal damage. BTE hearing aids can generate feedback when the earmold's tubing or the hearing aid's earhook are cracked or allow leakage of sound around their joints. Sometimes a hearing aid will squeal when the ear canal changes shape during the act of chewing or when the mold slips out because of similar jaw movements.

Hearing-impaired listeners should be able to set their hearing aids' volume as high as required to make voices comfortably loud. They should know that the volume setting must not be determined by the emission of feedback. If a desired setting cannot be reached because of feedback, the aid does not fit properly, and a new earmold or hearing aid cast must be obtained.

New users should realize that feedback is related to the amount of power needed, so the greater the power used, the tighter the fit of the earmold must be. Furthermore, users should understand that the closer the microphone is to the sound outlet, or the more open the fitting is, the greater the chances are of getting feedback. Of course, this means that while a vented or wide open earmold is more comfortable than a full and closed one, a mold or its vent cannot be more open than is necessary to avoid feedback at the desired use levels.

In cases of profound high-frequency hearing loss, feedback squeal is often inaudible to the user of the device, but it is highly annoying to those nearby. Even if no one is bothered by this high-pitched sound, it must be avoided simply because it introduces distortion and consumes power without any positive purpose.

It is important to remember that short, simply written materials, such as the example shown in Figure 3-1, facilitate a clearer understanding of the problem of feedback, its causes, and the solutions available.

Changing Batteries

Most individuals can easily learn to change batteries. Others, however, because of poor sight or insufficient dexterity, may not be able to master this task and will need help from others. It is important to make sure that no one leaves the office without having practiced taking batteries out of the hearing aid and replacing them correctly, or that there will be someone at home to help in this task. It is a good idea to suggest to clients that batteries should always be changed while sitting next to a table, preferably over a tray covered with a soft cloth or towel, and in the best possible light. Anyone who has dropped a small

---

Hearing aids often produce a loud, high-pitched whistle that can be extremely annoying to you and to others around you. This loud noise is produced by amplified sound that escapes from your ear canal and "feeds back" into the aid's mike, becoming amplified again and again.

You may hear that whistle when you touch the aid or place your hand close to it, or when you forget to turn off the aid before taking it out or putting it in your ear. Also, your aid may whistle if it is not correctly inserted in your ear.

If you cannot set your aid's volume to make it sound as loud as you want because it starts to whistle, check first whether you have pushed the aid or the earmold in as far as it should be. If you cannot make the aid stop whistling, let us know as soon as you can.

We may have to remake your earmold or your aid so that a better fit can be achieved, or perhaps a reduction in the vent's diameter will solve the problem. In one way or another, we will have to solve your problem.

You cannot go on using an aid that is constantly *whistling!*

FIGURE 3-1. If Your Aid Whistles. Sample of instructional material on hearing aid feedback.

battery and had it hide behind the least likely object knows the reason for such precautions. Figure 3–2 shows a practical way of presenting this type of information for further reading at home.

For many hearing aid users, rechargeable batteries are a practical option, and their advantages or disadvantages should be discussed. One advantage of this option is that built-in batteries do not have to be changed. A disadvantage is that they need to be recharged regularly. A common misunderstanding about this type of hearing aid has been caused by advertisements that claim "a hearing aid without batteries" when the instrument is actually an aid with a built-in rechargeable cell. Rechargeable batteries that are removable and can be replaced by regular batteries are also available. This option solves the problem of

---

As you probably know, all batteries have a *negative* (−) and a *positive* (+) side. The battery drawer door in your hearing aid shows the (+) side with a small red cross. Be sure to place your battery so that the two (+) signs match. If the battery is placed in the wrong direction, the aid will not work.

The positive side in hearing aid batteries is usually flat and shows the (+), while the negative side has rounded edges, like this:

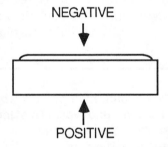

The bottom or negative side of the battery drawer is also rounded so that the battery fits snugly only when it is inserted in the correct direction. In many aids, if the battery is placed incorrectly the battery door cannot be closed.

To insert the battery you can grasp it between your thumb and index finger, with the positive side touching the thumb. Push the battery through the front or through the larger opening. If the battery door does not close easily, do not force it shut! The battery must be in the wrong direction. When the battery is in the correct position, the door should close easily.

In some cases, the battery door may stop just short of being fully closed and you need to give it one more firm push until it clicks in. Otherwise the aid will not work.

FIGURE 3–2. Changing the Batteries. Sample of instructional material on how to change hearing aid batteries.

rechargeable batteries that run down when least expected, and its availability should be made known to hearing aid users.

Questions about batteries such as "When should I change it?" or "How long should it last?" should also be answered. Figure 3–3 presents answers to common questions about batteries in a handout form that can be used to reiterate the information that has been given orally. The audiologist or the hearing aid dispenser also needs to explain the difference between air and so-called mercury batteries and to provide information about purchasing batteries (how many at a time, where). Sources of mail order distribution, such as the American Association of Retired Persons (AARP), should be discussed. The effects of humidity, the use of battery meters and their availability, the need to make sure that the hearing aids are turned off when not in use, and that the battery door should be left open during the night are topics that must be cov-

ered. An extremely important warning must be given regarding the proper way to dispose of dead batteries to avoid danger to children, pets, and the environment. An example of such a warning is shown in Figure 3–4.

Care of the Instrument

There is a natural fear of damaging such a small and expensive instrument. Users should learn to handle their aids only over soft floors or carpets. Taking aids out of the ear or trying to put them in over tile or other hard surfaces should be avoided. If a hearing aid is dropped on the living room carpet, damage is not likely to occur. If it falls on the bathroom floor, sink, or tub, the impact can cause serious damage.

New hearing aid users need to be cautioned about allowing their aids to come into contact with water, hair spray, per-

---

You know that a battery is dead when you turn up the aid's volume and you cannot hear any amplified sound. If your aid is on your hand, the battery is dead if the aid does not "whistle."

You have to be sure, however, that the battery is inserted in the correct position, that the battery door is fully closed, and that the aid is turned full-on. If your aid has an "on-off" switch, it must be set to "M" (for microphone).

If you insert a new battery and the aid still does not work, then the problem is different. Either you have the on-off switch in the wrong position (it may be set to "T" for telephone, or on "O" for off), or you placed the battery upside down, or did not close the battery door completely.

Another possibility is that the sound outlet is plugged with earwax. Look closely at the tip-end of your aid or your earmold, and see if it needs cleaning.

Of course, if none of the above conditions exists, the aid may not be working and you need to call us as soon as possible. Before you give up, try again! Check all of the above-mentioned problems.

FIGURE 3–3. When to Change Your Batteries. Sample of instructional material on when to change hearing aid batteries.

Hearing aid batteries are *dangerous when swallowed.* Children and pets have been hurt seriously, and even fatal results have been recorded.

If a battery has been swallowed, see a doctor immediately, and call: **National Button Battery Hotline, (202) 625-3333,** collect.

To avoid such accidents, keep batteries and hearing aids away from children and pets. If children are old enough, warn them about their danger.

Because of their mercury content, batteries are also *dangerous to the environment.* Do not throw them away; save them in a jar or an envelope, and mail them every year or two to your supplier, or to:

CENTRAL INSTITUTE FOR THE DEAF
818 South Euclid Avenue
St. Louis, MO 63110

FIGURE 3-4. A Very Important Warning About Batteries. Sample of instructional material on precautions in storing and disposing of hearing aid batteries.

fume, or talcum or face powder. Hearing aids should never be handled over a bowl of soup or a cup of coffee. Vaseline and other oily substances, which may be used to ease the insertion of earmolds or aids, can plug up the sound outlets and damage the hearing aid enough to require professional repair. The removal of earwax from the sound-outlet of an ITE or a canal hearing aid, even when using the proper tool, can be dangerous if not done carefully. Hearing aids should always be handled with clean, dry hands, and proper cleaning procedures should be demonstrated. Written information (see Figure 3-5) can be important reinforcement to the spoken word.

In addition to making sure that the client knows the warranty terms extended by the manufacturer, the availability of insurance against damage, loss, and theft should be explained, and its importance discussed.

Written Reinforcement of Instructions

The items discussed in this chapter do not exhaust the enormous amount of in-

formation the first-time hearing aid user needs to know. Obviously, no normal human being will be able to assimilate all of it in a short session. Although the audiologists or the hearing aid dispensers must cover these areas, no one should assume the information has been understood and will be remembered. Written repetition of the information that has been given orally is indispensible.

The first written communication that customers should receive is a report of the results of the post-fitting tests. Figure 3-6 is an example of such a letter. Another very important follow-up is a set of written cards, or individual sheets, that deal with one topic at a time. These should be given to the client with the suggestion that he or she read one each day and keep them for repeated perusal and use when needed. Information handouts will be more effective if they include illustrations, even if they are not professionally drawn. Material of this type is not written up separately for each individual, but is enclosed with or referred to in the individual report letter sent immediately after the hearing aid fitting session.

Hearing aids are well-built instruments, but they can be damaged if you drop them on hard surfaces. Always handle them when you are sitting down or standing over a rug, never when you are over a tile floor.

Be sure that your hands are dry and clean when you handle your aids. Water can ruin them, and oily creams or Vaseline can plug up their sound inlet or outlet ports. Never spray your hair or powder your face when you have an aid in your ear. Always take off your aids when you take a bath, shave, or wash your face.

Never loan your aid to anyone. It will not fit anybody else's ear correctly. Because of this it can make a loud squeal or whistle that is not only bothersome but also dangerous. If your aid is very powerful, it could even damage somebody's hearing.

Do not leave your aid where a child or a pet can grab it. Put it away every night in the same place, preferably, its original box, and leave the battery door open, If it is a very humid time of the year, use a dehumidifier pack. Never leave your aid inside the glove compartment of your car.

Never stick anything into the aid's sound outlet port or into the mike's opening. If you have trouble with earwax, use the brush you were given and a soft tissue.

Keep your ears free of earwax as much as you can. If needed, see your physician regularly and have your ears cleaned.

FIGURE 3–5. Taking Care of Your Hearing Aids. Sample of instructional material on proper care of hearing aids.

Figures 3–1 through 3–6 are examples of the type of written information that should be provided.

Most hearing aid manufacturers include excellent descriptions of the hearing aid, instructions for its use, handling of the controls, precautions, and trial strategies. It is important to be aware of their recommendations and to review them with the client. Furthermore, clients should be encouraged to read these pamphlets with care within the first few days of the trial period. Two examples of manufacturer's instructions are shown in Figures 3–7 and 3–8.

THE TRIAL PERIOD

Whether a hearing aid dispenser subscribes to the full-refund, one-month trial period, or offers a partial refund or some type of rental option that gives the buyer a chance to experience the effects of amplification before making a final decision, it is important to supervise and encourage a fair and efficient trial effort. This effort does not, or should not, mean the use of subtle pressure to complete a sale without regard for the user's satisfaction, but rather a professional effort to achieve the client's optimal satisfaction *whether or not* the hearing aid is finally purchased. The following strategies are some of the many ways to increase the probabilities of achieving client satisfaction.

First Use of the Hearing Aid

There are several ways to approach the problem of how much and when to use the

Dear Mr. Jones:

This letter is to remind you of the explanation I gave you regarding your "audiogram." I hope it makes sense to you.

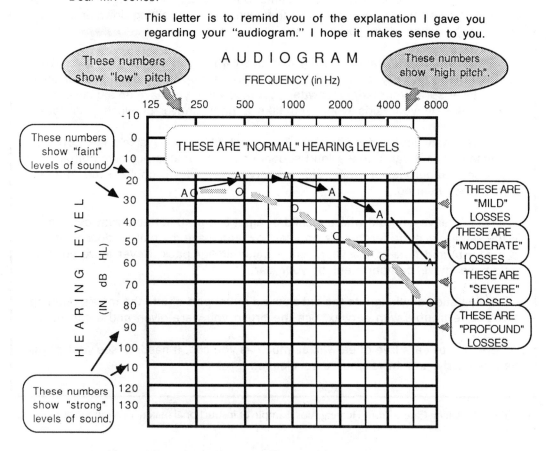

The line that is connected by the letter (O) represents the faintest levels of sound that you were able to hear with your RIGHT EAR, and WITHOUT YOUR HEARING AID.

As you can see, the levels that you heard in the low-pitch range show hearing that is near the "normal" range. However, your hearing for the higher-pitch sound shows losses that range from "mild," to "moderate," to "severe." With this amount of hearing, we calculate that you are able to hear 70% of the sound available in face-to-face conversations.

The line that connects the letter (A) shows the fainter levels of sound that you were able to hear WITH YOUR HEARING AID, worn on the right ear. As you can see, these "aided" levels are much closer to the normal hearing range: with this comfortable amount of amplification, you can hear *as much as 94% of the sound available in face-to-face conversations.*

If you have any questions, do not nesitate to call me.

David P. Pascoe
AUDIOLOGIST

FIGURE 3-6. Sample of a post-fitting report letter.

Care and Maintenance of Your Aid

Keep your aid clean by wiping it periodically with a dry tissue or cloth. When you remove your aid, check to see if any wax particles are lodged in the receiver or vent opening and, if so, brush gently with the cleaning brush provided with your aid.

To avoid any possibility of damage to the receiver, do not insert anything more than ⅛ of an inch into the receiver opening. If you experience any difficulties in removing the wax, you should consult your hearing aid dispenser.

How to Change the Battery in Your Aid

Insert fingernail in fingernail projection of battery compartment and gently swing the compartment open. Turn aid upside down and the old battery will drop out. Turn aid back to upright position and insert new battery from above, making sure plus (+) side is up (as illustrated) and corresponds to (+) on battery compartment.

If the battery compartment does not easily close DO NOT FORCE IT CLOSED but check to make sure that the battery is not upside down or improperly seated in the compartment. If compartment still will not close easily, trying inserting a different battery — as sometimes batteries can swell due to chemical reactions within the battery itself.

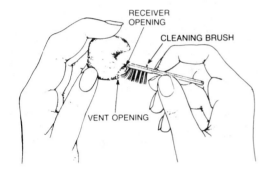

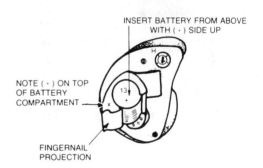

FIGURE 3–7. Sample of a hearing aid manufacturer's operating instructions. (Courtesy of Qualitone Hearing Aids and Audiometers.)

hearing aid in the beginning. Commonly, clients are advised to start with only a few minutes of use in quiet surroundings and then to gradually increase the time the aid is worn and begin to use it in more difficult listening situations. Another approach is to advise the client to use the aid as much as possible, resting only when, and if, fatigue or nervousness are experienced. New users can also be advised to begin by setting the volume of the hearing aid to low loudness levels and then gradually increase it to higher and possibly more useful setting.

Even though the strategies mentioned are commonly recommended, there are no data to support any one of them as the "best," or the only way to begin. The best solution may be to discuss the various alternatives with clients and let them try them with an open mind. If someone turns on a hearing aid and finds that it sounds wonderful, should it be taken off after a few minutes merely to follow the dispenser's instructions? If the aid hurts, either from auditory or physical causes, should it be kept in the ear simply because "you told me to do

THE GAIN CONTROL

The gain control enables you to adjust the amount of amplification provided by your CE-6. You may wish to change it as you encounter different listening situations.

To change the level, use the tip of one finger to rotate the gain control. To make the sound louder, rotate the control forward. To make it softer, turn the control backwards.

As you adjust the gain control, you may hear a whistling noise called *feedback*. This is caused by amplified sound that escapes the ear and is reflected by your hand back into the microphone. The feedback should cease when you take your hand away.

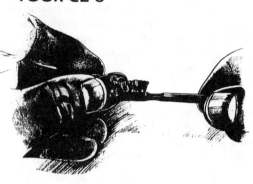

TAKING CARE OF YOUR CE-6

When not wearing your CE-6, be sure to remove the battery from its compartment to prevent an excessive reduction in battery life. If your CE-6 will not be used for an extended period of time, place it in the carrying case and store in a cool, dry place.

The Brush-aide is provided to help you keep your hearing aid clean. Use the Brush-aide daily to remove earwax or other particles which may have accumulated on the canal end of the aid or around the gain control and battery compartment. A careful brushing accompanied by gentle wiping with a soft cloth will keep your CE-6 clean.

TELEPHONE USE

When using a telephone, your CE-6 works best by holding the receiver close, but not pressing against your ear. If you hear a whistling noise, tilt the receiver at an angle until the noise stops. Experiment until you find the best position for listening.

FIGURE 3–8. Sample of a hearing aid manufacturer's operations manual. (Courtesy of Starkey Labs, Inc.)

it?" Obviously not. Chances are that each person will react and adjust to amplification individually, and what works for one may not work for another.

Judging the Hearing Aid's Effectiveness

Comparing the quality of sound, or the difficulty of various listening situations, is not an easy thing to do. Nevertheless, listeners should be encouraged to compare their satisfaction in the same situations with and without aids. The best situations to test are those in which the listener is passive. It is important to be able to listen for a few minutes without the aids and then for a similar period with them on. If the set is not turned up to strong levels, listening to the television news, can be a good test. In this situation, it is better to ask someone else, a friend or relative with good hearing, to set the volume to a "normal" level.

Listeners should be encouraged to keep a diary of their experiences with the new hearing aid, or aids, during the trial period. The following questions can be asked: How long did you use your aids today? Where did you use them? What sounds have you heard that you have not heard recently? Have conversations been easier to follow? Did you hear as well, better, or worse with the hearing aids? What problems did you notice? Did you have to change the volume often, or were you able to forget about it? Providing clients with a notebook in which to keep a daily diary of their new experiences with amplified sound is helpful. In addition to questions about daily use, the notebook can include other reminders of some of the information discussed with the client.

Clients should also be advised to keep a record of dates batteries are changed since radical changes in battery life can mean that the aid is not functioning well or that the hearing aid is not being turned off overnight. Figure 3–9, is an example of a simple, weekly diary.

When two hearing aids are being tried, the comparison should include the contrast between using both and only one. In such cases, monaural listening can also be compared between ears. The availability of these comparisons is a good argument for binaural trial. Undoubtedly, this is the most valid way of deciding whether two hearing aids are really better than one, and if one hearing aid appears to be sufficient, in which ear the instrument gives the greatest satisfaction.

Maintaining Contact with the Client

There are several ways of increasing contact with the new users during a trial period. A simple method, of course, is to remind the client to call when problems arise or if he or she has questions. The dispenser's telephone number and the most appropriate hours to call can be written on a business card, or included in the notebook mentioned above. A less frequently used method is to put the client's name on a telephone call list and assign specific dates to call so that contact can be made at least once or twice during the trial period.

Two or three group sessions that include the new users as well as one or two family members or friends can be offered, either free or for moderate fees. In these sessions, the fitter of the hearing aids can present the same information that has been given, but now in general form. These sessions can also be to practice the development of visual attention and auditory awareness. The exchange of information and concerns between individuals who are facing a common challenge can be encouraged.

Instructional sessions can be extended past the trial period, but they are especially important during the first month of hearing aid use because these are the days when avoidable failures occur. Many individuals are either unable or unwilling to attend classes. Others probably do not need much help or supervision. Everyone, however, must receive sufficient information to understand the problems of hearing impairment and to ease the acceptance of hearing aids.

For some people, either because of distance or lack of mobility, something equivalent to a correspondence course can be an answer. Short, single topic letters can be sent periodically. Sample topics include: What is "lip reading"? What can you expect from visual attention? How does a hearing aid work? What makes a listening situation difficult? What sounds can be confused with each other? How can you improve the clarity of your speech and that of others? How to improve sound in your home? Why are two hearing aids often better than one? Why does your hearing aid whistle?

Obtaining Support from Relatives or Friends

Some individuals do not need help from others, and may not even want anyone to notice that they are using hearing aids. Others, however, may have trouble inserting the hearing aid correctly or be unable see well enough to change the batteries. These people need help every day, at least until those tasks are learned. In these cases, a husband, son or daughter, good friend, neighbor, or nurse or therapist should be instructed in these procedures so that the hearing aids are used and used properly.

When people who are nervous and not enthusiastic about using hearing aids start to learn how to handle them, they often give up after the first few minutes with comments like: "I cannot do it." "I am too dumb, too old." These individuals need to relax, to go home and try the hearing aid again without the tension of doing it in front of a stranger, no matter how friendly that strang-

NAME: _____

Date trial started: _____

SECOND WEEK

1. Have you changed batteries yet? If so, write down the date you changed it (them): _____

2. How long have you been using the aid(s) every day?

   _____

3. List the places or situations in which you have been using the aid(s):

   _____

   _____

   _____

4. Have you had any problems? If yes, please write them down:

   _____

   _____

   _____

5. In what situation have you noticed that you heard better because of your hearing aid(s)?

   _____

   _____

   _____

REMINDER:

Do not forget to turn off the aid and open the battery door every night. In fact, you should do this whenever you are not using your aid(s) for any length of time. ***This will save your battery's life.***

FIGURE 3–9. Sample of a hearing aid trial journal.

er may be. But they also need someone there to encourage them, to confirm their impressions, and to provide a friendly voice to listen to. These difficulties are normal; everyone feels awkward when handling something so small for the first time. These feelings must be created, and no one can do it better than an understanding friend.

Unfortunately, all too often people who are close to a person with a hearing impairment not only do not understand the depth of the problem, but also may contribute to the anxiety and the frustration felt by the client. Wives, husbands, children, and grandchildren can have false expectations. They may believe that the hearing aid should easily solve the problem: "Now you will hear." "You are not trying." "You are just being stubborn." Attitudes like these are not likely to help. These people are important and indispensable factors in successful hearing aid use, and they should be included in counseling strategies.

Supportive Literature

Many pamphlets and books have been written precisely to convey the information discussed here. Besides manufacturer's pamphlets, there are others that can be used. Suggested reading materials and where they may be obtained are presented later in this chapter.

End of the Trial Period

A postcard should be sent, or a telephone call should be made, a few days before the end of the agreed-on trial period. The client should be encouraged to retain the hearing aid, or aids, if he or she is satisfied or to return it or them if not satisfied. If there are problems that should be inspected, the client should be invited to come in. If a major alteration or hearing aid remake must be done, the trial period should be extended, and its duration should be stated in writing. Strong efforts should be made to

avoid the sale or purchase of hearing aids that will not be used. Such sales tend to increase negative customer attitudes and create adverse publicity. Clients who are satisfied with honest and sincere efforts to help, rather than merely to sell, will return and will recommend friends who need help.

FOLLOW-UP

Once the trial period is over and a client has decided to keep the hearing aid, several strategies for continued contact must be established. Some clients will not need further supervision, other than possible trouble-shooting, for several years. Others, however, because of their greater hearing loss or because of greater feelings of insecurity, will need practical schemes of short- or long-term aural rehabilitation.

Periodic Hearing and Hearing Aid Measurements

Clients who kept their hearing aids, as well as those who did not, should be encouraged to return every year for a hearing test. A special calendar can be maintained to which names are constantly added so that reminder notes are sent at the proper times. Special retest prices can be established to encourage clients to return.

Visual inspection and electronic measurements of the hearing aids should be done once a year. Maintenance tasks, such as changing tubing, cleaning battery contacts, clearing vents, checking dampers, and listening for noisy controls, can be recorded on cards and made part of the customer's record.

Information Updates

From time to time, there are interesting articles that should be shared will all customers. These articles may include information about new products, such as television caption decoders, cochlear implants, medical advances, new styles of instruments, or digital hearing aids. Newsletters related to services, group meetings, and visiting personalities may also be sent to clients. With the advent of word processing equipment, which can enable us to maintain contact and distribute information in simple and economic ways, contacts like these are now more feasible.

Peer Groups

Clients should be encouraged to participate in groups such as SHHH (Self Help for Hard of Hearing People, Inc.), which was organized by hearing-impaired individuals to achieve the goal stated in the group's name. This national organization promotes the creation of local autonomous groups. These groups formed by hearing-impaired individuals meet periodically to discuss and share experiences related to their hearing problems. Their primary purpose is to educate themselves, their relatives, and their friends about the causes, characteristics, problems, and possible remedies for hearing loss. (The address of the national office is 7800 Wisconsin Avenue, Bethesda, MD 20814; [301] 657-2248 for voice calls; [301] 657-2249 for TTY or TDD calls.)

SHHH publishes a bi-monthly magazine called Shhh, which prints articles of practical, scientific, legal, and organizational interest to members. Anyone may subscribe to it by becoming a member of SHHH and paying a yearly fee. Membership is not limited to hearing-impaired individuals. Clinics and business organizations dealing with the hearing impaired should join and place this magazine in their waiting room reading racks.

The National Association of the Deaf (814 Thayer Avenue, Suite 301, Silver Spring, MD 20004), is another peer group organization. It is directed toward profoundly deaf individuals whose hearing losses are of congenital or pre-lingual

origin. This organization also publishes a journal, Deaf American.

Other Sources of Information

In addition to the previously mentioned groups, other organizations dealing with the dissemination of information about hearing problems include:

National Association for Hearing and Speech Action, 10801 Rockville Pike, Rockville, MD 20852. Helpline: 1-(800) 638-8255 (during office hours, EST).

National Hearing Aid Society, 20361 Middlebelt, Livonia, MI 48152. Telephone: 1-(800) 521-5247.

Better Hearing Institute, 1430 K Street, N.W., Suite 600, Washington, DC 20005. Telephone: 1-(800) 424-8576.

Alexander Graham Bell Association for the Deaf, Inc., 3417 Volta Place, N.W., Washington, DC 20007. Telephone: 1-(202) 337-5220 (voice and TDD calls).

Although it is not an organization specifically devoted to the hearing impaired, the AT&T National Special Needs Center provides information about telephonic aids to improve communication (1-[800] 233-1222, for voice calls; 1-[800] 833-3232, for TDD or TTY calls).

Recommended Reading Materials

Here are a few of the more recent books dealing with the auditory problems of adult individuals:

Adjustment to Adult Hearing Loss by Harold Orlans (Ed.). College-Hill Press, Boston, MA. 1985. 204 pages.

Coping with Hearing Loss, A Guide for Adults and their Families by Susan V. Rezen and Carl Hausman. Dembner Books, New York. 1985. 191 pages.

Helping the Older Adult with an Acquired Hearing Loss by Joan M. Sayre. (Suggestions and techniques for clinicians, audiologists and others working with the adult hearing impaired). 56 pages. Also, by the same author, *Handbook for the Hearing-Impaired Older Adult* (an individualized program). 70 pages. Both booklets published by The Interstate Printers and Publishers, Inc., Danville, IL. 1980.

Excellent pamphlets are also distributed by several sources. A few are listed below.

Hearing Aids — A Guide to Their Wear and Care, published by the Patient Information Library, Krames Communications (312-90th Street, Daly City, CA 94015). 16 pages.

All About Hearing Aids, published by the Alexander Graham Bell Association for the Deaf. 12 pages.

Hearing Loss. Hope Through Research, published by the U.S. Department of Health and Human Services, National Institute of Health, Publication No. 82-157. 35 pages.

Neglected Facts About Hearing, Sears, Roebuck and Co., 1980. 20 single-column pages.

Hearing Health Care, a set of pamphlets, published by courtesy of the Oticon Corporation and distributed by the New York League for the Hard of Hearing, that includes reprints from articles of various institutions and journals. Includes titles such as: "Which hearing aid for me?" "Help! There's something wrong with my hearing aid!" "Hearing loss in the elderly" and "You know I can't hear you when the water's running . . . ."

Hearing Aid Care, Hearing Aid User's Guide, Suggestions For The Family, Aural Rehabilitation Review and many more titles distributed by the Starkey Laboratories, Inc.

Learning to Hear Again, published by Audiotone. Although meant for Audiotone distributors, this is a well-written pamphlet dealing with strategies for initial hearing aid use.

Batteries and Other Supplies

Many hearing aid distributors organize purchasing clubs, which supply batteries to customers at reasonable prices. These clubs provide an excellent way to maintain regular contact with customers, and also provide an ongoing opportunity for supervision. Clients who belong to the AARP should be reminded that their association distributes batteries at very low prices. Anyone 50 years old or older can join, and for people in this age range, the availability of low-cost hearing aid batteries is reason enough to do so. (Write to: AARP, Membership Processing Center, 3200 E. Carson Street, Lakewood, CA 90712.) Local groups, like SHHH chapters, can also organize their own purchasing clubs.

New Hearing Aids, Additional Hearing Aids, and Changes of Hearing Aid Type

People are often interested in new products, even when they are satisfied with what they have. Hearing aid dispensers must be careful not to exaggerate the possible value of a new type of hearing aid but clients should be provided with the facts to make intelligent decisions.

Other devices designed to assist the hearing impaired are available. Audiologists and hearing aid dispensers serve as sources of information about these specialized instruments (e.g., those that provide better television reception such as the infra-red light transmitters, which are now becoming available even in theaters). Adaptors that improve telephone coupling are available, as are sound-to-light or sound-to-vibration transducers, which allow the profoundly deaf to respond better to simple acoustic signals such as alarm clocks, door bells, and smoke alarms. There are also the television decoders for closed-caption reception and TTY or TDD receiver-transmitters, which enable telephone communication for the severely or profoundly deaf. Sources of information or catalogs of assistive devices for the hearing impaired include:

Special Devices for Hard of Hearing, Deaf, and Deaf-Blind Persons, by J. Hurvitz and R.

Carmen. Little, Brown and Company, Boston, MA. 1981. 297 pages.

Harc Mercantile, Ltd., 3130 Portage, Kalamazoo, MI 49003.

Hal-Hen Co., 35-53 24th Street, Long Island City, NY 11106.

Sound Resources, Inc., 201 Ogden, Hinsdale, IL 60521.

Trouble Shooting, Repairs, and Loaner Hearing Aids

Although audiologists and hearing aid dispensers can solve some hearing aid problems in the office, a hearing aid must sometimes be sent back to the manufacturer or to a repair facility. In these situations, the dispenser should be able to fit acceptable "loaner" aids. In the case of BTE hearing aids, an acceptable loaner hearing aid can easily be fitted, making sure that its power level is not greater than the hearing aid it replaces. For canal or ITE aids, small units of the same style can be fitted snuggly to any ear with "instant" earmold material. The availability of power and tone controls, even in canal size hearing aids, gives the dispenser sufficient versatility to fit most hearing problems, at least temporarily. Of course, instant earmolds and BTE loaner aids can be provided to clients who are willing to use them.

Client awareness of basic trouble-shooting strategies should be encouraged. This objective can be pursued through trouble-shooting charts, such as the ones shown in the Appendix. These charts are meant to be used as references by hearing aid users, to help them look for possible causes and solutions to common problems they may encounter.

The topics covered in this chapter are of great importance and have not been covered exhaustively. If each professional can add items provided by her or his experience, the goal of improving the chances of success in hearing aid usage will be achieved.

The inclusion of activities in this chapter does not imply that all of them can or should be carried out. They are ideas and frames of reference that can serve as guides in the organization of individual programs. How much is included in a program depends both on individual needs and on practical aspects related to time, distance, and cost. Nevertheless, the guiding principle should be that no matter how much the audiologist or the hearing aid dispenser does, it probably will not be enough.

APPENDIX

Trouble-Shooting Chart

Symptom	Possible Causes	Solutions
1. No sound, hearing aid does not seem to work WARNING! Never ask others to listen to your hearing aid by placing it directly in their ear. Since your hearing aid will not fit anyone else correctly, it will probably "whistle" and this sound may be dangerous to their hearing. It is all right to listen for the whistle when the hearing aid is not in the ear.	A. On-off switch in wrong position. Your hearing aid may or may not have an on-off switch. It may be part of the volume control or be separate. Your hearing aid may use the battery door to turn the hearing aid on and off. To do this you may have to open the door in a different direction, opposite than when you change the battery. B. The battery door may not be firmly closed or the battery is in the wrong position.	With the hearing aid on your hand, turn the volume control full-on and flip the on-off switch to "M." Listen for the feedback whistle. Or with the hearing aid in your ear flip the switch back-and-forth, listen for the sound to appear. Be sure you know how your hearing aid's switches work. If you are not sure, ask your hearing aid counselor. First make sure that the battery is inserted in the correct direction. The battery's "+" side should match correctly with the "+" sign in the battery drawer. Then push the hearing aid's battery door in firmly, until you feel a click. If you cannot see the "+" symbols, either use a looking-glass or ask someone else to look for them. WARNING! If you force the door shut when the battery is in the wrong position, you can damage the hearing aid!
	C. Battery is dead or too weak.	If you have a battery meter, check the battery and see if it still reaches the "green" or acceptable level. Otherwise, simply try a new battery. If the hearing aid works, retire the old battery in the correct manner. (See the special warning about correct ways to dispose of batteries.)
	D. Battery contacts may be dirty or the battery surfaces may be greasy.	Remove the battery and clean surfaces with a clean cloth. Cleaning the battery contacts is best left for the professional.

(continued)

APPENDIX *(continued)*

Symptom	Possible Causes	Solutions
1. No sound, hearing aid does not seem to work *(continued)*	E. The sound outlet hole of your hearing aid or of your earmold may be plugged up with earwax.	Examine the outlet carefully under a good light. Use the tool that came with your hearing aid (a small brush or a wire loop) to remove the wax. Do not insert pins or wires more than one-eighth of an inch into the hole. You may damage the receiver or earphone. If you cannot clean the hearing aid, take it to your hearing aid counselor.
	F. With behind-the-ear or eyeglass hearing aids, the tubing that connects the hearing aid to the earmold may be plugged with humidity, or it may be twisted.	If your hearing aid does not "whistle" when it is in your hand and you turn it on, disconnect the earmold and see if the whistle starts. This would show that the problem is either in the earmold or the tubing. Check both for dirt, and after washing them in warm, soapy water, blow air through the tubing to make sure that it is completely dry. When you replace the earmold, be sure to connect the tubing to the hearing aid correctly, so that the earmold faces in the right direction and does not have to be twisted to enter your ear canal.
	G. In the case of pocket or body hearing aids, the cord or wire that connects the hearing aid to the receiver may be broken or defective. It may also be poorly connected at either end.	After making sure that both plugs are well connected, move the cord up and down to see if the hearing aid whistles. This would show that the cord is defective and needs replacement. If you have a spare cord (which you should), try changing it to see what happens.
	H. Your ear canal may be totally plugged by earwax.	If you do not hear any sound from your hearing aid but other people can hear it whistle when it is out of your ear, you should see your physician and as him or her to check your ears. Do not attempt to clean deep into your ears. If there is enough wax to close the ear canals, they should be cleaned under the supervision of a physician.

Symptom	Possible Causes	Solutions
	I. Your hearing may have gotten worse.	See your physician or ask your audiologist to retest your hearing. He or she should then make the proper recommendations.
	J. In the case of body hearing aids, the contact between the earmold and the receiver may not be sufficiently tight.	A thin plastic washer can be placed in this joint, to improve the seal. If this is not sufficient, either the receiver or the earmold will have to be changed.
2. Hearing aid whistles, squeals, or howls The hearing aid's amplified sound feeds back into the microphone.	A. Hearing aid is turned on and is not in the ear.	This is perfectly normal and shows that the hearing aid is working.
	B. The hearing aid or the earmold is not fully or properly inserted into the ear.	First turn the volume down to stop the whistling. Then with your fingers feel around the rim of the hearing aid or the earmold to see if any parts are sticking out of place. You may have to twist the earmold, or pull your ear back, while you push the earmold farther in. When you have it reset, turn the volume up again to the level you normally use.
	C. There is too much earwax in your ear canal.	Earwax may force you to set your hearing aid to a stronger level. This may be sufficient to cause "feedback." You should follow the recommendations made in 1H.
	D. The squeal may occur only when you have your hand near the hearing aid, or when you lean your head against a pillow. A hat close to the hearing aid can also cause this problem.	If your earmold or hearing aid is correctly inserted, and you are bothered by this occasional squeal, consult your hearing aid counselor to see what can be done.
	E. If your hearing aid or earmold has a "vent" (this is a simple hole or tube that goes through the earmold into the ear canal), and the vent had a plug to either close or reduce its size, the vent plug may have fallen out.	You have to take your hearing aid back to the seller, so that the vent plug can be reinserted.

(continued)

APPENDIX *(continued)*

Symptom	Possible Causes	Solutions
2. Hearing aid whistles, squeals, or howls *(continued)*	F. Your ear may have stretched, or the earmold may have shrunk so that the hearing aid or earmold do not fit tightly anymore.	You probably need a new earmold impression, unless your hearing aid counselor can improve the fit by increasing the size with a plastic additive.
	G. In the case of "behind-the-ear" hearing aids (also eyeglass aids), the earmold tubing may have sprung a leak. The tubing may have become too stiff and may have cracked.	Your hearing aid counselor will have to replace the tubing. This is a simple procedure and should not take much time. Tubing should be changed periodically.
	H. If none of the above conditions applies, it is possible that the hearing aid is damaged and has an internal problem.	If your hearing aid squeals even when you plug the sound outlet, the feedback is internal, and it should be sent in for repair.
3. Sound is not strong enough	A. Often the hearing aid has sufficient power, but you cannot raise it to the level you want because it begins to whistle.	Check section 2. Consult your hearing aid counselor. If nothing can be done to improve the hearing aid or earmold fit, a new impression may have to be made.
	B. The battery may be getting low.	Try a new battery and see if the problem disappears.
	C. Your ear canal may be plugged with earwax.	See your physician.
	D. Your hearing may have changed.	Have your hearing retested. See your audiologist or your physician.
	E. The entry port to your hearing aid's microphone may be dirty.	Unless you can clearly see some dirt or fuzz over the microphone's entrance that can be cleaned with your small brush, take your hearing aid to your hearing aid counselor.
	F. The weather has been very cold or extremely humid.	Batteries, especially the "air" type, can react both to extreme cold and to excessive humidity. Take the battery out, and either wipe it with a clean cloth or let it warm up.

Symptom	Possible Causes	Solutions
	G. In the case of "behind-the-ear" and "eyeglass" hearing aids, the earmold's tubing may be bent or twisted.	Check this condition and reinsert earmold carefully.
	H. The earmold or the tubing may be plugged, either by earwax or by drops of humidity. This can happen, especially with the "Libby" horn tubing.	Disconnect earmold from hearing aid and blow through tubing, preferably with the "forced-air bulb" to avoid breath humidity. If needed, wash the earmold with warm, soapy water and dry it carefully. If you prefer not to deal with this, take the hearing aid to your hearing aid counselor.
	I. The acoustic "damper" inserted into the tubing may be plugged.	This element cannot be washed, so if air alone does not do the job, you must take the hearing aid back to the hearing aid counselor.
4. Sound stops and starts intermittently	A. There may be dirt in the volume control or in the battery contacts.	There are special sprays for electronic circuits. Your hearing aid counselor will be able to take care of this problem.
	B. In the case of "body" or "pocket" type hearing aids, the cord may be defective, or its contacts may be loose.	If you have a spare cord, try it and see if the problem disappears. Otherwise you will have to take your hearing aid to the counselor.
	C. The problem may be a loose internal component.	This will require professional repair.
5. Hearing aid sounds "funny" The sound is distorted or scratchy There is a buzz or a hum constantly	A. The battery may be running low.	Change battery and see if problem disappears.
	B. The switch may be set to "T" and the microphone is thus disconnected.	Check switch position and see if problem disappears.
	C. Your hearing aid may be working at a level that is too close to its maximum power output.	Your hearing aid counselor will have to deal with this. It may be possible to adjust the hearing aid's power, or the hearing aid will have to be changed.

(continued)

APPENDIX *(continued)*

Symptom	Possible Causes	Solutions
5. Hearing aid sounds "funny" *(continued)*	D. Dirt in the volume control may produce a scratchy sound when you adjust it.	See 4A above.
	E. Your hearing aid may have too much power in the higher-pitch sound region. If your hearing for these sounds is very poor, what you hear may sound distorted.	Your hearing aid's "frequency response," which is the way in which your hearing aid responds to various "tones," may have to be changed. See your hearing aid counselor.
	F. Your hearing aid may be damaged internally.	Take your hearing aid back and your hearing aid counselor will check it to decide about needed repair.
Your voice sounds "hollow," or you hear an "echo" when you speak	G. Your earmold is probably too tight and does not allow any sound pressure to escape.	This problem may be solved by "venting" your earmold or your hearing aid, but whether this is possible or not will have to be decided by your hearing aid counselor.
6. Your hearing aid or your earmold hurts	A. The pain or discomfort may be "physical." In other words, your ear canal or your outer ear hurts because your hearing aid or your earmold is too tight or has an edge that pushes against your skin.	If the pain does not seem to decrease with time but on the contrary, it gets worse, take the hearing aid off and call your hearing aid counselor. Try to pinpoint the place where it hurts so that your counselor can decide whether it can be fixed by buffing, or whether a new hearing aid or earmold must be made.
	B. Your discomfort may be "acoustic," in other words, due to the impact of sound on your hearing.	Your hearing aid counselor will have to test you and measure the sound produced by your hearing aid, preferably in your ear. Your hearing aid or your earmold and tubing may have to be adjusted to reduce the source of discomfort. If this cannot be done, a new hearing aid may have to be tried.

Symptom	Possible Causes	Solutions
7. Your batteries are not lasting very long In order to know how long your batteries last, you need to keep track, on paper, of when you change them.	A. You may be forgetting to turn off your hearing aid at night or when you are not using it (or them).	Since in some cases, it is difficult to know if the hearing aid is "off," it is better to open the battery drawer at night and whenever you put your hearing aid away. This disconnects the battery and prolongs its life.
	B. You may have bought a defective batch of batteries.	Batteries that have been kept too long on the shelf may have lost some of their life. If kept in their plastic cases and not opened, "air" batteries, will last much longer. Try a battery from a different batch and keep track of the starting date.
8. You cannot use your hearing aid on the telephone	A. If your hearing aid has a "T" switch, your telephone may not be compatible.	Some telephones do not have enough magnetic field leakage to drive your hearing aid's "T" coil. Ask your counselor about special telephone couplers.
	B. You may not be placing the telephone in the best position over your hearing aid.	Try moving the telephone around your ear and see if the sound increases. Also, once you set your hearing aid on "T," you can increase the hearing aid's volume.
	C. If you do not use or do not have a "T" switch, you may be placing the telephone too close to your ear. This causes feedback.	When you use the telephone through the hearing aid's microphone, you must keep the receiver slightly away from the hearing aid. Use one finger to keep the telephone just away from your ear.

4

■ HEARING AID AMPLIFICATION AND CENTRAL PROCESSING DISORDERS

BRAD A. STACH ■

*T*he use of a hearing aid may enable a person to overcome a peripheral sensitivity loss, but this benefit may be compromised by concomitant central auditory processing disorder (CAPD). Elderly patients, who constitute the largest number of hearing aid users (Cranmer, 1985), often have hearing problems characterized by both peripheral and central components (Pestalozza & Shore, 1955; Schuknecht & Igarashi, 1964; Jerger, 1973; Jerger & Hayes, 1977a, 1977b; Hayes, 1980; Otto & McCandless, 1982; Welsh, Welsh, & Healy, 1985). If central disorder adversely affects hearing aid use, then its effects must be understood and quantified before the communication disorder can be ameliorated. Similarly, identification of children with specifically auditory central processing disorder is increasing rapidly (Jerger, Johnson, & Loiselle, 1988). The possible adverse effect of amplification on individuals with both central and peripheral hearing disorder warrants careful attention.

Perhaps an even greater challenge than delineating the relationship between hearing aid use and central auditory disorder is developing beneficial amplification strategies. Merely amplifying sound to overcome a peripheral hearing loss may provide little, if any, advantage to a young or aging auditory system that requires an enhanced signal-to-noise (S/N) ratio because of central auditory disorder. Remote-microphone assistive listening devices and better noise reduction circuitry in conventional hearing aids are two developments that hold promise as effective intervention strategies for individuals with central processing disorder.

THE NATURE OF CAPD

Peripheral auditory function involves the outer ear, middle ear, cochlea, and eighth nerve. Central auditory function involves structures of the brainstem, midbrain, and cerebral cortex. Functionally, the peripheral mechanism is responsible for auditory sensitivity and for basic frequency, amplitude, and temporal coding. The central mechanism processes information from the peripheral mechanism into meaningful percepts. A disorder of the peripheral mechanism results in a loss of auditory sensitivity as measured by pure-tone threshold audiometry and can, by distortion of incoming signals, result in decreased speech understanding. Conversely, a disorder of the central mechanism results in reduced capability in the processing of auditory information.

Disorders of the peripheral mechanism are relatively well understood. Abnormality of the outer or middle ear results in a conductive sensitivity deficit, with little effect on suprathreshold speech understanding. Abnormality of the cochlea results in a sensorineural sensitivity deficit. Speech understanding, as conventionally measured by single-syllable phonetically balanced (PB) words presented without background competition, is usually reduced to an extent that can be explained by the degree and configuration of the sensitivity loss. Central auditory function, if measured with tests that are relatively immune to peripheral sensitivity loss, will not be affected by the cochlear disorder. Abnormality of the eighth nerve may or may not result in peripheral sensitivity loss but can affect speech understanding to varying degrees.

Disorders of central auditory processing are manifested by two fundamental characteristics. First, auditory sensitivity loss rarely results from CAPD. Pure-tone thresholds, in the absence of other deleterious factors, are usually normal in patients with CAPD. Second, the most pervasive characteristic of CAPD is poor speech understanding. Although performance is typically quite normal on tests in which unaltered speech materials, such as PB words, are presented in quiet, performance is reduced on complex speech tasks that stress the processing of auditory information.

The existence of CAPD is often a source of controversy. In a general sense, CAPD can be thought of as a diminished ability of the central nervous system to process auditory information. The most common operational definition of CAPD is a reduction in ability to understand speech, especially when speech is altered in the temporal or frequency domain or when competing signals are present. Clinical measurement of central processing ability is based on speech audiometric techniques, many of which have been validated on patients with neurologic disorders (Lynn, Benitez, Eisenbrey, Gilroy, & Wilner, 1972; Jerger & Jerger, 1975; Jerger, 1987; Musiek & Baran, 1987). By inference, then, a patient whose poor performance on speech audiometric tasks resembles that of a neurologically impaired patient is said to have a processing disorder at the level of the central auditory nervous system, or CAPD.

Because the diagnosis of CAPD has been so dependent on behavioral, speech-based techniques, its very existence has been questioned. A deficit in speech understanding in a child, for example, has often been considered to be an artifactual manifestation of a language deficit, an attentional deficit, or a memory deficit. That is, test results may be explained as easily by these non-auditory factors as by the existence of a true auditory deficit (Rees, 1973). Similarly, in the elderly, decline in memory, speed-of-information processing, and peripheral hearing sensitivity have all been implicated as the cause of reduced speech understanding (Working Group on Speech Understanding and Aging, 1988). However, recent evidence suggests that neither cognitive decline, language deficit, nor peripheral hearing loss can be invoked as the simple explanation for the decline in speech processing that characterizes CAPD. Indeed, in both children (Jerger, Martin, & Jerger, 1987; Jerger, Johnson, & Loiselle, 1988) and the elderly (Jerger, Jerger, Oliver, & Pirozzolo, 1989; Jerger, Stach, Pruitt, Harper, & Kirby, 1989), auditory processing disorders that cannot be explained on the basis of these non-auditory factors have been isolated.

Central auditory processing ability can be measured in a number of ways (see, for example, Jerger & Hayes, 1977a; Noffsinger & Kurdziel, 1979; Tallal, 1980; Keith, 1982; Jerger & Jerger, 1983; Spitzer, 1983; Musiek & Baran, 1987). One method is to use distorted speech materials such as low-pass filtered speech (Bocca, 1958) or time-compressed speech (Beasley, Forman, & Rintelmann, 1972). Numerous studies have shown abnormal processing of these "sensitized" speech materials by patients with auditory central nervous system disorder (Jerger, 1960; Calearo & Antonelli, 1968; Kurdziel, Noffsinger, & Olsen, 1976). Another way to measure central function is by use of dichotic tests such as the Staggered Spondaic Word (SSW) test (Katz, 1962), dichotic consonant-vowel test (Berlin & Lowe, 1972), Dichotic Sentence Identification (DSI) test (Fifer, Jerger, Berlin, Tobey, & Campbell, 1983), competing sentence test (Willeford, 1977), and dichotic digits test (Kimura, 1961). Still another method is to measure speech understanding in the presence of a background competing message or noise. Tests such as PB words in noise (Olsen, Noffsinger, & Kurdziel, 1975), the Synthetic Sentence Identification (SSI) test (Jerger, Speaks, & Trammel, 1968), and the Pediatric Speech Intelligibility (PSI) test (Jerger, Lewis, Hawkins, & Jerger, 1980; Jerger, Jerger, & Abrams, 1983) fall into this category. Another approach is to measure speech understanding across a range of intensities and quantify *rollover,* the paradoxically poorer performance with increasing intensity (Jerger & Jerger, 1971).

Although all of these strategies have been found to be more or less sensitive as measures of central auditory ability, problems in interpretation of many of the strategies can occur if a peripheral hearing loss, a language disorder, or a cognitive deficit is present. That is, performance on such tests can be affected by other auditory and nonauditory factors, and differentiation of peripheral or cognitive components from central components can be difficult. These confounding variables either need to be controlled during the test session or their influence on tests results must be quantifiable.

GROUPS AT SPECIAL RISK FOR CAPD

Children

Many children with language and learning deficits have been found to have auditory perceptual impairment (Pinheiro, 1977; Willeford, 1977; Freeman & Beasley, 1978; Willeford & Billger, 1978; Farrer & Keith, 1981; Johnson, Enfield, & Sherman, 1981; Lubert, 1981). However, because of a wide range of tests designed to measure auditory perception, a large number of classification schemes for children with disorders of this nature, varied educational strategies used for intervention, philosophical differences among professionals involved, and the tendency toward multimodality deficits in these children, the nature and scope of CAPD has not been altogether clear. Despite this confusion, evidence continues to accumulate, from both clinical and research settings, attesting to the reality of what so many clinicians have for so long suspected: that some children may have a problem as a result of a specific deficit in auditory processing and that such deficits may co-exist with peripheral hearing loss or may exist independently of any actual sensitivity deficit.

Clinical and research experience with both children and elderly adults has convinced my colleagues and I of the reality of CAPD and the need to take seriously the implications of its impact on communication. For example, I see increasing evidence of a population of children with isolated CAPD. In almost a syndrome-like manner, these children have a history of chronic otitis media and parental and teacher complaints of inattentiveness, distractibility, and difficulty hearing in the presence of background noise. Clinical manifestations include normal hearing sensitivity, normal performance on single-syllable word tests presented in quiet, and an assortment of deficits on tests of central auditory processing.

Elderly Population

Also at risk for CAPD is the elderly population. Although the effects of aging on the peripheral auditory mechanism and age-related changes in central auditory structure and function are well known, these latter changes, so-called central presbycusis, appear to be less well understood and are certainly less often measured.

Numerous histopathologic and morphologic studies have documented structural degeneration in the neurologic pathways of the auditory system as a result of the aging process. Evidence of neural degradation has been found in the auditory nerve (Schuknecht, 1964; Krmpotic-Nemanic, 1971) and at the level of the auditory brainstem and cortex (Brody, 1955; Hinchcliffe, 1962; Kirikae, Sato, & Shitara, 1964; Hansen & Reske-Nielsen, 1965; Corso, 1976).

The effect of structural changes in the auditory periphery is to attenuate incoming sound. For the most part, speech understanding deficits can be explained by the degree of loss and shape of the audiometric contour (Goetzinger, Proud, Dirks, & Embrey, 1961; Jerger & Hayes, 1977a; Mills, 1978). In contrast, the major effect of structural changes in the central auditory pathways is one of degradation of speech processing (Hinchcliffe, 1962; Lutterman, Welsh, & Melrose, 1966; Sticht & Gray, 1969; Antonelli, 1970; Bergman, 1971; Bergman, Blumfield, Cascardo, Dash, Levitt, & Marguiles, 1976; Konkle, Beasley, & Bess, 1977; Orchik & Burgess, 1977; Arnst, 1982; Bosatra & Russolo, 1982; McCroskey & Kasten, 1982). Aging patients have been shown to perform more poorly than would be predicted on

the basis of the audiogram alone on tests that incorporate distorted and time-altered speech materials or speech presented in a background of noise (Pestalozza & Shore, 1955; Goetzinger et al., 1961; Konig, 1969; Jerger, 1973; Shirinian & Arnst, 1982; Hayes, 1984). Because age related changes can occur throughout the auditory system, many patients with presbycusis will demonstrate behavior suggestive of both peripheral and central auditory disorder.

The implications of these observations for intervention, in both children and the elderly, are important. If a patient has CAPD, conventional approaches to amplification may be inadequate or even inappropriate. One must determine whether a hearing aid is the best strategy for someone whose primary problem is not a loss of sensitivity, but rather a decrement in speech understanding.

AMPLIFICATION AND CAPD

Amplification and CAPD in Children

While benefit from hearing aid use in children with both hearing loss and central disorder has eluded careful study, attempts have been made to use amplification systems in children with educational handicaps who have normal hearing or mild hearing loss and who are not considered by traditional criteria to be candidates for hearing aids. The underlying assumption of these studies is that educational deficits are often related to auditory deficits. Alteration of auditory information with amplification, therefore, should enhance auditory processing and have a positive effect on educational intervention.

Sarff (1981) and Sarff, Ray, and Bagwell (1981) described a program entitled Mainstream Amplification Resource Room Study (MARRS) in which 110 children from grades 4, 5, and 6 were selected for study. Each child in the group had an academic deficit and auditory thresholds of no better than 15 dB HL and no poorer than 35 dB HL. Although central processing ability was not measured directly, the educational difficulties of these children were presumed to relate directly to auditory deficits resulting from minimal hearing loss.

Students from the MARRS study were assigned to one of two groups. The intervention procedure for one group was in the form of special help in a learning disabilities resource room as an adjunct to the traditional classroom setting. The other group had no special resource room. Instead, the students were confined to a standard classroom in which amplification equipment was installed. The teacher wore a microphone and wireless transmitter coupled to two loudspeakers. The teacher's lectures and instructions were thus amplified before being presented to the students.

Preceding and following these intervention strategies, student competency in various academic areas was measured. Results showed increased academic achievement for both groups and a tendency for greater achievement by students in the amplified classroom. Apparently, the enhancement of S/N by amplification intervention altered the classroom listening environment enough to reduce the negative educational effect of auditory deficits.

These positive results may well have resulted simply from overcoming the mild peripheral hearing loss present in these children. An alternative explanation is that many of these children with minimal hearing loss and educational deficits had CAPD, although auditory processing ability was not measured directly. If so, then it would follow, based on the MARRS study, that amplification intervention on a group or an individual basis might prove to be a beneficial strategy for children with such an auditory disorder.

Shapiro and Mistal (1985) also provided evidence supporting a proactive amplification approach to educationally impaired children. On the assumption that one characteristic of reading-disabled chil-

dren is their relative inability to process rapid speech formant transitions, the authors suggested that such children would have difficulty with perception of high-frequency consonant information. They hypothesized that fitting these otherwise normal-hearing children with mild-gain, high-frequency, in-the-ear (ITE) hearing aids would provide the additional information necessary for good speech perception. Four illustrative cases demonstrated improvement in areas such as auditory memory, complex word repetition, and intelligibility of PB words.

These findings are intriguing in terms of the potential for benefit from amplification in children with auditory processing deficits. However, large deficiencies remain in understanding of candidacy, measurement techniques, and appropriateness of amplification arrangements.

Children with central processing disorders may or may not have concomitant peripheral hearing loss. Similarly, children with peripheral hearing loss may or may not have central processing disorder. As a result, few children with central disorder are fitted with amplification. Consequently, the effect of amplification on central disorder in this population is not well known. Such is not the case, however, in the aging population. Many individuals in the geriatric age group have peripheral hearing loss that is amenable to amplification intervention, and many have concomitant central auditory disorder. Thus, it is in this population that the greatest strides have been made in understanding the relationship between amplification and central disorder.

Amplification and CAPD in Aging

However well substantiated the phenomenon of central presbycusis appears to be, the question of its effect on hearing aid use remains unclear. Some studies have suggested that elderly patients are generally less satisfied with amplification than younger patients (Jerger & Hayes, 1976; Berger & Hagberg, 1982), but it is not clear whether this dissatisfaction is related to nonauditory aging problems or central auditory aging. Two areas of research have addressed this question. The first is the relationship between central auditory disorder and clinical performance with amplification, and the second is the relationship between central auditory disorder and satisfaction with or benefit from hearing aid use.

Central Presbycusis and Hearing Aid Performance

If central processing disorder affects hearing aid use, then the elderly patient with central presbycusis should perform more poorly during hearing aid evaluations. Hayes and Jerger (1979) studied performance with hearing aids of 154 patients age 60 years or older. They divided the patients into three groups based on comparison of speech intelligibility scores for PB words presented in quiet and SSI sentences presented in competition. The peripheral group had SSI scores that were equal to or better than PB scores, the intermediate group had SSI scores that were poorer than PB scores by no more than 20 percent, and the central group had SSI scores at least 20 percent poorer than PB scores.

Comparison of aided performance was based on a hearing aid evaluation procedure in which the SSI was presented at various message-to-competition ratios (MCR) for aided and unaided conditions (Jerger & Hayes, 1976). Figure 4–1 shows the results of aided performance for the three groups. The group with central disorder performed more poorly than the other groups at all MCRs. A systematic decline in performance also occurred as the central component increased. The authors further divided the groups to match for age and degree of sensitivity loss in an attempt to rule out any possible contribution of these factors to the performance differences. Even with age and degree of hearing loss accounted for, the

group with central auditory disorder performed more poorly.

The authors concluded that central processing disorder has a detrimental effect on performance with hearing aids in the clinical setting. Since the evaluation procedure used has been suggested to be a valid measure of hearing aid user satisfaction (Jerger & Hayes, 1976; Gerber & Fisher, 1979; Hayes, Jerger, Taff, & Barber, 1983), it is reasonable to assume that the deleterious effect of central disorder shown in the clinic would manifest itself as reduced benefit to the user in everyday life situations.

Central Presbycusis and Hearing Aid Satisfaction and Benefit

Several studies have reported on the relationship between central presbycusis and hearing aid user satisfaction. Jerger and Hayes (1976) sent questionnaires to patients seen for hearing aid evaluations. The authors asked the patients to rate their hearing aid use as satisfactory, sometimes helpful, or unsatisfactory. Of 47 respondents who had purchased hearing aids, 72.3 percent rated the hearing aid as satisfactory, 14.9 percent as sometimes helpful, and 12.8 percent as unsatisfactory. To determine whether the groups exhibited differences in central auditory ability, the authors studied aided sound-field performance on the SSI at three MCRs. Results showed little difference in performance between groups at an easy MCR (+10 dB), but a progressive separation of groups as the listening condition became more difficult. At a difficult listening condition (−10 dB), aided performance for the unsatisfactory group was substantially poorer than aided performance for the satisfactory group.

McCandless and Parkin (1979) classified 140 hearing aid users into site-of-lesion categories based on 12 audiologic measures. Criterion for successful hearing aid use was total daily wearing time. The authors considered a successful user to be anyone who wore the hearing aid for 8 hr a day or longer. A moderately successful user

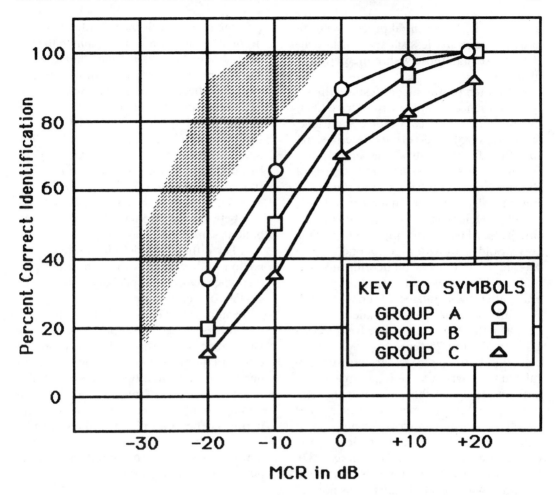

FIGURE 4–1. Aided performance in the sound field for three groups of elderly subjects: Group A = peripheral, Group B = intermediate, Group C = central, MCR = message to-competition ratio. From Hayes & Jerger, 1979. Reprinted with permission.

wore the aid for 4 to 8 hr, whereas anyone who wore the aid fewer than 4 hr was placed in the category of poor fit. Individuals who did not wear the hearing aid at all were placed in the rejection category. Of all hearing aid users with central site of lesion, only 11 percent were classified as successful users, and 89 percent rejected hearing aid use. In contrast, 84 percent of users with middle ear site and 71 percent of users with cochlear site were considered successful. The authors cautioned that the groups with the higher rejection rates were comprised mostly of aging patients and that general decline with aging could not be ruled out as a causative factor.

In another study relating hearing aid performance to hearing aid user satisfaction, Hayes and colleagues (1983) surveyed 78 hearing aid users who had been fitted based on hearing aid evaluation with the SSI procedure. Users were asked to judge their satisfaction based on a 4-point scale. Aided results in a difficult listening condition (−10 MCR) were 30 percent poorer for those in the unsatifactory and sometimes helpful categories than for those in the very helpful category. It appears that hearing aid users who have central processing difficulty are generally less satisfied with hearing aid use than those with more peripheral losses.

An attempt was made to study directly the influence of central disorder on hearing aid benefit (Krisco, Lesner, Sandridge, & Yanke, 1985). The authors described results from four patients whose central auditory function was classified on the basis of PB-SSI discrepancy. They used the Hearing Aid Performance Inventory (HAPI) (Walden, Demorest, & Hepler, 1984) to define successful use of amplification. One 66-year-old man with a peripheral pattern was judged as a successful hearing aid user, and one 77-year-old patient with a peripheral pattern was judged as unsuccessful. Similarly, one 67-year-old patient with a central pattern was considered a successful user, and one 72-year-old patient with a central pattern was considered unsuccessful. On the basis of these four subjects, the authors concluded that there was no relationship between perceived hearing aid benefit and central auditory function. In an expanded study of 24 adult male subjects (Krisco, Lesner, Sandridge, & Yanke, 1987), the authors reported that the HAPI score of the group with a central pattern was not significantly different than that of the group with a peripheral pattern. Interestingly, HAPI scores also could not be used to differentiate between groups that were formed on the basis of degree of peripheral hearing loss or on the basis of subject age. This apparent lack of sensitivity of the HAPI to these important factors may be reflected in the central versus peripheral comparison as well.

One of the most challenging aspects of hearing aid research has been the validation of fitting techniques. The difficulty has always been the means of quantifying user satisfaction. The audiologist likes to define hearing aid benefit as the amplification arrangement that will best maximize use of residual hearing. Thus, the best aided performance in the clinical setting should pro-vide the patient with the audiologist's definition of benefit, and consequently, the patient should be satisfied with hearing aid use. Yet patients' definition of benefit can be quite different, and their reasons for satisfaction or dissatisfaction can be unrelated to the actual quality of sound (Kapteyn, 1977; Cunningham, Merle, & Drake, 1978; Surr, Schuchman, & Montgomery, 1978; Brooks, 1985; Franks & Beckmann, 1985). Indeed, Berger and Hagberg (1982) suggested that there is no well-defined connection between help from the hearing aid and patient satisfaction.

The difficulty of defining patient satisfaction and relating it to hearing aid performance can be especially difficult in studies of central presbycusis. Aging patients appear to be less satisfied with hearing aid use in general (Berkowitz, 1975). How much of this dissatisfaction is related to sound quality is not altogether clear. Patients who perform more poorly on auditory tasks because of reduced central processing ability or, conversely, patients who perform better, may or may not relate satisfaction to this performance. Thus, some patients who *benefit* from amplification may not be *satisfied* with amplification.

Report of a Study

To evaluate further the question of hearing aid benefit in patients with CAPD, the author and his colleagues carried out a small study using an interviewing technique in an attempt to circumvent some of the problems associated with patients' definitions of satisfaction (Stach, Jerger, & Smith, 1986). We tried to focus, not on whether the patient was satisfied with hearing aid use, but on the extent to which the patient benefitted from the use of amplification. The underlying assumption was that a patient who might actually benefit from hearing aid use in certain situations might still be dissatisfied with the hearing aid due to any number of factors not related to aided performance. Two groups of patients with hearing loss, one with speech audiometric patterns suggesting peripheral disorder and the other with patterns suggesting mixed peripheral and central disorder, were formed. Benefit from hearing aid use was then determined by telephone interview.

Procedure

Files of 158 patients with sensorineural hearing loss who purchased hearing aids from The Methodist Hospital Audiology Service in Houston, Texas were reviewed. Based on results of the SSI obtained during routine, unaided speech audiometry, patients were placed into either a central group or a peripheral group. Criterion for inclusion in the central group was a maximum SSI score of 60 percent or less that could not be explained on the basis of peripheral sensitivity loss. Inclusion in the peripheral group required a maximum SSI score of 70 percent or better with rollover of no more than 20 percent. Only those patients with obvious, bilateral central or peripheral patterns were included. Two groups of 15 patients each were then matched on the basis of age and degree of peripheral sensitivity loss. In all, 30 patients were selected for study.

To determine hearing aid benefit, each patient was contacted by telephone. The caller was an audiologist who was blind to both the study design and the group to which each patient was assigned. The audiologist was instructed to inform the patient that she was doing a routine follow-up on selected hearing aid users. She did not use a formal questionnaire. Rather, she attempted to engage the patients in conversation about how they were functioning with their hearing aids, the types of problems they were having, and the benefit they were receiving in common listening situations. The patient was purposely not asked to rate hearing aid satisfaction. Immediately following the conversation, the audiologist rated her perceptions of the patient's use of the hearing aid on a 5-point scale from very helpful (rating of 5) to no benefit (rating of 1).

In all, 25 patients were contacted successfully. One patient in the central group was removed from the study because the unsatisfactory rating assigned to her resulted from her failure to wear the hearing aid because of earmold discomfort. Results from 12 patients in each group remained for analysis.

Results

Figure 4–2 shows the age and degree of hearing loss of the two groups. Although the patients in the peripheral group were slightly older and had slightly more hearing loss, there were no statistically significant differences between groups. Maximum SSI scores from the ear fitted with a hearing aid were averaged for each group and are shown in Figure 4–3. Mean SSI score for the central group was 32.5 percent and for the peripheral group it was 83.3 percent. Also shown in Figure 4–3 is aided performance of the two groups on the SSI procedure at an MCR of −10 dB. The central group performed more poorly with hearing aids, as indicated by a mean score of 67.5 percent as opposed to the peripheral group mean score of 81.7 percent. Length of hearing aid use was similar in the two groups. Mean length of use was 10.3 months for the central group and 9.6 months for the peripheral group. Length of hearing aid use ranged from 6 months to 13 months for all patients. Binaural hearing aids were worn by 4 patients in each group. All others wore only one hearing aid. The central group was comprised of 6 males and 6 females, and the peripheral group was comprised of 8 males and 4 females.

Benefit ratings assigned to the central group were poorer than those assigned to the peripheral group. The mean rating for the central group was 3.0, and the mean rating for the peripheral group was 4.0. While the mean difference was small, the distribu-

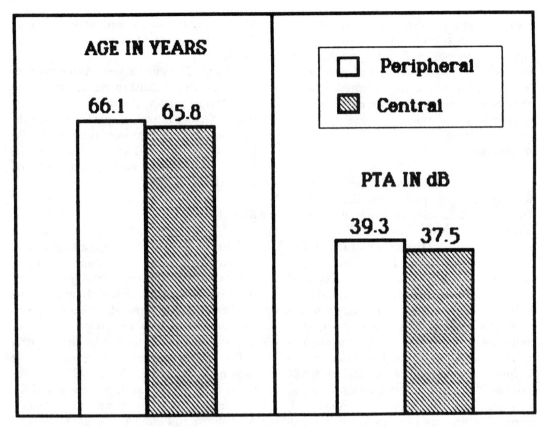

FIGURE 4-2. Mean age and pure-tone average (PTA) for central and peripheral groups.

tion of ratings for the two groups was strikingly different. Figure 4-4 shows these distributions. Ratings for the peripheral group were distributed in a manner that was not unexpected. Most of the patients reported hearing aid use that was rated by the examiner as either very helpful or often helpful. None of the patients in the peripheral group reported usage consistent with no benefit. Ratings from the central group, however, were fairly evenly distributed across the rating range. While some reported usage consistent with a very helpful rating and most reported usage consistent with a helpful rating, 33 percent of the patients reported usage consistent with no benefit from hearing aid use.

In an attempt to identify factors contributing to the lack of benefit for certain patients in the central group, the 3 patients with a rating of 5 (very helpful) were compared with the 4 patients with a rating of 1 (no benefit). The patients who did not experience aided benefit had a mean age of 68 years while patients who did had a mean age of 56 years. The configuration of the peripheral hearing loss was also different between the two groups. Figure 4-5 shows the mean pure-tone audiograms for the two subgroups. The ear chosen to compute the mean was either the aided ear or, in the case of those with binaural hearing aids, the better ear. The group that reported hearing aids to be very helpful had a flatter audiometric configuration, and the group that did not benefit from hearing aids had a more steeply sloping configuration. It is of interest that audiometric slope was not re-

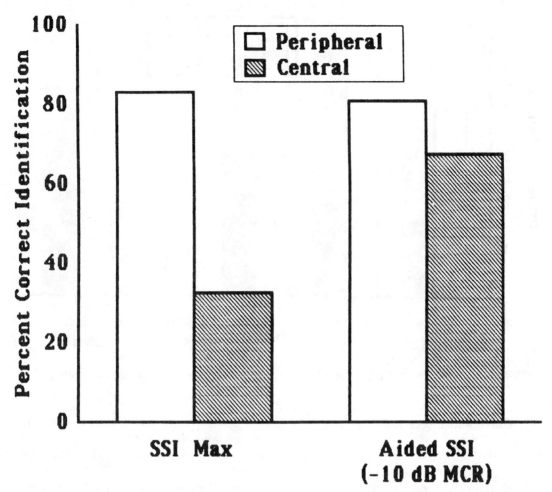

FIGURE 4–3. Mean unaided and aided Synthetic Sentence Identification (SSI) scores for central and peripheral groups. MCR = message-to-competition ratio.

lated to benefit rating in the peripheral group. Correlation between rating and slope of hearing loss (difference between puretone thresholds at 500 and 4000 Hz) was 0.61 for the central group but only 0.04 for the peripheral group.

Discussion

These results are quite interesting from a clinical perspective. In general, patients with central auditory disorder were not judged to be receiving as much benefit from hearing aid use as patients with peripheral hearing loss. Patients with central auditory disorder also did not perform as well as a group on aided measures of speech understanding in difficult listening situations.

Of even greater interest was the finding of a large disparity among individual benefit ratings within the central group. It appears that, while central processing disorder does not necessarily contraindicate hearing aid use in an individual patient, there is a reasonably high probability that a patient with central disorder will not receive optimal amplification benefit. This range of benefit may help to explain the findings of Kricos and colleagues (1985).

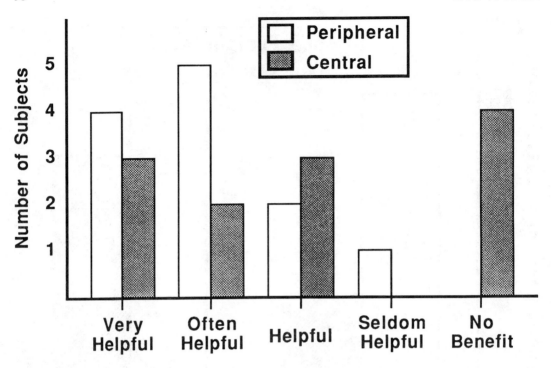

FIGURE 4–4. Distribution of reported benefit ratings of hearing aid use for peripheral and central groups.

Cause and Effect Relationship?

Central processing disorder can result from aging. These senescent changes in central ability are quite likely to progress with increasing age. Cross-sectional data suggest a relationship between dissatisfaction with hearing aid use and central presbycusis. Various studies have shown that groups of patients who are less satisfied with hearing aid use do not perform as well as satisfied groups on aided measures, and also that groups of patients with suspect central auditory integrity generally experience less benefit from hearing aid use. These data suggest the hypothetical possibility that a satisfied hearing aid user could become dissatisfied as the pattern of auditory aging changes over time from peripheral to central. If there truly is a relationship between central processing ability and hearing aid benefit, then the insidious progression of central auditory aging might result in a progressive decline in ability to use amplification successfully.

Stach, Jerger, and Fleming, (1985) reported audiologic findings in an elderly patient over a 9-year period. The patient was first seen at the age of 70. Figure 4–6 shows results of pure-tone and speech audiometry. The sensitivity loss was mildly sloping and symmetrical. Speech audiometry was slightly asymmetrical. The right ear was characterized by a small PB–SSI discrepancy and slight rollover of the SSI function. At the time, the patient noted significant communication difficulty but did not feel that it warranted the use of amplification.

The patient returned at the age of 75 with increased communication complaints. Pure-tone sensitivity and PB scores were essentially unchanged, but results from the SSI showed a decrease in the maximum score and significant rollover on both ears. The patient was fitted with a hearing aid on the right ear at that time. Over the next 4 years, the patient reported successful hearing aid use in quiet listening conditions, but increasing difficulty understanding speech in noisy situations.

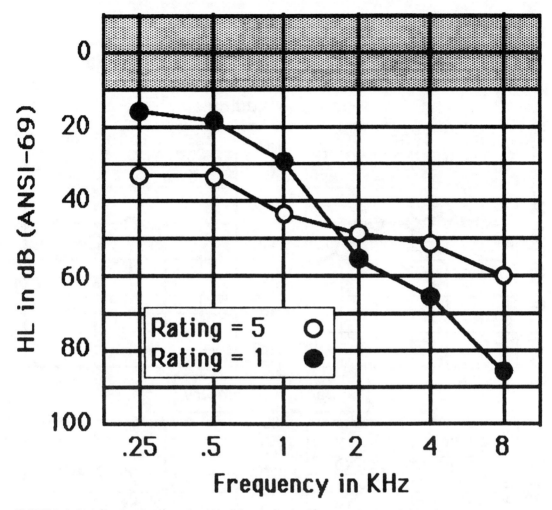

FIGURE 4–5. Mean audiograms for two subgroups of subjects with central disorder. One group had a benefit rating of 5 (very helpful), and the other group had a benefit rating of 1 (no benefit).

At the age of 79, the patient returned to the clinic because he felt that his hearing aid was no longer working appropriately. He reported the hearing aid to be increasingly less useful and finally quit wearing it altogether. One day when the patient tried it again, he was convinced that it had ceased functioning. He reported that it still seemed to amplify sound but that the clarity was very poor. A routine electroacoustic analysis of the hearing aid showed it to be functioning within manufacturer's specifications and unchanged from the original analysis.

On the assumption that his peripheral sensitivity must have changed during the intervening years, the patient was re-tested during that visit. Figure 4–7 shows the audiologic results. Pure-tone sensitivity was relatively unchanged, as was maximum performance for PB words. Performance on the SSI, however, had decreased dramatically. Figure 4–8 shows pure-tone sensitivity and maximum PB and SSI scores on four occasions over the 9-year period. While sensitivity and ability to understand speech in quiet had changed little, understanding of speech presented in competition showed a progressive and substantial decline.

My colleagues and I believe that the decline in central auditory function, appar-

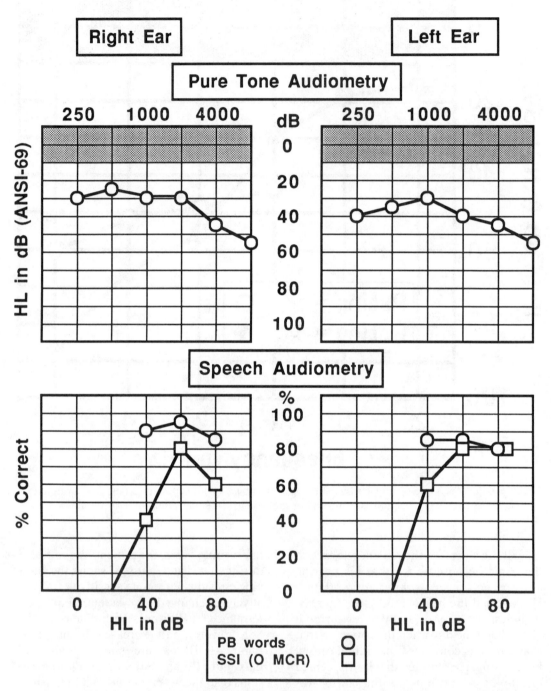

FIGURE 4–6. Pure-tone and speech audiometric results in a patient with presbycusis at age 70 years. Speech audiometry results are for PB words presented in quiet and SSI at 0 dB MCR. From Stach, Jerger, & Fleming, 1985. Reprinted with permission.

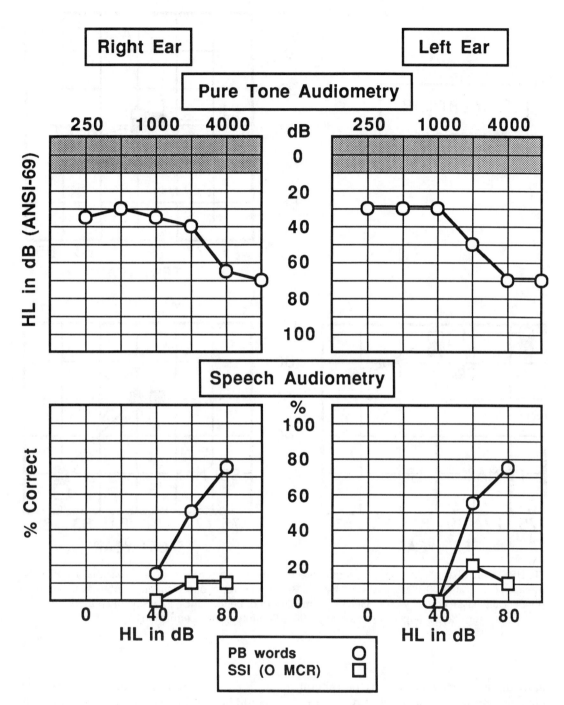

FIGURE 4-7. Pure-tone and speech audiometric results in a patient with presbycusis at age 79 years. Speech audiometry results are for PB words presented in quiet and SSI at 0 dB MCR. From Stach, Jerger, & Fleming, 1985. Reprinted with permission.

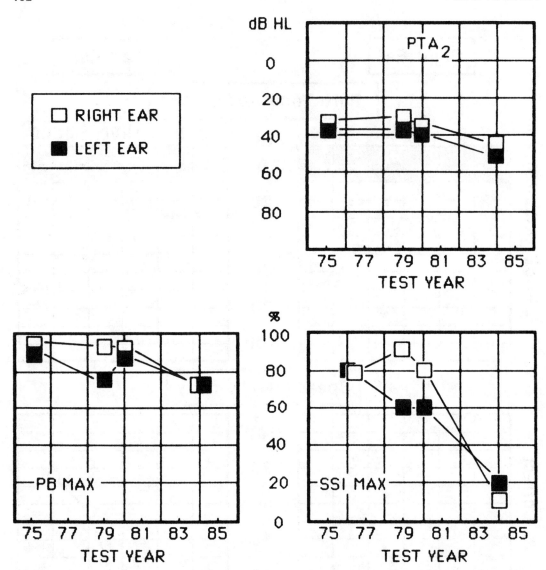

FIGURE 4–8. Changes in pure-tone and speech audiometric scores over a 9-year period. PTA2 = average of HTLs at 1000, 2000, and 4000 Hz. PB MAX = maximum of performance–intensity function for phonetically balanced (PB) words. SSI MAX = maximum of performance–intensity function for synthetic sentences. From Stach, Jerger, and Fleming, 1985. Reprinted with permission.

ently quite independent of any peripheral changes, resulted in a parallel decline in benefit from hearing aid use. We could find no evidence of significant general cognitive decline or any other intervening factors to explain the progression away from satisfactory use of amplification.

By conventional criteria, this patient could be considered an excellent candidate for successful amplification. The sensitivity loss was relatively mild, and the maximum PB scores were nearly 80 percent. The fact that the patient was an unsuccessful user strengthens the argument that central processing disorder can have substantial impact on benefit from hearing aid use.

SUCCESSFUL AMPLIFICATION STRATEGIES IN CAPD

Evidence of decreased hearing aid performance resulting from central auditory disorder is interesting and could certainly help guide the professional in terms of patient counseling about reasonable expectations and optimal listening conditions and strategies. Yet it would be disappointing at best if a more active approach to amplification could not be taken to help ameliorate the communication difficulty resulting from central processing disorder.

Electroacoustic Alteration of Conventional Hearing Aids

If patients with CAPD are to have even a chance of successful hearing aid use, alterations that reduce background noise and enhance S/N are critical. The presence of background noise is probably more detrimental to patients with CAPD than to any other group of hearing aid users. It is even quite likely that hearing aid amplification of background noise makes hearing aid use counterproductive for some of these patients. The same electroacoustic modification strategies that are used to reduce noise for patients with peripheral hearing loss are even more critical for patients with central disorder. As adaptive signal processing technology advances, the likelihood of increased amplification benefit for people with CAPD will undoubtedly improve.

Theoretical Value of Assistive Listening Devices

Since specifically auditory central processing disorder is most often characterized by difficulty processing speech in the presence of background noise, my colleagues and I have recently begun to recommend the use of remote microphone systems, such as personal FM assistive listening devices (ALDs), to children and adults with central deficits (Stach, Loiselle, Jerger, Mintz, & Taylor, 1987). The ALDs most commonly recommended are quite similar to those traditionally used in classrooms for the hearing impaired. The speaker wears a microphone that is attached to an FM transmitter. The listener wears an FM receiver tuned to the transmitter frequency, and the signal is delivered to the ear in one of two ways. For cases in which the hearing loss has both a peripheral and central component, hearing aids are recommended to overcome the peripheral loss and are used in conjunction with FM systems for the central loss. Transduction of signals is typically done through the hearing aid telecoil and ALD neck-loop. In cases in which the disorder is primarily central only the FM system is recommended, and the signal is transduced via an insert receiver or lightweight headphones.

Illustrative Cases

Judging from reports in the literature and from clinical experience, the number of children and elderly adults with CAPD seems to be substantial. A recent estimate by my colleagues and I determined that after degree of hearing loss is accounted for, as many as 80 percent of clinical patients ranging in age from 75 to 79 years have some degree of central presbycusis (Spretnjak, Stach, & Jerger, 1988). The following two cases serve as illustrative examples of the kinds of patients we have seen. Patients were evaluated and managed by the clinical staff of The Methodist Hospital Audiology Service at the Neurosensory Center of Houston, Texas. The patients are representative of the success we have experienced with the application of FM assistive devices to people with central auditory disorder.

Case No. 1

Patient M.S. had a history of chronic otitis media that lasted until he was 4 years of age. At age 6 years, he was exposed to a gun-shot that reportedly left him with a hearing loss for approximately 48 hours. Audiologic testing at that time showed a mild sensorineural hearing loss with a notch at 4000 Hz. When he was 11 years old, his parents again sought audiologic consultation for behaviors that included the inability to simultaneously write and listen and a propensity for turning up the television volume control. By this time he was in the fifth grade, and although results of educational testing had always placed him in the above average categories, he was diagnosed as having auditory retention and recall difficulties. His teachers assigned him preferential seating in the classroom because of what they described as an inability to pay attention and a mild degree of recalcitrance. He was seen by another audiology facility one month earlier and was fitted with hearing aids. Because of his complaints about increased listening difficulty while wearing the hearing aids, the parents came to us for a second opinion.

Figure 4–9 shows results from our audiologic evaluation. M.S. had a peripheral, mild-to-moderate, sensorineural hearing loss and normal middle ear function. Results of speech audiometry were characterized by a PB–SSI discrepancy that could not be explained by the configuration of the sensitivity loss. Further, the SSI function showed significant rollover. These speech results suggested to us that he had a concomitant central auditory disorder and that the disorder was exacerbated at higher intensities. Auditory evoked potential measures helped to confirm these central findings. The auditory brainstem response was well-formed, with peak latencies and inter-peak intervals within normal limits. Late latency responses were also present and well-formed. Middle latency responses, however, were abnormal bilaterally.

We hypothesized that the patient's problems with traditional amplification resulted from an increased difficulty understanding speech in competition when the hearing aids amplified sound to these higher levels. Figure 4–10 shows results of the hearing aid evaluation. Speech understanding of synthetic sentences was measured at several MCRs with no hearing aid, with his own hearing aid (Hearing Aid 1), with a hearing aid that we predicted might be more appropriate for his sensitivity loss (Hearing Aid 2), and with a personal FM system. Results showed very minor aided improvement and only in easy and average listening conditions. However, he showed substantial improvement in performance, especially in difficult listening conditions, when the S/N ratio was made more favorable by use of an ALD.

M.S. has now used his ALD for over a year. He wears it at all times in the classroom and finds it particularly useful at home during conversations at dinner and while watching television. Anecdotal parent and teacher reports have been extremely positive, and his grades in school have improved substantially.

Case No. 2

S.B. is a 75-year-old man with a long history of progressive hearing loss and hearing aid use. While he still found his hearing aids to be beneficial in quiet situations, he complained of increasing difficulty at his weekly lunch meetings and other social occasions. His wife reported that he was becoming increasingly withdrawn socially because he was no longer able to communicate effectively with his friends.

Figure 4–11 shows results of the audiologic evaluation. The hearing loss was sensorineural and moderate-to-severe in degree. Understanding of PB words presented in quiet was depressed, consistent with the configuration of the peripheral hearing loss. SSI results were disproportionately depressed, consistent with CAPD.

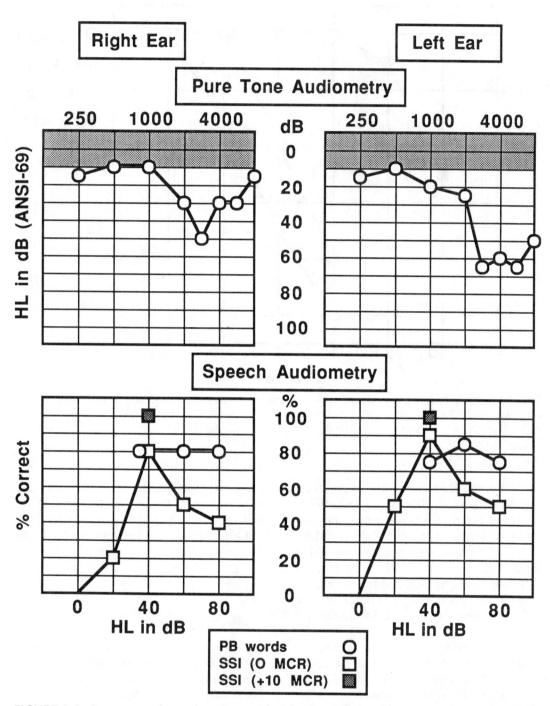

FIGURE 4–9. Pure-tone and speech audiometric results in an 11-year-old patient with central auditory disorder. Speech audiometry results are for PB words presented in quiet, SSI at 0 dB MCR, and SSI at +10 dB MCR.

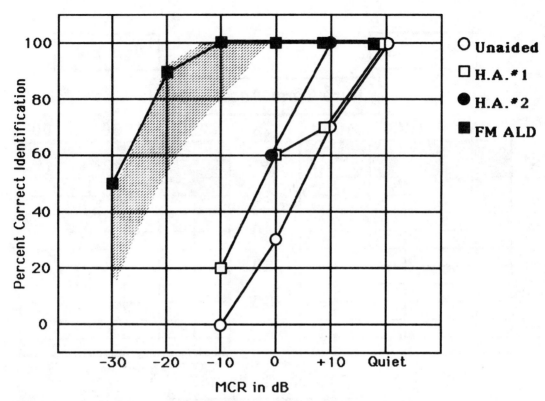

FIGURE 4-10. SSI hearing aid evaluation results from an 11-year-old patient with central auditory disorder with two different hearing aids (H.A. #1 and H.A. #2) and with an FM assistive listening device (FM ALD). Shaded area represents range of performance for normal listeners. MCR = message-to-competition ratio.

Figure 4–12 shows results of the hearing aid evaluation. Despite our best efforts, we could not find a hearing aid that outperformed his own, nor could we show binaural advantage. Yet even his best aided performance was relatively depressed in difficult listening situations. When an FM system was used in conjunction with his own hearing aid, performance increased dramatically.

We offered to loan S.B. the ALD for a trial period to determine whether he would find it to be of benefit under everyday circumstances. He refused, however, and insisted on immediate purchase. At his follow-up visit, his wife described what she considered to be a rebirth in S.B.'s social activity level. It appears that, in the case of S.B., the amplification arrangement

necessary for benefit was one that not only overcame the attenuation deficit resulting from a peripheral sensitivity loss, but also one that provided the needed S/N advantage that had been reduced by central presbycusis.

SUMMARY

For many patients with CAPD, hearing aid amplification provides only marginal benefit. It is also quite possible for a previously satisfied hearing aid user to become progressively dissatisfied as central disorder progresses.

For both children and adults with central processing disorders, prosthetic devices that go beyond mere amplification of

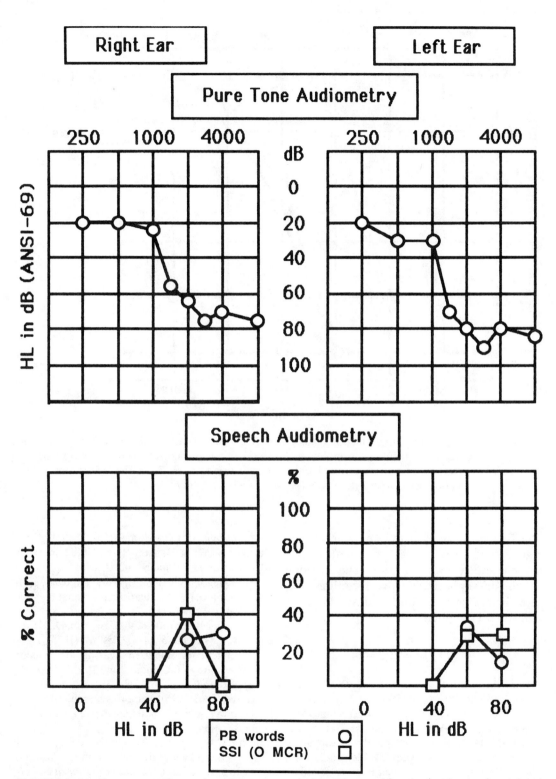

FIGURE 4–11. Pure-tone and speech audiometric results in a 75-year-old patient with mixed peripheral and central presbycusis. Speech audiometry results are for PB words presented in quiet and SSI at 0 dB MCR.

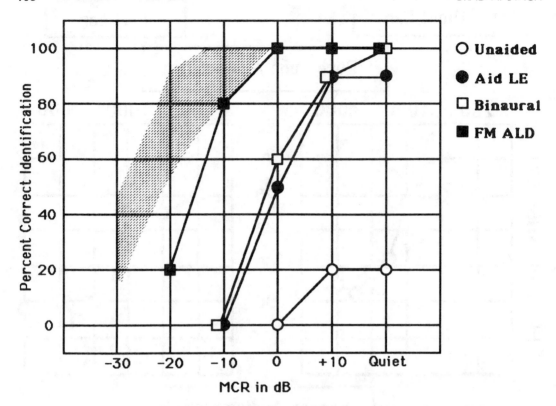

FIGURE 4-12. SSI hearing aid evaluation results from a 75-year-old patient with mixed peripheral and central presbycusis with a hearing aid on the left ear (Aid LE), hearing aids on both ears (binaural), and with an FM assistive listening device coupled to the left ear hearing aid (FM ALD). Shaded area represents range of performance for normal listeners. MCR = message-to-competition ratio.

sound may be needed to overcome communication disorder associated with poor speech understanding ability. The use of remote-microphone assistive listening devices is a promising amplification alternative for this population.

REFERENCES

Antonelli, A. (1970). Sensitized speech tests in aged people. In C. Rojskjaer (Ed.), *Speech audiometry* (pp. 66–79). Second Danavox Symposium. Odense, Denmark: Danavox.

Arnst, D. (1982). Staggered spondaic word test performance in a group of older adults. A preliminary report. *Ear and Hearing, 3,* 118–123.

Beasley, D. S., Forman, B., & Rintelmann, W. F. (1972). Intelligibility of time-compressed CNC monosyllables by normal listeners. *Journal of Auditory Research, 12,* 71–75.

Berger, K. W., & Hagberg, E. N. (1982). Hearing aid users' attitudes and hearing aid usage. *Monographs in Contemporary Audiology, 3*(4).

Bergman, M. (1971). Hearing and aging. *Audiology, 10,* 164–171.

Bergman, M., Blumfield, V., Cascardo, D., Dash, B., Levitt, H., & Marguiles, M. (1976). Age-related decrement in hearing for speech: Sampling and longitudinal studies. *Journal of Gerontology, 31,* 533–538.

Berkowitz, A. (1975). Audiological rehabilitation of the geriatric patient. *Hearing Aid Journal, 8,* 30–34.

Berlin, C. I., & Lowe, S. S. (1972). Temporal and dichotic factors in central auditory testing. In J. Katz (Ed.), *Handbook of clinical audiology* (pp. 280–312). Baltimore: Williams & Wilkins.

Bocca, E. (1958). Clinical aspects of cortical deafness. *Laryngoscope, 68,* 301–309.

Bosatra, A., & Russolo, M. (1982). Comparison between central tonal tests and central speech tests in elderly subjects. *Audiology, 21,* 334–341.

Brody, H. (1955). Organization of the cerebral cortex, III: A study of aging in human cerebral cortex. *Journal of Comparative Neurology, 102,* 551–556.

Brooks, D. N. (1985). Factors relating to the under-use of postaural hearing aids. *British Journal of Audiology, 19,* 211–217.

Calearo, C., & Antonelli, A. R. (1968). Audiometric findings in brainstem lesions. *Acta Otolaryngologica, 66,* 305–319.

Corso, J. (1976). Presbyacusis in noise-induced hearing loss. In D. Henderson, R. P. Hamernik, D. S. Dosanjh, & J. H. Mills (Eds.), *Effects of noise on hearing* (pp. 497–524). New York: Raven Press.

Cranmer, K. S. (1985). Hearing aid dispensing — 1985. *Hearing Instruments, 36,* 6–14.

Cunningham, D. R., Merle, K. S., & Drake, J. (1978). Users' satisfaction with hearing aids. *Journal of the American Auditory Society, 4,* 81–85.

Farrer, S. M., & Keith, R. W. (1981). Filtered word testing in the assessment of children's central auditory abilities. *Ear and Hearing, 2,* 267–269.

Fifer, R. C., Jerger, J. F., Berlin, C. I., Tobey, E. A., & Campbell, J. C. (1983). Development of a dichotic sentence identification test for hearing-impaired adults. *Ear and Hearing, 4,* 300–305.

Franks, J. R., & Beckmann, N. J. (1985). Rejection of hearing aids: Attitudes of a geriatric sample. *Ear and Hearing, 6,* 161–166.

Freeman, B. A., & Beasley, D. S. (1978). Discrimination of time-altered sentential approximations and monosyllables by children with reading problems. *Journal of Speech and Hearing Research, 21,* 497–506.

Gerber, S. E., & Fisher, L. B. (1979). Prediction of hearing aid users' satisfaction. *Journal of the American Auditory Society, 5,* 35–40.

Goetzinger, C., Proud, G., Dirks, D., & Embrey, J. (1961). A study of hearing in advanced age. *Archives of Otolaryngology, 73,* 662–674.

Hansen, C., & Reske-Nielsen, E. (1965). Pathological studies in presbyacusis: Cochlear and central findings in 12 aged patients. *Archives of Otolaryngology, 82,* 115–132.

Hayes, D. (1980). Central auditory problems and the aging process. In D. S. Beasley & G. A.

Davis (Eds.), *Aging communication processes and disorders* (pp. 257–266). New York: Grune & Stratton.

Hayes, D. (1984). Hearing problems of aging. In J. Jerger (Ed.), *Hearing disorders in adults* (pp. 311–337). Boston: College-Hill Press.

Hayes, D., & Jerger, J. (1979). Aging and the use of hearing aids. *Scandinavian Audiology, 8,* 33–40.

Hayes, D., Jerger, J., Taff, J., & Barber, B. (1983). Relation between aided synthetic sentence identification scores and hearing aid user satisfaction. *Ear and Hearing, 4,* 158–161.

Hinchcliffe, R. (1962). The anatomical locus of presbycusis. *Journal of Speech and Hearing Disorders, 27,* 301–310.

Jerger, J. (1960). Audiological manifestations of lesions in the auditory nervous system. *Laryngoscope, 70,* 417–425.

Jerger, J. (1973). Audiological findings in aging. *Advances in Oto-Rhino-Laryngology, 20,* 115–124.

Jerger, J., & Hayes, D. (1976). Hearing aid evaluation: Clinical experience with a new philosophy. *Archives of Otolaryngology, 102,* 214–225.

Jerger, J., & Hayes, D. (1977a). Diagnostic speech audiometry. *Archives of Otolaryngology, 103,* 216–222.

Jerger, J., & Hayes, D. (1977b). Hearing and aging. In S. S. Han & D. H. Coons (Eds.), *Special senses in aging* (pp. 109–118). Ann Arbor: University of Michigan Press.

Jerger, J., & Jerger, S. (1971). Diagnostic significance of PB word functions. *Archives of Otolaryngology, 93,* 573–580.

Jerger, J., & Jerger, S. (1975). Clinical validity of central auditory tests. *Scandinavian Audiology, 4,* 147–163.

Jerger, J., Jerger, S., Oliver, T., & Pirozzolo, F. (1989). Speech understanding in the elderly. *Ear and Hearing, 10,* 79–89.

Jerger, J., Speaks, C., & Trammel, J. (1968). A new approach to speech audiometry. *Journal of Speech and Hearing Disorders, 33,* 318–327.

Jerger, J., Stach, B., Pruitt, J., Harper, R., & Kirby, H. (1989). Comments on "speech understanding and aging." *Journal of the Acoustical Society of America, 85,* 1352–1354.

Jerger, S. (1987). Validation of the pediatric speech intelligibility test in children with central nervous system lesions. *Audiology, 26,* 298–311.

Jerger, S., & Jerger, J. (1983). Neuroaudiologic findings in patients with central auditory disorder. *Seminars in Hearing, 4,* 133–159.

Jerger, S., Jerger, J., & Abrams, S. (1983). Speech audiometry in the young child. *Ear and Hearing, 4,* 56–66.

Jerger, S., Johnson, K., & Loiselle, L. (1988). Pediatric central auditory dysfunction. Comparison of children with confirmed lesions versus suspected processing disorders. *The American Journal of Otology, 9*(Suppl.), 63–71.

Jerger, S. Lewis, S., Hawkins, J., & Jerger, J. (1980). Pediatric speech intelligibility test. I. Generation of test materials. *International Journal of Pediatric Otorhinolaryngology, 2,* 217–230.

Jerger, S., Martin, R. C., & Jerger, J. (1987). Specific auditory perceptual dysfunction in a learning disabled child. *Ear and Hearing, 8,* 78–86.

Johnson, D. W., Enfield, M. L., & Sherman, R. E. (1981). The use of staggered spondaic word and the competing environmental sounds test in the evaluation of central auditory function of learning disabled children. *Ear and Hearing, 2,* 70–77.

Kapteyn, T. S. (1977). Rejection of hearing aids: Attitudes of a geriatric sample. *Ear and Hearing, 6,* 161–166.

Katz, J. (1962). The use of staggered spondaic words for assessing the integrity of the central auditory nervous system. *Journal of Auditory Research, 2,* 327–337.

Keith, R. (1982). Central auditory tests. In N. Lass, L. McReynolds, J. Northern, & D. Yoder (Eds.), *Speech, language, hearing: Volume III. Hearing disorders* (pp. 1015–1038). Philadelphia: W.B. Saunders.

Kimura, D. (1961). Some effects of temporal lobe damage on auditory perception. *Canadian Journal of Psychology, 15,* 156–165.

Kirikae, I., Sato, T., & Shitaro, T. (1964). Study of hearing in advanced age. *Laryngoscope, 74,* 205–221.

Konig, E. (1969). Audiological tests in presbycusis. *International Audiology, 8,* 240–259.

Konkle, D., Beasley, D., & Bess, F. (1977). Intelligibility of time-altered speech in relation to chronological aging. *Journal of Speech and Hearing Research, 20,* 108–115.

Kricos, P. B., Lesner, S. A., Sandridge, S. A., & Yanke, R. B. (1985). Influence of central auditory function on perceived amplification benefits in the elderly: Case reports.

Journal of the Academy of Rehabilitative Audiology, 18, 871–875.

Krmpotic-Nemanic, J. (1971). A new concept of the pathogenesis of presbycusis. *Archives of Otolaryngology, 93,* 161–166.

Kurdziel, S., Noffsinger, D., & Olsen, W. (1976). Performance of cortical lesion patients on 40% and 60% time-compressed materials. *Journal of the American Auditory Society, 2,* 3–7.

Lubert, N. (1981). Auditory perceptual impairments in children with specific language disorders: A review of the literature. *Journal of Speech and Hearing Disorders, 46,* 3–9.

Lutterman, D., Welsh, O., & Melrose, J. (1966). Responses of aged males to time altered speech stimuli. *Journal of Speech and Hearing Research, 9,* 226–230.

Lynn, G., Benitez, J., Eisenbrey, A., Gilroy, J., & Wilner, H. (1972). Neuroaudiological correlates in cerebral hemisphere lesions. *Audiology, 11,* 115–134.

McCandless, G. A., & Parkin, J. L. (1979). Hearing aid performance relative to site of lesion. *Otolaryngology Head-Neck Surgery, 87,* 871–875.

McCroskey, R., & Kasten, R. (1982). Temporal factors and the aging auditory system. *Ear and Hearing, 3,* 124–127.

Mills, J. H. (1978). Effects of noise on young and old people. In D. Lipscomb (Ed.), *Noise and audiology* (pp. 229–241). Baltimore: University Park Press.

Musiek, F. E., & Baran, J. A. (1987). Central auditory assessment: Thirty years of challenge and change. *Ear and Hearing, 8,* 22S–35S.

Noffsinger, P. D., & Kurdziel, S. A. (1979). Assessment of central auditory lesions. In W. F. Rintelmann (Ed.), *Hearing assessment* (pp. 351–377). Baltimore: University Park Press.

Olsen, W. O., Noffsinger, D., & Kurdziel, S. (1975). Speech discrimination in quiet and in white noise by patients with peripheral and central lesions. *Acta Otolaryngologica, 80,* 375–382.

Orchik, D., & Burgess, J. (1977). Synthetic sentence identification as a function of age of the listener. *Journal of the American Audiology Society, 3,* 42–46.

Otto, W. C., & McCandless, G. A. (1982). Aging and auditory site of lesion. *Ear and Hearing, 3,* 110–117.

Pestalozza, G., & Shore, I. (1955). Clinical evaluation of presbycusis on the basis of different tests of auditory function. *Laryngoscope, 65,* 1136–1163.

Pinheiro, M. L. (1977). Tests of central auditory function in children with learning disabilities. In R. W. Keith (Ed.), *Central auditory dysfunction* (pp. 223–256). New York: Grune & Stratton.

Rees, N. (1973). Auditory processing factors in language disorders: The view from Procruste's bed. *Journal of Speech and Hearing Disorders, 38,* 304–313.

Sarff, L. S. (1981). An innovative use of free field amplification in regular classrooms. In R. J. Roeser & M. P. Downs (Eds.), *Auditory disorders in school children* (pp. 263–272). New York: Thieme-Stratton.

Sarff, L. S., Ray, H. R., & Bagwell, C. L. (1981). Why not amplification in every classroom? *Hearing Aid Journal, 34,* 11.

Schuknecht, H. (1964). Further observation on the pathology of presbycusis. *Archives of Otolaryngology, 80,* 369–382.

Schuknecht, H., & Igarashi, M. (1964). Pathology of slowly progressive sensorineural deafness. *Transactions of the American Academy of Ophthalmology and Otolaryngology, 68,* 222–242.

Shapiro, A. H., & Mistal, G. (1985). ITE-Aid auditory training for reading and spelling-disabled children. Clinical case studies. *The Hearing Journal, 38,* 26–31.

Shirinian, M., & Arnst, D. (1982). Patterns in performance intensity functions for phonetically balanced word lists and synthetic sentences in aged listeners. *Archives of Otolaryngology, 108,* 15–20.

Spitzer, J. B. (1983). A central auditory evaluation protocol: A guide for training and diagnosis of lesions of the central system. *Ear and Hearing, 4,* 221–228.

Spretnjak, M. L., Stach, B. A., & Jerger, J. F. (1988). The prevalence of central presbyacusis in a clinical population. *ASHA, 30*(10)

143 (abstract).

Stach, B. A., Jerger, J. F., & Fleming, K. A. (1985). Central presbyacusis: A longitudinal case study. *Ear and Hearing, 6,* 304–306.

Stach, B. A., Jerger, J. F., & Smith, S. L. (1986). Central auditory disorder and hearing aid satisfaction. *ASHA, 28*(10), 69 (abstract).

Stach, B. A., Loiselle, L. H., Jerger, J. F., Mintz, S. L., & Taylor, C. D. (1987). Clinical experience with personal FM assistive listening devices. *The Hearing Journal, 10*(5), 24–30.

Sticht, T., & Gray, B. (1969). The intelligibility of time-compressed words as a function of age and hearing loss. *Journal of Speech and Hearing Research, 12,* 443–448.

Surr, R. K., Schuchman, G. I., & Montgomery, A. A. (1978). Factors influencing use of hearing aids. *Archives of Otolaryngology, 104,* 732–736.

Tallal, P. (1980). Auditory processing disorders in children. In P. Levison & C. Sloan (Eds.), *Auditory processing and language. Clinical and research perspectives* (pp. 81–100). New York: Grune & Stratton.

Walden, B., Demorest, M., & Hepler, E. (1984). Self-report approach to assessing benefit derived from amplification. *Journal of Speech and Hearing Research, 27,* 49–56.

Welsh, L. W., Welsh, J. J., & Healy, M. P. (1985). Central presbyacusis. *Laryngoscope, 95,* 128–136.

Willeford, J. (1977). Assessing central auditory behavior in children: A test battery approach. In R. W. Keith (Ed.), *Central auditory dysfunction* (pp. 43–72). New York: Grune & Stratton.

Willeford, J. A., & Bilger, J. M. (1978). Auditory perception in children with learning disabilities. In J. Katz (Ed.), *Handbook of clinical audiology* (2nd ed.). Baltimore: Williams & Wilkins.

Working Group on Speech Understanding and Aging. (1988). Speech understanding and aging. *Journal of the Acoustical Society of America, 83,* 859–894.

5

PEDIATRIC CONSIDERATIONS IN SELECTING AND FITTING HEARING AIDS

JERRY L. NORTHERN ■

SANDRA ABBOTT GABBARD ■

DEBORAH L. KINDER ■

*I*mpairment of hearing is a serious handicap in the development of a young child. Undetected, or untreated, hearing impairment in children can impede intellectual development, create poor speech and language patterns, and result in a severe communication handicap. The identification of hearing loss in children is not an easy task, and the hearing-impaired child may present a confusing clinical picture. Delays in the identification of children with hearing loss are still not uncommon, creating irretrievable loss of time for the habilitation of the child's problems. On the other hand, developments in hearing aid evaluaton procedures during the past decade have provided more scientific approaches to selecting and fitting hearing aids in children.

Accurate quantification and evaluation of a child's hearing impairment is important to assure optimal management of the problem. Early diagnosis and early use of amplification is critical to later edu-cational management. Determination of the degree of hearing impairment in the young child is an ongoing process that requires an experienced audiologist. The hearing aid fitting in each child is also an ongoing procedure, and each person involved must understand that every decision is tentative and will be subject to change as new information becomes available. Matkin (1984) described three major problems currently in need of correction pertaining to the use of hearing aids by children: (1) many children with substantiated hearing loss are not using adequate amplification; (2) insufficient real-ear aided testing is done with children who wear hearing aids; and (3) research studies verify that many hearing aid instruments worn by children are not functioning properly because of inadequate routine maintenance.

One of the biggest problems in fitting hearing aids to hearing-impaired children is the unacceptable delay in time between identification of the hearing loss and the actual implementation of amplification for the child (Bergstrom, 1976; Shah, Chandler, & Dale, 1978). Simmons (1980) reviewed records of 42 babies fitted with hearing aids at an average age of 22 months. Although it may seem to some that having a hearing aid in place on a youngster as young as 22 months is admirable, it must be pointed out that nearly all of these children were suspected to have hearing loss *prior* to their discharge from the newborn nursery. Simmons summarized reasons for the lengthy delay in fitting of hearing aids to these children as (1) referral back to the primary care physician for ear examination and medical clearance accompanied by long, silent intervals of time without action; (2) multiple physical and developmental problems of the child in which hearing impairment was only part of the total concern of the parents; and (3) parental disbelief or avoidance of the fact that their child indeed had a significant hearing loss. In view of these factors, it is important for the audiologist to be ever vigilant and concerned for the hearing-impaired child's welfare and to persist with whatever steps are necessary to ensure that amplification is appropriately fitted and utilized at as early an age as possible. A recent editorial by Upfold (1988) forecasts new emphasis on the fitting of hearing aids to children with mild and conductive impairments in the future.

In this chapter attention focuses on pediatric auditory status assessment, rationale for hearing aid selection with children, and suggestions for fitting strategies and management concerns. Children require special consideration since they cannot verbally describe the qualities of the amplified sound they perceive through their hearing aids. Accordingly, the selection, fitting, verification, and management procedures for amplification need to be modified to meet the needs of this special population. For purposes of this chapter, the focus will be on the pediatric popula-

tion less than 4 years of age, and severe-to-profound deaf children who have limited verbal capabilities. Older, school-age children can usually participate in the audiologic evaluation procedures traditionally described for adults.

EVALUATION OF HEARING IN CHILDREN

The principles of normal childhood development of auditory and speech functions form the basis for evaluating hearing in infants and children. The audiologist must possess substantial experience in evaluating hearing in normal children to develop the clinical insight and keen observation skills required to note the discrepant responses of children with auditory handicaps. There is no specific testing technique to fit all children all of the time. Flexibility, patience, understanding, and persistence are the watchwords of successful hearing testing with children.

Numerous techniques are available to evaluate the hearing of children. Since the auditory evaluation is an ongoing process, the various techniques are utilized with full consideration of the child's maturational development. Difficult-to-test children should be evaluated with as many techniques as possible to confirm questionable hearing test results. A thorough description of the auditory evaluation of children is presented by Northern and Downs (1984) and Wilson and Thompson (1984).

Conditioned Orientation Reflex (COR) Audiometry

When a visual or auditory stimulus is presented to an infant or a young child, the child will reflexively turn his head toward the source of the stimulus in an "orienting" response. Also known as "visual reinforcement audiometry," the technique employs classical conditioning practices to condition the orientation response. A light, or a lighted transparent toy, is flashed simultaneously with the presentation of a sound-field auditory signal. After a few conditioning trials, presentation of only the auditory stimulus causes the child to orient toward the sound source, a response that is reinforced by illuminating the toy or flashing the light. Threshold levels may be established with sound-field warble tone signals, narrow bands of noise, or speech signals. This procedure is particularly useful for children between 12 months and 3 years of age. The testing procedure is relatively simple and quick, is usually accomplished in 10 minutes or less, and produces valid results in the majority of children. This technique is often used with young children to establish functional gain of hearing aids by comparing unaided and aided sound-field thresholds.

Behavioral Play Audiometry

Three and 4-year-old children are often evaluated through a play-conditioning technique that utilizes some motivational activity such as putting rings on a tower, dropping blocks in a can, or building a peg-board fence with pegs. The advantage of this procedure is that it is used with earphones so that responses from each ear of the child are established independently. The youngster is conditioned to hold a block above a box until a loud tone is presented. The child is taught to drop the block immediately when the sound is heard, and the action is appropriately rewarded by the examiner. When the child is able to perform the activity without help, an entire audiogram can be obtained for air- and bone-conduction across the frequency range, even when masking in the opposite ear is necessary. This procedure is especially useful to establish unaided and amplified thresholds at each frequency for each ear.

Speech Audiometry

Jerger (1987) pointed out that some form of speech-based measurement should be included in each hearing aid evaluation. Speech audiometry may be more difficult to administer to children, but the purpose of the hearing aid is to optimize auditory perception for hearing-impaired children to learn speech and language. Speech audiometry in its simplest form with a cooperative youngster approximately 3 years old directs the child at controlled intensity levels to follow simple spoken commands, identify body parts, and point out common toys. Utilizing these tasks with the sound-field system or under earphones, the speech reception threshold (SRT) can be established for each ear. Many young children may be too shy to repeat words verbally, but they will often follow simple speech identification tasks.

The 4-year-old with adequate speech and language patterns may cooperate with tests of speech recognition (discrimination). If the child will repeat words, special children's discrimination word lists are available. When possible, speech recognition scores are especially valuable in assessing hearing aid performance. Closed-set pictures presented on cards are also useful; children point to the appropriate object representing the perceived word. The challenge is to select a discrimination test equal to the child's receptive language level (Jerger, Lewis, & Hawkins, 1980; Jerger, Jerger, & Lewis, 1981). Jerger, Jerger, and Fahad (1985) described the use of the Pediatric Speech Intelligibility (PSI) sentence materials to carry out hearing aid evaluations on a 3-year, 6-month-old child who was too immature to be tested with conventional speech tests.

Immittance Audiometry

No hearing evaluation in a young child is complete without inclusion of immittance audiometry. Although not a test of hearing per se, immittance audiometry is a technique for evaluating the physiologic function of the middle ear system and is extremely valuable in differentiating between normal and pathologic middle ears. The immittance audiometry test battery in children should include tympanometry and acoustic reflex threshold determination. Tympanometry, including the measurement of middle ear pressure, is an extremely useful technique for identifying and monitoring the pathophysiology of the middle ear and the concurrent presence of conductive hearing loss. More elaborate evaluation of the stapedial reflex with an acoustic immittance meter may be used to estimate sensorineural hearing sensitivity (Northern, 1988).

Cooper, Langley, Meyerhoff, and Gates (1977) examined 1133 children with negative pressure tympanograms between −150 and −400 mm H_2O and noted their hearing threshold levels to be elevated by as much as 25 dB. Norris, Jirsa, and Skinner (1977) concluded that audiologists should expect conductive loss of approximately 8 dB in the speech frequency range with a middle ear pressure of −100 mm H_2O and approximately 20 dB when negative middle ear pressure reaches −400 mm H_2O. This study points out that the greatest threshold shift as a consequence of negative middle ear pressure occurs at the midpoint of the speech frequency range, a fact that has considerable significance for hearing aid users with poor Eustachian tube function. As the hearing aid gain is increased to compensate for the increased hearing loss, acoustic feedback as well as distortion may decrease hearing aid performance.

Rubin (1980) cited the importance of impedance measurements with deaf children because of the high incidence of middle ear pathology in that population. She reported that, in one year, 50 percent of the hearing-impaired toddlers and infants in the Lexington Infant Center demonstrated middle ear pathology. Accordingly, all infants should be evaluated with immittance testing during each session of the hearing aid evaluation procedure and fitting to identify the presence of intermittent middle ear negative pressure. Acoustic im-

mittance measurements play an important role in monitoring the effectiveness of hearing aids with children, and should be a part of every routine clinical visit from a child wearing amplification.

HEARING AID EVALUATION IN CHILDREN

Obviously, hearing aid evaluation techniques that are easily used with adults, who can respond verbally about the quality of amplification provided, cannot be used without modification with hearing-impaired children. Considerable controversy exists among hearing professionals about the "best" hearing aid evaluation procedure, and accordingly, a wide variety of procedures exist from which to choose (Gwyn, 1988). However, with children, rigidity in the hearing aid evaluation is not possible since every child presents with unique problems, different maturation levels, variance in cooperative abilities, and often limited audiometric information. It behooves the audiologist to become familiar with numerous hearing aid evaluations and techniques and to be prepared to use the most appropriate procedure to match the individual needs of each child (Lewis, 1985). It is not within the scope of this chapter to review the extensive literature in this area, but an overview of the more common approaches to selection and evaluation of hearing aids in children follows.

An important principle to apply in pediatric hearing aid evaluation is the concept of establishing a *target response* that can be met with amplification. Prior to selection of specific hearing aids for the hearing-impaired child, consideration must be given to the optimal frequency response and output to be achieved with the amplification devices. Then the evaluation procedure should be carried out in such a manner that the audiologist is able to compare the real-ear amplified response with the target response. If the real-ear amplified response is less than, or exceeds, the target response, the audiologist must be skilled in modifying the amplification system under evaluation to meet the target criteria.

Many audiologists turn to a prescriptive approach to selecting hearing aid electroacoustic parameters with children since air conduction thresholds may be the only available audiologic information. The use of prescriptive measures utilizing a formula technique has become a common practice during the last decade. A clear and concise summary of seven commonly used prescriptive methods for hearing aid selection has been published by Davis and Mueller (1987).

Numerous studies have been conducted to evaluate and compare various prescriptive techniques with hearing-impaired adults. In general terms, no single prescriptive technique withstands serious scrutiny (Schwartz, 1982). Curran (1988) stated that the most popular prescriptive methods for hearing aid selection are based on puretone thresholds and fail to take into account individual differences or the effects of coupling configuration. Studies that have compared various formulae techniques on the same hearing-impaired patients have found either that each formula produces different results (Byrne, 1987; Byrne & Tonisson, 1976), or that no significant differences can be consistently identified among the methods (Humes, 1986; Sullivan, Levitt, Hwang, & Hennessey, 1988).

Functional Gain

Functional gain is the difference between *unaided* and *aided* minimal response levels. The purpose of functional gain measurement is to compare unaided and aided responses under identical conditions. The young child is seated on the parent's lap between two loudspeakers. Minimal response levels are then obtained for speech signals and test frequencies, or narrow bands of noise, of 250 through 8000 Hz

without the hearing aids. Visual response audiometry (VRA) can be applied as necessary. With the hearing aids in place on the child and the gain controls set at preselected levels, minimal response levels are again obtained for speech and narrow band noise. The difference between the aided and unaided minimal response levels is the functional gain. If the functional gain is different from the target gain, appropriate adjustments should be made. Schwartz and Larson (1977) correctly pointed out that a major disadvantage with functional gain procedures is that the sound-field audiogram reflects performance only at threshold levels, and thus there is no assurance that the child will receive meaningful perception of speech at intensities sufficiently above threshold. Rines, Stelmachowicz, and Gorga (1984) suggested that minimal response levels in sound field underestimate functional gain when unaided hearing levels are near normal limits.

Uses for functional gain measurements include comparing the performance of hearing aids with different internal settings, obtaining information regarding various types of earmolds, monitoring stability of the young child's amplification system over time, and demonstrating improvement in unaided versus aided conditions (Ross & Tomasetti, 1980). However, since functional gain measurements are typically made in 5 dB intervals, smaller differences due to hearing aid adjustment may not be noticeable with functional gain measurements.

Computerized Probe Microphone Real-Ear Measurements

Computerized real-ear probe microphone hearing aid analysis offers an important opportunity to improve hearing aid fittings with children. This technique utilizes a soft silicone tube that is inserted into the ear canal with the hearing aid and earmold in place. The amplified sound in the ear canal is picked up by a probe microphone through the silicone tube and is subjected to signal processing by a special purpose computer and presented on a visual display or printout. It is now possible for the audiologist to know precisely the aided frequency response and amplified signal intensity in the child's ear canal. For many years it has been necessary to estimate ear canal sound pressure at each frequency by interpolating data obtained from a 2 cc cavity, and utilizing correction factors as a mathematical means to determine real-ear specifications.

The major advantage of the computerized probe microphone real-ear measuring device is that the entire amplification system is evaluated so the effects of tubing, earmold, filters, and so forth can be acknowledged. Physiologic differences among children, such as the length, diameter, and shape of the ear canal, which are extremely important considerations in fitting hearing aids with children, are taken into account in real-ear probe microphone measurements. Real-ear computerized measurements provide quick, objective data regarding insertion gain, in-situ response, and relative gain, as well as the telemagnetic response of the hearing aid. The measurements may be read in 1 dB intervals; even this small change made with hearing aid adjustment will be clearly noted. This information is valuable during the hearing aid selection, fitting verification, and postfitting management of the hearing-impaired child. Most real-ear measurement equipment also includes a "listening" system, through high-fidelity lightweight earphones, so that the amplified sounds can be monitored easily by the child's parents, who thereby gain full appreciation of exactly how their youngster's hearing aids amplify environmental and speech sounds.

An important aspect of this revolutionary new equipment is the ability to plot visually on the video screen a target amplified hearing aid response. The hearing aid fitter is able to use any method of gain prediction (i.e., the half-gain rule, POGO,

and so forth) to achieve the best amplified responses for each child. Then, acoustic measurements performed in the ear canal with probe microphone systems can provide information regarding the total effect of the hearing aids, earmold plumbing, and sound-field effects with minimal patient cooperation (Libby, 1987). It is important to note that probe-microphone measurements in infant ear canals have documented that the fundamental resonance frequency of the external ear decreases from approximately 6000 Hz at birth to the adult resonance value of 2700 Hz by the second year of age (Kruger, 1987). This information is of value in selecting appropriate hearing aid frequency characteristics in babies.

Comparison of the real-ear response with the target amplification response permits manipulation of the acoustic coupling system with predictable effects on the frequency range to be modified. Earmold venting may be used to suppress low-frequency output, reduce the "fullness" sensation, and eliminate tolerance problems by reducing amplified output. Acoustic dampers may be used as mid-frequency controls to smooth out the amplified frequency response between 1000 and 3000 Hz and to reduce hearing aid output and insertion gain. Acoustic horn effects are often used to extend the amplified high frequency response out to 4000 Hz to improve speech intelligibility. Following each acoustic modification it is a simple matter to verify the result of manipulation.

The use of this technology in fitting hearing aids and managing amplification with hearing-impaired children should have widespread application. The real-ear response in no way can be construed to represent what the child hears, which requires cerebral integration. Probe-microphone evaluation gives audiologists confidence in their selection and fitting of hearing aids to this difficult-to-test population. We are currently using the real-ear probe microphone system with all of our pediatric hearing aid patients.

The initial step in our hearing aid procedure is the preselection of the desired hearing aid frequency response, gain, and output characteristics based on available audiometric information. *All* aspects of the pediatric audiometric test battery are utilized to obtain *as much audiometric information as possible* regarding the child's hearing loss. Clinical selection of the hearing aid is made to achieve the optimal insertion gain required by the patient. To these values are added the effect of tubing and earmold modifications. These target results are plotted in advance and stored on the video screen of the real-ear analyzer.

The second step in the fitting procedure is to determine the insertion gain with the hearing aid, tubing, and earmold in the child's ear canal with real-ear probe microphone measurements. This step may be conducted with more than one hearing aid, and a variety of earmold modifications, to determine which of the available hearing aids and coupling systems best fits the target preselected frequency response. During the "acoustic tuning" implementation phase of the procedure, the hearing aid is modified until the insertion gain response noted on the real-ear analyzer most closely approximates the preselected curve stored on the video screen. Modifications may include adjustments of the hearing aid internal trimmers, volume control, or other aspects of the acoustic plumbing. Repeated evaluation with the real-ear probe system clearly shows the effects of each and every acoustic modification.

Hard copy of the final fitting result is recorded by the computer's printer and is useful for future comparison and evaluation of hearing aid performance. Comparative real-ear measurements, as well as speech audiometry, when possible, are performed at each of the child's routine return visits or when difficulties with the hearing aid are reported by the parents.

Aided Auditory Brainstem Evoked Response (ABR)

Audiologists often look for an objective approach to hearing aid selection, especially with young children. Numerous authors have suggested using aided ABR measurements because patient participation is not necessary. Aided ABR evaluation for hearing aid fitting can be implemented with appropriate younger children. However, questions have been raised about the accuracy of ABR hearing aid measurements, as well as genuine concerns about the lengthy time and high expense of the procedure. Another major limiting factor is that the ABR technique does not provide specific frequency information.

In reviewing literature on aided ABR procedures, there is no agreed-on evaluation technique. Mahoney (1985) proposed the following protocol: (1) At 50 dB SPL, begin the aided ABR with a high gain hearing aid, and if there is no response, increase the click stimulus; (2) following an aided ABR recording, increase the gain until Wave V latency and amplitude stabilize; and (3) establish a latency-intensity function at varying frequency and compression settings. Kiessling (1982, 1983) utilized aided ABR amplitude intensity information to determine appropriate hearing aid settings. He offered a mathematical technique for optimal hearing aid fitting from unaided earphone-stimulated ABR intensity amplitude curves. The computation includes the intensity in dB of the stimulus and the amplitude of the ABR Wave V in nanovolts. The hearing aid components calculated are average gain in dB, dynamic range in dB, compression factor, and type of compression. The steepness of the ABR intensity-amplitude curve dictates the amount of compression that is needed. Cox and Metz (1980) suggested that the gain of the hearing aid be adjusted to the level where additional increases in gain no longer produce further decreases in ABR Wave V latency. They reported that the accuracy rate of hearing aid prescription by ABR may be as much as 75 percent of the accuracy rate of traditional hearing aid fitting procedures. The authors concluded that accuracy is associated with the configuration of the hearing loss, with greater accuracy for flat and precipitous losses than for gradually sloping losses. They also believe that clicks, in addition to tone pips, yield greater accuracy in hearing aid fittings.

HEARING AID SELECTION

Type of Instrument

The preselection procedure begins with consideration of the type of hearing aids to be utilized. Body-type hearing aids are now less often recommended for children because of technological improvements in ear-level hearing aids, especially in terms of adjustment, flexibility, and amount of power. Ear-level aids are lightweight, have no external wires or tubes, do not amplify clothing noise, and, most importantly, provide hearing reception at the natural position on the head. Ear-level hearing aids are the general choice for most children, with the exception of the multiply handicapped child with poor head control that may lead to persistent feedback problems when ear-level aids are utilized.

In-the-ear (ITE) hearing instruments have not been widely used with children according to a survey reported by Curran (1985). Although tremendous strides have been made in the technology of ITE hearing aids, their major limitations for children involve their inability to provide direct audio input and poor telecoil response. These limitations prohibit the use of personal FM systems and assistive listening devices with the child's hearing aid. Until the addition of direct audio input and improved telecoil response in ITE hearing aids, it seems likely that ITE hearing aids will be recommended only for children with mild hearing losses. The problem of a child outgrowing the ITE hearing aid is actually easily solved by simple recasing of the instrument as often as necessary.

Bone-conduction hearing aids are rarely used these days except for infants or young children with conductive-type hear-ing loss due to congenital anomalies such as microtia of the pinnae or atresia of the external ear canal.

Monaural Versus Binaural Hearing Aids

Children have a critical need for hearing because of the interdependence of the auditory sense with the development of speech and language. Although considerable controversy has existed over the years relative to the merits of binaural versus monaural amplification, our policy is that *all children should be fitted with binaural hearing aids whenever possible* to maximize optimal hearing potential. It is well acknowledged that binaural amplification results in improved speech discrimination skills, especially in the presence of background noise, and improved auditory localization abilities. Another positive feature of binaural hearing aid fittings is the psychoacoustic phenomenon of loudness summation, which makes it possible to use less gain in each hearing aid (Ross, 1980).

Traditional candidates for binaural hearing aids are children with bilateral, symmetrical hearing loss. However, asymmetrical hearing loss should not be a contraindication to binaural amplification. The fitting of binaural amplification with all hearing-impaired children should prevail until contraindications (such as total deafness in one ear) are determined.

An interesting project conducted by Silman, Gelfand, and Silverman (1984) studied auditory deprivation in monaural and binaural aided adult males. The auditory performance of the subjects prior to the use of hearing aids was compared to their auditory performance after 4 to 5 years of hearing aid use to determine whether the unaided ear would show effects of auditory deprivation. Over this period of time, no differences were found in pure-tone thresholds or speech recognition scores for the two groups. However, results revealed that speech recognition scores remained stable for the binaurally fitted patients, while the unaided ear of the monaurally fitted patients showed an auditory deprivation effect. This study has important implications that urge the binaural fitting of all children who need hearing aids. The attitudes of professionals dispensing hearing aids have been changing over the past decade in favor of binaural fittings (Mueller, 1986).

The Acoustic Coupling System

The earmold itself is an essential feature of the hearing aid system. It provides support for the hearing aid, directs the amplified sound into the ear canal, and when properly fitted prevents acoustic feedback.

Variations in earmold configuration can substantially alter the electroacoustic characteristics of the hearing aid. Accordingly, it is important to evaluate each hearing aid with the earmold that is to be used with it. This may require two or more sessions with the child: one session to take the earmold impression, and an additional session after the permanent custom earmold has been fabricated. It is particularly difficult to conduct hearing aid evaluations with children using stock earmolds, since they often do not fit well in the child's ear canal and most certainly do not represent how the hearing aid will perform when the child has his own earmold. The pinna continues to grow in size in children until about 9 years of age. Thus, earmolds should be remade every 3 to 6 months in the child's early years, or once a year after age 5, to ensure adequate fit.

The earmold may be crafted in many ways (with open vents, various tubing, filters, and so on) to enhance the hearing aid. The material of the earmold is relatively insignificant in terms of general acoustics. The most important factor about the earmold is that acoustic feedback must be prevented if the child is to obtain maximum benefit from the hearing aid.

Through developments in subminiature transducers and electronics, the physical performance of hearing aids has been vastly improved, and problems previously associated with the earmold and acoustic coupling are now sufficiently understood so that a smooth frequency response of the hearing aid, as perceived by the user, can be individually tailored in a highly predictable manner (Killion, 1982). One of the most important electroacoustic characteristics of a hearing aid is the absence of "peaks and valleys" in the frequency response curve.

The development of transducers with wideband capabilities, and the "stepped diameter" approach to the conventional acoustic coupling system, which can be extended to the earmold to improve the high frequency response of the aid, have had tremendous impact on the fidelity of amplification. Libby (1982) described various earmold and tubing construction to influence the electroacoustic frequency response of the hearing aid system in a predictable fashion. Venting the earmold is an effective technique to influence low frequency responses below 1000 Hz, which in effect reduces the patient's total sound pressure level exposure significantly (by as much as 20 dB at some frequencies). Damping is a useful technique to smooth the frequency range between 1000 and 3000 Hz, and the acoustic horn or stepped-diameter approach to the acoustic coupling system often extends the frequency response beyond 3000 Hz. Construction of the earmold becomes increasingly important to preserve the high frequency response of the hearing aid. To meet these needs, a one-piece tapered, internally stepped bore horn can be used effectively to conserve high frequency components of amplified sound, which are so important to hearing-impaired children in the learning of speech and auditory discrimination.

HEARING AID SELECTION

In general terms, the principles behind the selection of hearing aids for children are no different than hearing aid characteristics used by adults. Libby (1982) has summarized these considerations as follows: (1) select an amplification system with a smooth frequency response and no sharp peaks; (2) plan to compensate for the 10 to 15 dB insertion loss at 2700 Hz created by the occluding earmold; (3) ensure a wide frequency bandwidth to ensure greater fidelity for speech and music; (4) preserve an appropriate balance between high frequency amplification for speech recognition and low frequency energy for intelligibility and sound quality; and (5) the output of the hearing aid should not exceed the patient's loudness discomfort level.

Considerations Related to Age

The selection of a specific hearing aid for a hearing-impaired child challenges the skills of even the most experienced audiologists. When a child has both receptive and expressive speech and language, the selection of a hearing aid is certainly easier. It is the non-verbal child who poses problems, since this youngster is not capable of communicating with the audiologist about the quality of various hearing aids. Appropriate selection of the frequency response and output characteristics must be carefully considered in fitting amplification to children. A number of techniques, both behavioral and electroacoustic, have evolved as a means to select the optimal hearing aid for each patient. None of the methods provides exact, precise information that is valid for *every* hearing aid fitting, but each procedure provides direction about the appropriate range of performance that the hearing aid must encompass. Often, more than one hearing aid instrument will meet the appropriate gain and output requirements, and selection is then based on other considerations, such as hearing aid size, durability, cosmetics, ease of use, cost, and availability of service and insurance (Matkin, 1986).

It is common wisdom to select a hearing aid that has a broad range of adjustable controls that can provide flexibility for changing the response of the hearing aid as

necessary. As more data are accumulated and accuracy of test results improves as the child grows older and matures, changes in the hearing aid system will undoubtedly be necessary. Routine hearing aid assessment and alteration for all children using amplification is an important part of the process, and the audiologist must be prepared to make hearing aid response changes as often as necessary. We do not advocate any specific procedure because no single technique fits all circumstances for all children. The audiologist must be prepared and willing to utilize the technique that provides the most useful information in a reasonable time period.

An important concept relative to children's amplification introduced by Gengel, Pascoe, and Shore (1971) assumes that a positive correlation exists between aided speech discrimination performance and the area of speech spectrum received with amplification. Thus, the goal of hearing aid selection is to utilize a hearing aid that amplifies, at a comfortable gain setting, as much of the speech spectrum as possible. Bands of noise corresponding to the intensity of corresponding segments in normal conversational speech are used to compute average speech spectrum levels for octaves over the standard frequency range. Gengel and colleagues computed approximate average speech levels for bands of noise centered at five test frequencies, when the overall sound pressure level of the spectrum was 70 dB SPL, to be 60 dB at 250 Hz, 61 dB at 500 Hz, 58 dB at 1000 Hz, 54 dB at 2000 Hz, and 46 dB at 4000 Hz.

The protocol of this evaluation is to establish aided thresholds with these selected narrow bands of noise when the hearing aid is set at a comfortable listening level. To estimate the average levels above threshold at which the child receives the speech spectrum at conversational level, the aided threshold sound pressure levels are subtracted from the average speech spectrum levels. The difference values in dB represent the approximate sensation level at which each frequency band of speech will be perceived during normal conversation. Gengel and colleagues suggested that the hearing aid of choice is the unit that amplifies the widest possible speech spectrum 10 to 20 dB above the aided threshold. The authors proposed this procedure for evaluating and selecting hearing aids for children with severe-to-profound hearing loss. Schwartz and Larson (1977) confirmed the value of this procedure with severely hearing-impaired children.

The publications of Ross and Seewald (1988), Seewald and Ross (1988), and Seewald (1988) have continued to develop this suprathreshold approach to selection of hearing aids for hearing-impaired children. Their procedure has been to determine amplification target levels by using estimates of the average levels associated with the long-term speech spectrum relative to the child's unaided sound-field detection levels. Although some controversy exists among researchers as to the exact intensity levels representative of frequency segments within the long-term speech frequency spectrum (Olsen, Hawkins, & Van Tasell, 1987), the overall concept is to provide children with an amplified speech signal that is audible throughout the broadest frequency range possible. In general terms, the desired sensation level of the amplified speech decreases in an accelerated non-linear function with increasing hearing loss (Seewald, Ross, & Spiro, 1985). Although older children can be assessed with this technique through behavioral sound-field measures, probe microphone measurements provide information regarding the real-ear frequency characteristics quickly and easily in the child's ear canal.

Hawkins (1987a) described a similar procedure in which the child's auditory detection levels are determined in sound-field using behavioral techniques. Then, an unoccluded frequency specific stimulus is presented with the probe microphone in the child's ear canal, at the level at which threshold was obtained and ear canal SPL levels of the stimulus are recorded. With the probe tube in the same position, the hearing aid is fitted and real-ear aided responses (REAR) are determined with the input stimuli presented at levels determined by the long-term speech spectrum. By comparing the real-ear unoccluded response (REUR) at threshold levels with the REAR produced with the speech spectrum level input, an estimate can be made of the sensation level at each frequency of the amplified long-term speech spectrum.

Hearing Aid Output

Hearing aids should not be selected because of their power output — also known as saturated sound pressure level (SSPL), alone. After all, every hearing aid has a volume control that can be adjusted within the limits of the hearing aid. Although one would not purposefully choose a hearing aid with inadequate output, a common error is to "overfit" with too much power. Seewald, Ross, and Spiro (1985) pointed out that the selection of real-ear SSPL is a compromise. The SSPL must be high enough to provide adequate amplification without exceeding the saturation level frequently, yet the SSPL must not exceed the child's loudness discomfort level.

Clinicians must be aware that hearing aid specifications are reported relative to a 2 cc hard-walled cavity. A hearing aid coupled to a child's ear canal will enclose a cavity that is considerably less than 2 cc, resulting in increased sound pressure levels at the tympanic membrane. The average enclosed ear canal cavity volume, with an earmold in place is 1.0 to 1.4 cc for an adult, and only 0.8 to 1.0 cc for a child. In infants, the physical volume may be as small as 0.5 cc.

The ANSI hearing aid specifications relative to a 2.0 cc cavity are altered significantly when the hearing aid is coupled tightly to an ear canal that is less than 2.0 cc in volume. From physical acoustics it is well established that each time cavity volume is reduced by one-half, sound pressure within the cavity is increased 6 dB. Children with ear canal volumes approximately 0.5 to 1.5 cc may actually receive considerably more amplification than indicated by the hearing aid technical specification sheet; that is, an instrument with a high frequency average SSPL90 of 130 dB as measured in a 2.0 cc coupler may be capable of creating 142 dB SPL when coupled to an ear having a 0.5 cc space between the tip of the earmold and the eardrum.

McCandless and Miller (1972) described a technique for establishing hearing aid gain by use of acoustic reflex thresholds as measured with an immittance meter. With this procedure, the patient is fitted with a hearing aid to one ear and an immittance probe tip placed in the contralateral ear. Using constant sound pressure input of average environmental sounds or conversational speech, the gain control of the hearing aid is slowly raised until the acoustic reflex is barely observed in the contralateral ear. A gain setting is accomplished by adjusting the controls just below this level, which will be safely under the patient's loudness discomfort level. This technique appears to determine a gain level that provides maximum intelligibility for speech (Rappaport & Tait, 1976). In subjects with significant hearing loss, behavioral and acoustic reflex estimates of functional gains were found to be in good agreement (Rines, Stelmachowicz, & Gorga, 1984). Ross and Tomassetti (1980) suggested that the SSPL of the hearing aid should not exceed the SPL that elicits an aided stapedial reflex. They described a real-ear/2 cc coupler correction factor to be added to the acoustic reflex threshold for a particular frequency. For example, if at 2000 Hz the coupler overestimates the frequency response by 10 dB and the acoustic reflex sound-field threshold is 125 dB, then the coupler maximum output at 2000 Hz should not exceed 135 dB.

Unfortunately, the acoustic reflex is often absent in severe-to-profound sensorineural hearing loss. In addition, acoustic reflexes may be absent due to unilateral or bilateral middle ear effusion, a common finding in young children. Hall and Ruth (1986) reported that the acoustic reflex technique is probably useful in only 40 to 50 percent of the average pediatric population undergoing hearing aid evaluation.

In terms of frequency response of a hearing aid for a child, the primary objective is to obtain audibility of the speech spectrum. Ultimately, the desired frequency response should be based on the child's audiometric configuration, which may be estimated as minimal response levels for speech signals, narrow band noise stimuli, or warble tone signals (Stelmachowicz, Larson, Johnson, & Moeller, 1985). The primary energy for consonants and monosyllabic words is found in the higher frequencies. In most cases, low frequencies should not be amplified as much as the high frequencies due to the upward spread of masking phenomenon. That is, when low frequency environmental noise is amplified too much, the level of noise may be sufficiently intense to produce a masking effect that makes speech recognition more difficult. The use of real-ear measurements with a probe microphone in the child's ear canal is the most accurate method to determine the final frequency response of the amplified signal.

OVERAMPLIFICATION IN CHILDREN

Clinicians often worry that powerful hearing aids fitted to children may cause additional hearing damage due to overamplification. Many case studies have been published over the years showing that the use of a powerful hearing aid can indeed cause temporary and permanent threshold shift. In our opinion, the most common error made in selecting and fitting amplification for children is overamplification due to the increase in sound pressure level hearing aid ouput when the system is coupled tightly to the child's small ear canal. The current use of real-ear probe-microphone measurements, taken from the child's ear canal with the hearing aid in place, should be conducted at every opportunity to ensure that proper, and safe, amplification levels are maintained.

Rintelmann and Bess (1977) investigated the literature on documented threshold shifts from overamplification to establish maximum output levels. They cautioned that children with severe-to-profound sensorineural hearing losses who are fitted binaurally should not have SSPLs higher than 120 dB SSPL. They suggested that this group can safely tolerate monaural amplification above 120 dB SSPL, but SSPLs approaching 130 dB SPL should be recommended with caution. Based on their experiences, Heffernan and Simons (1979) offered a specific follow-up routine, including: (1) check of performance with the new hearing aid within 30 days of purchase, (2) electroacoustic analysis of the new hearing aid within 30 days of purchase, (3) monthly appointments thereafter to monitor hearing thresholds until the hearing levels have stabilized for at least 3 months of continual hearing aid use, (4) reevaluation at least every 3 months for the next calendar year, and (5) annual otologic and audiologic evaluations as long as the hearing aid is worn.

A number of reviews of studies dealing with potential hearing damage in children due to powerful hearing aids have been published in a variety of sources (Binnie, 1985; Humes & Bess, 1981; Mills, 1975; Rintelmann & Bess, 1988). In general, the results of these studies suggest that the routine use of a hearing aid is usually not associated with additional deterioration of hearing in most children. However, there is also no question that documented decreases in auditory sensitivity related to hearing aid amplification have been verified in specific cases (Hawkins, 1982; Heffernan & Simons, 1979; Jerger & Lewis, 1975). Practically speaking, it is helpful to select a hearing aid that has a gain control that is separate from the SSPL. The audiologist is then able to ensure adequate gain without overamplifying the child.

Sullivan (1987) described a procedure using the real-ear probe microphone system as a "safe" means to determine the aided SSPL90 response. The technique establishes probe microphone frequency responses for full-on gain and reference test gain (60 dB SPL input) in a closed 2 cc cavity. Then the probe microphone system is used in the wearer's ear to measure real-ear reference test gain with 60 dB SPL input. By subtracting the reference test gain measures obtained in the 2 cc cavity and in the wearer's ear, a transfer function can be applied to extrapolate the aided SSPL90 in the user's ear from the 2 cc aided full-gain response obtained in the initial step of this procedure. This indirect estimate of the aided SSPL90 response in the real ear may be of particular benefit in children when clinicians need to avoid potential acoustic trauma exposure.

AMPLIFICATION IN EDUCATIONAL SETTINGS

The primary concern for hearing aids on children in an educational setting is that the amplification devices function properly. Numerous studies have verified that hearing aids worn by children in schools are often malfunctioning, thereby providing limited or no auditory input for educational purposes (Northern, McChord, Fischer, & Evans, 1972; Zink, 1972). In spite of the availability of hearing aid monitoring information for classroom teachers (Potts & Greenwood, 1983), a recent study reported that teachers of hearing-impaired students believe that hearing aid malfunctions seldom occur, even though on-site data confirm that significant hearing aid problems are actually a common occurrence (Elfenbein, Bentler, Davis, & Niebuhr, 1988). Accordingly, each hearing aid worn by a child must be conscientiously monitored by everyone concerned — the parents, the teacher, the audiologist, and the child.

The use of amplification in the educational setting has been carefully scrutinized over the years due to the inherent problems of signal-to-noise ratio and reverberation in the classroom. The enactment of Public Law 94–142, the Education for All Handicapped Children's Act of 1975, resulted in increasing numbers of hearing-impaired children being mainstreamed into regular classrooms. The classroom environments include rooms that, for the most part, are designed with little attention to the problems of reverberation. These school facilities include the gymnasium, the assembly hall, the auditorium, and the open classroom. Finitzo-Hieber and Tillman (1978) demonstrated that reverberation times as short as 0.4 s adversely affect speech intelligibility for normal-hearing and hearing-impaired children. They also demonstrated that hearing-impaired students are more sensitive to the masking effects of noise than normal hearing students. According to Gengel (1971), a minimum signal-to-noise (S/N) ratio of +15 to +20 dB is necessary for hearing-impaired students to achieve maximum aided speech intelligibility. There is no doubt that everything possible should be done to reduce reverberations and to improve the S/N ratio in classrooms (Olsen, 1981). Overcoming poor classroom acoustics is an important consideration in the successful use of amplification by hearing-impaired children.

However, the easiest and best means of dealing with such problems often is through the use of FM amplification systems. The issue of which type of amplification system is most effective in eliminating these problems and in allowing the hearing-impaired student maximum educational success has been continually questioned. The types of traditional auditory training systems available include the hardwire system, the portable desk system, the loop induction system, the loop radio frequency system, the freefield (wireless) FM system, and the infrared system. All of these systems have the advantage of significantly reducing interference from reverberation and S/N ratios. However, their effectiveness has been criticized because the child is required to take off the hearing aids while the auditory training system is in place.

In an effort to allow students the use of their own hearing aids while still reducing the effects of reverberation and poor S/N characteristics of the classrooms, personal FM systems have become the choice of many school systems in recent years. The output, gain, and frequency response of the personal FM unit is dependent on the electroacoustic response of the personal hearing aids. A transmitter is worn by the speaker and a receiver is worn by the hearing-impaired individual. The hearing aids are coupled to the system by either direct audio input, neck loop, or silhouette. For many hearing-impaired students, this may be truly the "least restrictive environment."

Hawkins (1984) demonstrated that the FM advantage over a personal hearing aid was equivalent to a +15 dB improvement in S/N ratio in children with mild-to-moderate hearing impairment, and according to Steighner (1986), children in the mild-moderate hearing loss range have become more frequent users of FM classroom systems. Bess, Clee, and Culbertson (1986) successfully used FM systems with some children with unilateral hearing impairments. The goal is to reduce the adverse effects from poor S/N ratios, which affect children with unilateral losses more than normal hearing children.

Hawkins (1987b) described a procedure to measure the real-ear performance of an FM system using a probe microphone, ear canal technique. The procedure permits a rapid comparison of the real-ear hearing aid response and the real-ear response of the FM system. With the probe tube in the ear canal, measurements are made of the hearing aid alone with a 60 dB SPL input. Then the FM system is attached to the hearing aid (with the FM microphone attached next to the compression microphone of the real-ear system) and evaluated with an 80 dB SPL input to account for the higher input level created by an approximate 6-inch difference between the speaker's mouth and the FM microphone. Hawkins warned that the use of sweep frequency pure tones or warble tones in these measurements may compromise the accuracy of the frequency response in the low frequencies, and therefore recommended the use of bands of noise representing the aided long-term speech spectrum as input stimuli.

ALTERNATIVES TO TRADITIONAL AMPLIFICATION

Unfortunately, not every profoundly hearing-impaired child who is fitted with hearing aids benefits from them. What are the options for these children who exhibit no awareness to sound with hearing aids? What do we do with the young child who has had intensive auditory training, excellent family support, and appropriate hearing aid fittings for one year, but demonstrates no behavioral differences with or without hearing aids? There are some options available for this population. Tactile aids or cochlear implants should be considered for children who fail to benefit from hearing aids. The question is: Can the tactile aid provide optimal benefit without the risk of surgery and the higher cost of the cochlear implant?

Tactile Aids

Tactile aids consist of auditory signals that are changed into either vibratory or electrical patterns on the skin. The vibrotactile approach presents a vibration to the skin through a bone conduction vibrator, a small solenoid, or other mechanical transducer. The electrotactile approach presents the acoustic signal through the skin via an electrical current. As Roeser (1985) described it, "the goal of a tactile communication system is to extract relevant information from the acoustic signal and to present it to the individual in a tactile mode as a means of supplementing or replacing the auditory reception of the acoustic signal, with the successful reception of speech as the ultimate challenge."

Vibrotactile devices have been preferred over electrotactile due to the availability of vibrators and difficulties of applying an electrical current to the skin. Vibrotactile devices, however, have poor frequency response and high-power requirements. They also generate harmonic frequencies that produce an audible distraction to hearing persons. The high power requirements of vibrotactile aids have kept efficient wearable units off the market (Roeser, 1985).

Saunders, Hill, and Easley (1978), developed the Teletactor, a two-channel device that electrically stimulated the forehead. Later development of the Teletactor provided stimulation to the abdomen with 32 electrodes. Saunders and colleagues reported that extended use of the device showed no adverse effects from using electrical current to the skin and that intensity level was not influenced by perspiration. Sparks, Kuhl, Edmonds, and Gray (1978) developed the Multipoint Electrotactile Speech Aid (MESA) with 288 electrodes in a 36×8 array presented to the abdomen. They reported no side effects of pain or any other adverse reaction. Sachs, Miller, and Grant (1980) compared vibrotactile and electrotactile devices. Vibrotactile devices were more efficient in lower frequencies and electrotactile devices were more efficient in higher frequencies.

Investigations into the effect of tactile aids on speech production are encouraging. Goldstein and Stark (1976) analyzed consonant–vowel (CV) syllables of four profoundly deaf children using tactile, visual, and nonspeech displays. There was a significant increase in CV production in both the tactile and visual groups, while the control group demonstrated no significant change. Oller, Payne, and Gavin (1980) reported that several of their subjects demonstrated improvement in pronunciation of fricative and nasal consonants with tactile aid use. Friel-Patti and Roeser (1985) reported that their subjects increased vocalization and sign language with the vibrotactile aid and decreased vocalization and sign language without the tactile aid.

Cochlear Implants

A colloquium held in 1985 established minimum patient selection criteria for cochlear implants in children (Northern, 1986b). The recommended guidelines include a minimum age of 2 years; bilateral, profound, or total sensorineural deafness; completion of all pre-evaluation procedures; intelligence at least within normal limits; no additional handicaps that might adversely affect potential success with implant (such as autism or significant learning disabilities; strong evidence of family support; and team decision that satisfactory progress in auditory development is not being made despite effective training and appropriately fitted hearing aids. The colloquium also proposed a potential-for-success hierarchy with respect to the onset of profound, bilateral deafness, the duration of auditory deprivation, and the type of educational training the candidate has.

At the time of this writing, cochlear implants in children are still considered to be in the research stage. Only two cochlear implant devices have been approved by the Food and Drug Administration (FDA) for clinical investigation in children: The 3M/House cochlear implant was approved in 1981 by the FDA for children 2 years of age and older, and the Nucleus 22 device was approved by the FDA in 1986 for implantation in children at least 10 years of age.

MANAGEMENT OF THE HEARING-IMPAIRED CHILD

Medical Management

The medical evaluation of children with hearing impairment must be viewed as a critical prerequisite to the selection of amplification. Medical management includes determination of etiology of the hearing impairment, consideration for medical or surgical remediation when possible, and continued surveillance for middle ear dysfunction (Pappas, 1985). Medical management should be an ongoing process involving input from a wide range of medical specialists including geneticists, pediat-

ricians, otologists, radiologists, and others, as needed. The medical team often plays an important role in parental understanding and acceptance of the child's hearing impairment. The identification of specific syndromes or other significant health problems may influence the recommendations made by other professionals. For example, if the etiology of the hearing loss is attributed to intrauterine cytomegalovirus disease (CMV), progressive change in hearing sensitivity may be expected for several months; when opticochleodentate degeneration is identified, the progressive sensorineural hearing loss is accompanied by progressive visual loss and eventual blindness, which will significantly shape the audiologic, habilitative, and amplification recommendations for the child.

Consideration for possible medical or surgical intervention should be part of the otologic clearance obtained prior to selecting amplification for any child. It would be a disaster to fit hearing aids on a child whose hearing could be improved or returned to normal with medical intervention. With some potentially surgically correctable hearing losses, such as bilateral atresia, hearing aids are recommended until, when and if, surgical intervention is attempted and is successful.

The need for continued medical surveillance for middle ear dysfunction and progressive hearing loss is especially critical for children with hearing loss. Therefore, parents and professionals must be cognizant of the need for medical monitoring of the hearing-impaired child every 6 months until the age of 6 years. Routine medical management will take full advantage of improvements in techniques for treating deafness, such as improved versions of implantable hearing aids (Hough, Himelick, & Johnson, 1986).

Parent Management

The importance of parental involvement in the diagnostic and habilitative process of hearing-impaired children is crucial to the child's success with amplification. Unfortunately, there are no specific guidelines that can be followed when dealing with parents. Every child's parents have unique needs and must be dealt with on an individual basis. The parents' relationship with the audiologist begins with the first audiologic evaluation because it is often the audiologist who confirms that the child has hearing-impairment. Psychological reactions to crisis have been well documented by Shontz (1967), and he provided a useful model for the professional in recognizing the stages of parental reaction to the diagnosis. Lutterman (1979) described different counseling approaches and how the audiologist can help parents to cope with their child's special needs. He emphasized that the parents, not the professional, must make the decisions regarding their child's habilitation because they must take ultimate responsibility. For example, parents must accept and understand the need for amplification before hearing aids can be successfully placed on a hearing-impaired infant or child.

Once hearing aids have been recommended and selected, it is important for the parents to observe the child's aided and unaided responses in a sound-field situation to see for themselves that their child benefits from using personal amplification. This exercise helps establish realistic expectations from the parents, which are so important to habilitation of the hearing-impaired child. The parents must understand that, although personal amplification benefits their child greatly, hearing aids do not provide normal hearing.

Parental education is a continuing process. The initial stages of hearing aid fitting is a critical time for the exchange of accurate and complete information. Topics to be discussed with the parents include the advantages and limitations of hearing aid use, the importance of daily listening checks, guidelines for trouble shooting, the potential health hazards of battery ingestion, the initial adjustment to amplification, and the importance of close audiologic monitoring. The parents must understand that hearing aid selection and fitting in small children is always subject to change and that decisions are often tentative until complete information is available concerning the audiometric configuration of the child's hearing loss.

Of course, most information regarding use, care, and troubleshooting of hearing aids is the same for the pediatric and adult populations. Specific topic areas, such as initial adjustment to amplification, are unique to children and are usually age-related. According to Ross (1980), the initial adjustment period may be more of a problem for the parents rather than the hearing-impaired child. With small children, parents must learn to take control of when the hearing aids are worn rather than letting the child take the hearing aids off at will.

The audiologist's role in parental management has a significant impact on the overall management of a child with hearing loss. That role should include education, guidance, and counseling, since the *parents' attitude regarding amplification* may be the single most important factor in successful hearing aid use by the hearing-impaired child.

REFERENCES

Bergstrom, L. (1976). Congenital deafness. In J. Northern (Ed.), *Hearing disorders.* Boston: Little, Brown.

Bess, F. H., Clee, J. C., & Culbertson, J. C. (1986). Identification, assessment and management of children with unilateral sensorineural hearing loss. *Ear and Hearing, 7*(1), 43–51.

Binnie, C. A. (1985). Effects of amplification on the residual hearing of children. *Seminars in Hearing, 6*(3), 299–307.

Byrne, D. (1987). Hearing aid selection formulae: Same or different? *Hearing Instruments, 38*(1), 5–11.

Byrne, D., & Tonisson, W. (1976). Selecting the gain of hearing aids for persons with sensorineural hearing impairments. *Scandinavian Audiology, 5,* 51–59.

Cooper, J., Langley, L., Meyerhoff, W., & Gates, G. (1977). The significance of negative middle ear pressure. *Laryngoscope, 87,* 92–97.

Cox, L. C., & Metz, D. A. (1980). ABER in the prescription of hearing aids. *Hearing Instruments, 31,* 12–15, 55.

Curran, J. R. (1985). ITE aids for children: Survey of attitudes and practices of audiologists. *Hearing Instruments, 36*(4), 20–26.

Curran, J. R. (1988). Hearing aids. In N. Lass, L. McReynolds, J. Northern, & D. Yoder (Eds.), *Handbook of speech-language pathology and audiology* (pp. 1293–1314). Toronto: B. C. Decker.

Davis, J. W., & Mueller, H. G. (1987). Hearing aid selection. In H. G. Mueller & V. C. Geoffrey (Eds.), *Communication disorders in aging: Assessment and management* (pp. 408–436). Washington, DC: Gallaudet University Press.

Elfenbein, J. L., Bentler, R. A., Davis, J. M., & Niebuhr, D. P. (1988). Status of school children's hearing aids relative to monitoring practices. *Ear and Hearing, 9*(4), 212–217.

Finitzo-Hieber, T., & Tillman, T. W. (1978). Room acoustic effects on monosyllabic word discrimination ability for normal and hearing-impaired children. *Journal of Speech and Hearing Research, 21,* 440–448.

Friel-Patti, S., & Roeser, R. (1985). Evaluating changes in the communication skills of deaf children using vibrotactile stimulation. *Ear and Hearing, 4,* 31–40.

Gengel, R. W. (1971). Acceptable speech-to-noise ratios for aided speech discrimination by the hearing impaired. *Journal of Auditory Research, 11,* 219–222.

Gengel, R. W., Pascoe, D., & Shore, I. (1971). A frequency response procedure for evaluating and selecting hearing aids for severely hearing-impaired children. *Journal of Speech and Hearing Disorders, 36,* 341–353.

Goldstein, M. H., & Stark, R. (1976). Modifications of vocalizations of pre-school deaf children by vibrotactile and visual displays. *Journal of the Acoustical Society of America, 59,* 1477–1481.

Gwyn, R. D. (Ed.). (1988). Hearing aid fittings. *Seminars in Hearing, 9*(3), 167–251.

Hall, J. W., & Ruth, R. A. (1986). Acoustic reflexes and auditory evoked responses in hearing aid evaluation. *Seminars in Hearing, 6*(3), 251–277.

Hawkins, D. (1982). Overamplification: A well-documented case report. *Journal of Speech and Hearing Disorders, 47,* 376–382.

Hawkins, D. B. (1984). Comparisons of speech recognition in noise by children using hearing aids and FM systems. *Journal of Speech and Hearing Disorders, 49,* 409–418.

Hawkins, D. B. (1987a). Clinical ear canal probe tube measurements. *Ear and Hearing, 85,* 74–81.

Hawkins, D. B. (1987b). Assessment of FM systems with an ear canal probe tube microphone system. *Ear and Hearing, 8*(5), 301–303.

Heffernan, H., & Simons, M. (1979). Temporary increase in sensorineural hearing loss with hearing aid use. *Annals of Otology, Rhinology and Laryngology, 88,* 86–91.

Hough, J., Himelick, R., & Johnson, B. (1986). Implantable bone conduction hearing device: Audiant bone conductor. *Annals of Otology, Rhinology and Laryngology, 95,* 498–504.

Humes, L. E. (1986). An evaluation of several rationales for selecting hearing aid gain. *Journal of Speech and Hearing Disorders, 51,* 272–281.

Humes, L. E., & Bess, F. (1981). Tutorial on the potential deterioration in hearing due to hearing aid usage. *Journal of Speech and Hearing Research, 46,* 3–15.

Jerger, J. (1987). On the evaluation of hearing aid performance. *Asha, 29*(9), 49–51.

Jerger, J., & Lewis, N. (1975). Binaural hearing aids: Are they dangerous for children? *Archives of Otolaryngology, 101,* 480–483.

Jerger, S., Jerger, J., & Fahad, R. (1985). Pediatric hearing aid evaluation: Case reports. *Ear and Hearing, 6*(5), 240–244.

Jerger, S., Jerger, J., & Lewis, S. (1981) Pediatric speech intelligibility test: II. Effect of receptive language age and chronological age. *International Journal of Pediatric Otorhinolaryngology, 3,* 101–118.

Jerger, S., Lewis, S., Hawkins, J., et al. (1980). Pediatric speech intelligibility: I. Generation of test materials. *International Journal of Pediatric Otorhinolaryngology, 2,* 217–230.

Kiessling, J. (1982). Hearing aid selection by brainstem audiometry. *Scandinavian Audiology, 11,* 269–275.

Killion, M. (1982). Transducers, earmolds and sound quality considerations. In G. Studebaker & F. Bess (Eds.), *The Vanderbilt hearing aid report: Monographs in contemporary audiology* (pp. 104–111). Upper Darby, PA.

Kruger, B. (1987). An update on the external ear resonance in infants and young children. *Ear and Hearing, 8*(6), 333–336.

Lewis, N. (1985). Behavioral assessment technique for the selection of hearing aids in children. *Seminars in Hearing, 6*(3), 239–245.

Libby, E. R. (1982). In search of transparent insertion gain hearing aid responses. In G. Studebaker & F. Bess (Eds.), *The Vanderbilt hearing aid report: Monographs in contemporary audiology* (pp. 112–123). Upper Darby, PA.

Libby, E. R. (1987). Real ear considerations in hearing aid selection. *Hearing Instruments, 38*(1), 14–16.

Lutterman, D. (1979). *Counseling parents of hearing-impaired children.* Boston: Little, Brown.

Mahoney, T. (1985). Auditory brainstem response hearing aid applications. In J. Jacobson (Ed.). *The auditory brainstem response* (Chap. 19). Boston: College-Hill Press.

Matkin, N. (1984). Wearable amplification: A litany of persisting problems. In J. Jerger (Ed.), *Pediatric audiology.* Boston: College-Hill Press.

Matkin, N. D. (1986). Hearing aids for children. In W. R. Hodgson (Ed.), *Hearing aid assessment and use in audiologic habilitation* (3rd ed., pp. 170–190). Baltimore: Williams & Wilkins.

McCandless, G., & Miller, D. (1972). Loudness discomfort and hearing aids. *National Hearing Aid Journal, 25,* 7–32.

Mills, J. H. (1975). Noise and children: A review of the literature. *Journal of the Acoustical Society of America, 58,* 767–779.

Mueller, H. G. (1986). Binaural amplification: Attitudinal factors. *Hearing Journal, 39*(11), 7–10.

Norris, T., Jirsa, R., & Skinner, B. (1977). *The effect of pressure on pure tone thresholds.* Read before the annual meeting of the American Audiology Society, Miami, FL.

Northern, J. L. (1986). Selection of children for cochlear implantation. *Seminars in Hearing, 7*(4), 341–347.

Northern, J. (1988). Recent developments in acoustic immittance measurements with children. In F. H. Bess (Ed.), *Hearing impairment in children* (pp. 176–189). Parkton, MD: York Press.

Northern, J., & Downs, M. (1984). *Hearing in children* (3rd ed.). Baltimore: Williams & Wilkins.

Northern J. L., McChord, W., Jr., Fischer, E., & Evans, P. (1972). Hearing services in residential schools for the deaf. *Maico Audiological Library Series, 11,* 4.

Oller, D. K., Payne, S. L., & Gavin, W. J. (1980). Tactual speech perception by minimally trained deaf subjects. *Journal of Speech and Hearing Research, 23,* 769–778.

Olsen, W. O. (1981). The effects of noise and reverberation on speech intelligibility. In F. Bess, B. Freeman, & C. Sinclair (Eds.), *Amplification in education* (pp. 151–163). Washington, DC: Alexander Graham Bell.

Olsen, W. O., Hawkins, D. B., & Van Tasell, D. J. (1987). Representations of the long-term spectra of speech. *Ear and Hearing, 8*(5), 100S–108S.

Pappas, D. (1985). *Diagnosis and treatment of hearing impairment in children.* Boston: College-Hill Press.

Potts, P., & Greenwood, J. (1983). Hearing aid monitoring. *Language, Speech and Hearing Services in Schools, 14,* 163.

Rappaport, B., & Tait, C. (1976). Acoustic reflex threshold measurement in hearing aid selection. *Archives of Otolaryngology, 102*(3), 129–132.

Rines, D., Stelmachowicz, P., & Gorga, M. (1984). An alternate method for determining functional gain of hearing aids. *Journal of Speech and Hearing Research, 27*(4), 627–633.

Rintelmann, W. F., & Bess, F. H. (1977). High-level amplification and potential hearing loss in children. In F. H. Bess (Ed.), *Childhood deafness: Causation, assessment and management* (pp. 267–293). New York: Grune & Stratton.

Rintelmann, W. F., & Bess, F. H. (1988). High-level amplification and potential hearing loss. In F. H. Bess (Ed.), *Hearing impairment in children* (pp. 278–309). Parkton, MD: York Press.

Roeser, R. J. (1985). Tactile aids for the profoundly deaf. *Seminars in Hearing, 6*(3), 279–298.

Ross, M. (1980). Binaural versus monaural hearing aid amplification for hearing impaired individuals. In E. R. Libby, *Binaural hearing and amplification* (Vol. 2). Chicago: Zenetron.

Ross, M., & Seewald, R. C. (1988). Hearing aid selection and evaluation with young children. In F. Bess (Ed.), *Hearing impairment in children* (pp. 190–213). Parkton, MD: York Press.

Ross, M., & Tomassetti, C. (1980). Hearing aid selection for preverbal hearing-impaired children. In M. C. Pollack (Ed.), *Amplification for the hearing impaired* (2nd ed., pp. 213–253). New York: Grune & Stratton.

Rubin, M. (1980). Management of amplification for infants. *Seminars in Speech, Language and Hearing, 1,* 231–237.

Sachs, R. M., Miller, J. D., & Grant, K. (1980). Perceived magnitude of electroacoustic pulses. *Perceptual Psychophysics, 28,* 255–262.

Saunders, F. A. (1973). An electrotactile sound detector for the deaf. *IEEE Transactions of Audio and Electroacoustics, 21,* 285–287.

Schwartz, D. M. (1982). Hearing aid selection: An enigma. In G. A. Studebaker & F. H. Bess (Eds.), *The Vanderbilt hearing aid report: Monographs in contemporary audiology* (pp. 180–187). Upper Darby, PA.

Schwartz, D. M., & Larson, V. D. (1977). A comparison of three hearing aid evaluation procedures for young children. *Archives of Otolaryngology, 103,* 401–406.

Seewald, R. C. (1988). The desired sensational level approach for children: Selection and verification. *Hearing Instruments, 39*(7), 18–20.

Seewald, R. C., & Ross, M. (1988). Amplification for young hearing-impaired children. In M. C. Pollack (Ed.), *Amplification for the hearing-impaired* (3rd ed., pp. 213–267). New York: Grune & Stratton.

Seewald, R. C., Ross, M., & Spiro, M. K. (1985). Selecting amplification characteristics for young hearing-impaired children. *Ear and Hearing, 6*(1), 48–53.

Shah, C. P., Chandler, D., & Dale, R. (1978). Delay in referral of children with impaired hearing. *Volta Review, 80,* 207.

Shontz, F. (1967). Reactions to crisis. *Volta Review, 69,* 405–411.

Silman, S., Gelfand, S., & Silverman, C. (1984). Late-onset auditory deprivation: Effects of monaural versus binaural hearing aids. *Journal of the Acoustical Society of America, 76*(5), 1357–1362.

Simmons, F. B. (1980). Diagnosis and rehabilitation of deaf newborns, Part II. *Asha, 22,* 475.

Sparks, D., Kuhl, P., Edmonds, A., & Gray, G. (1978). Investigating the MESA (Multipoint Electrotactile Speech Aid): The transmission of segmental features of speech. *Journal of the Acoustical Society of America, 63,* 246–257.

Steighner, R. L. (1986, Fall). FM: An innovative perspective. *Rocky Mountain Journal of Communication Disorders, 2,* 12–14.

Stelmachowicz, P. G., Larson, L. L., Johnson, D. E., & Moeller, M. P. (1985). Clinical model for the audiologic management of hearing-impaired children. *Seminars in Hearing, 6*(3), 223–237.

Sullivan, J.A., Levitt, H., Hwang, J. Y., & Hennessey, A. M. (1988). An experimental comparison of four hearing aid prescription methods. *Ear and Hearing, 9*(1), 22–32.

Sullivan, R. F. (1987). Aided SSPL 90 response in the real ear: A safe estimate. *Hearing Instruments, 38*(10), 36.

Upfold, L. J. (1988). Children with hearing aids in the 1980s: Etiologies and severity of impairment. *Ear and Hearing, 9*(2), 75–80.

Wilson, W., & Thompson, G. (1984). Behavioral audiometry. In J. Jerger (Ed.), *Pediatric audiology* (pp. 1–44). Boston: College-Hill Press.

Zink, G. D. (1972). Hearing aids children wear: A longitudinal study of performance. *Volta Review, 74,* 41–51.

6

CONSIDERATIONS FOR THE SELECTING AND FITTING OF AMPLIFICATION FOR GERIATRIC ADULTS

ROBERT E. NOVAK ■

ARAM GLORIG ■

The process of aging can be divided into three related fields: biologic aging, the physiologic changes that occur at all levels of the individual organism and in all of its functions; psychologic aging, the age-related changes that occur in the behavior of the individual (i.e., perceiving, feeling, thinking, acting, and reacting); and social aging, the changing roles of the individual in society as a result of age-related biologic and psychologic changes.

In establishing a clinical procedure for the evaluation, selection, and fitting of hearing aid devices for the elderly, as well as in creating an effective patient management strategy, the audiologist or the dispenser must be conversant with the processes of aging. Unique skills and sensitivity are required to recognize the differences between geriatric patients and other people who need hearing aid amplification. The elderly often undergo biologic, physiologic, and psychologic changes at acceler-ated rates compared to younger popula-tions. These changes in function present constant challenges to professionals who not only make decisions regarding appro-priate hearing aid function but also provide follow-up care in which changes in per-formance may require modification of the instrument's output characteristics as well as alteration of counseling strategies.

This chapter offers an analysis of age-related changes in the hope that an ex-panded awareness of these changes will create an appreciation of the dynamics as-sociated with hearing aid utilization in the elderly population. The chapter is not intended to be an exhaustive analysis of the physiologic or neurologic changes that ac-company aging. However, specific changes and their probable etiologies and behav-ioral consequences are discussed to the ex-tent that such information may add to the knowledge of professionals working with the amplification needs of older persons.

Similarly, this chapter presents a sociological and psychological perspective of aging to better acquaint the reader with the unique dynamics often found in the aging population. Awareness of these processes leads to a more informed approach to ameliorating problems often identified with older hearing-impaired individuals.

The first part of this chapter is concerned in part with the aging process in the auditory system. Technically, this is defined as hearing loss due to biologic and physiologic changes that are strictly a function of the cell and its organisms. It is impossible to extract age-related cellular changes from changes facilitated by the addition of environmental stressors (e.g., noise, disease, iatrogenesis). The fact that one ages physiologically and biologically also means that there are effects of changing environments over the aging period. Any study of aging and its effects must assume that the effects that are found are a combination of intrinsic biologic factors and extrinsic environmental factors. At best, the selection of amplification systems is not a simple task, and the probable effects of aging in the selection process should be evaluated.

PRESBYCUSIS

Pathologic Considerations

High-frequency hearing loss associated with aging was first described in 1891, as was the term presbycusis (Zwaardemaker, 1891). The original spelling was presbyacusis, however, presbycusis has become the preferred spelling. Pathologic studies have failed to identify anything pathognomonic of presbycusis. It appears to be a collection of different entities that occur in various combinations and affect the entire auditory system from the middle ear up to and including the central nervous system. There are predictable changes in function and such changes require special consideration in the evaluation, selection, and fitting of hearing aid devices.

If one looks at the external ear in the aged, one finds that it has become flabby, the earlobe has become larger and loose, and the ear canal has become quite flexible and has sometimes partially collapsed. These changes are due to changes in the elasticity of the skin as well as the cartilaginous framework. Cartilaginous changes introduce a special concern when fabricating the earmold impression. The obvious problem presented is that, in order to make an acceptable impression, one must manipulate the ear in a manner that permits a canal opening adequate to allow the finished earmold, in-the-ear aid (ITE) or canal aid to pass amplified sound from the hearing aid earphone through the canal bore of the earmold, ITE, or canal hearing aid and, subsequently, to the eardrum.

Insertion of the earmold or hearing aid device into the external canal may produce soreness or irritation at the canal opening due to the sensitivity of the canal tissue when pressure is applied by the physical presence of the earmold or the canal portion of a hearing aid. These cartilaginous changes are so pronounced for some geriatric patients that the entrance to the canal is extremely narrow.

When the earmold impression is taken, the opening to the canal must be of sufficient size to permit effective use of the earmold. While taking the impression of the external ear canal, the pinna must be manipulated so that the narrow entrance to the canal opening is expanded to permit the impression material to be introduced and a usable ear impression to be taken. Sometimes, in an effort to make the opening as favorable as possible in the ear impression process, too much pressure is exerted against the canal wall when the finished product is inserted. It is this constant pressure that creates soreness or irritation and subsequent rejection of the device if early resolution is not provided.

Similar changes may occur in the structures of the middle ear, with associated changes in the sound transmission characteristics of the ossicles. This was demonstrated by Nixon and Glorig (1962) in a study of air and bone conduction thresholds as a function of age. They found an air-bone gap at 4000 Hz in many 55 year and older individuals. Air-bone gaps also were discovered by Rosen, Bergman, Plester, El Mofty, and Sotti (1962) in their study of elderly members of the Mabaan tribe in rural Sudan.

Glorig and Davis (1961) reported that they believed that an air-bone gap of this kind could also be caused by an inner ear conductive hearing loss as the result of changes in the basilar partition of the inner ear. These changes, which include the lessening of elastic tissue and the stiffening of the remaining components, have been identified via microscopic analysis. It is unclear what, if any, role these air-bone gap phenomena play in the determination of the recommended frequency-intensity response characteristics of the hearing aid. Their presence may account for a higher than expected most comfortable listening level (MCL) at frequencies where air-bone gaps occur. Higher MCLs may translate into higher gain prescriptions for older adults who have these air-bone gaps compared to other older and younger clients who have similar air conduction thresholds but an absence of high frequency air-bone gaps.

Schuknecht (1974) described four types of inner ear loss in presbycusis: sensoripresbycusis, neuropresbycusis, striapresbycusis, and inner ear conductive presbycusis. Glorig and Davis (1961) suggested a similar classification based on their own theoretical constructs.

Sensoripresbycusis is characterized by slowly progressive, bilaterally symmetrical high-frequency sensorineural hearing loss, with good single syllable word identification. The primary histopathologic finding is an absence or reduction of hair cells, primarily in the basilar portion of the cochlea.

Neuropresbycusis is characterized by high frequency sensorineural hearing loss with poor single syllable word identification. Atrophy of the spiral ganglion and nerves of the osseous spiral lamina, mainly in the basal corridor, are the most consistent histopathologic finding with this type of presbycusis.

Striapresbycusis or *metabolic presbycusis* is characterized by a slowly progressive, flat, bilaterally symmetrical sensorineural hearing loss starting in the third through sixth decades. Single syllable word identification is good, and there is usually no recruitment. The pathophysiology of striapresbycusis is related to the atrophy of the stria vascularis and a general reduction in sensitivity of all hair cells due to the meta-bolic changes of the endolymph.

Inner ear conductive presbycusis has been suggested by several authors (Glorig & Davis, 1961; Mayer, 1970; Schuknecht, 1974). Schuknecht (1974) described changes in the cochlear ducts that cause changes in the mass, stiffness, and friction of the moving membranes, thus affecting the transmission of acoustic energy. Mayer (1970) described thickening and hyalinization of the basilar membrane and calcium deposits located mainly in the basal coil. He suggested that the aging process of the basilar membrane causes stiffness and decreased mobility. The hypothesis of functional hearing loss due to increased stiffness of the basilar membrane correlates with its anatomical shape. The basilar membrane is narrow and thin at the basal coil and wide and relatively thick at the apical turn. The basal portion of the basilar membrane is more prone to loss of elastic properties due to aging, thus accentuating hearing loss at the high frequencies.

Figures 6–1 through 6–6 are diagrammatic representations of pathology found in microscopic studies of the temporal bones in individuals over 65 years of age. They are accompanied by pure-tone air conduction audiograms and word identification scores obtained by using phonetically balanced (PB) words. The diagrammatic cochlea shows hair cell rows. Open circles indicate cells that are pathologic. Note the correlation with the dark areas in

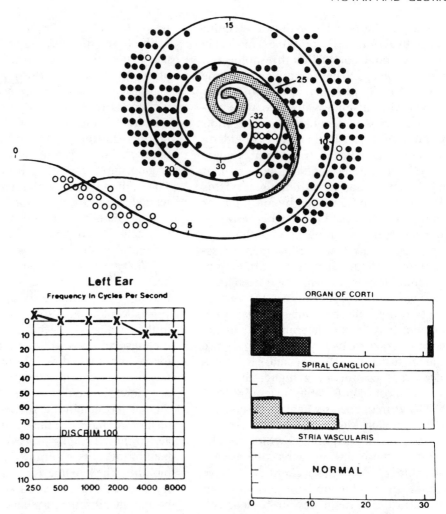

FIGURE 6-1. Pathology evident in a patient with primarily cochlear hair cell loss. Some damage also is evident in the spiral ganglia. Open circles indicate areas of hair cell loss.

the organ of Corti shown in the rectangles. Figures 6-1 and 6-2 show findings in patients with primarily cochlear pathology like that found with sensoripresbycusis. Figure 6-3 shows a patient with basal cochlear pathology and significant damage to the spiral ganglion. Note that, although pure-tone thresholds are normal through 2000 Hz, the PB score in quiet is only 82 percent.

Figure 6-4 shows more diffuse hair cell loss with spiral ganglion damage throughout the cochlea. These findings are consistent with the neuropresbycusis

classification. Note the very poor (55%) PB-word identification score and compare it to the relatively good identification score of 80 percent in Figure 6-2, which depicts similar pure-tone threshold results but minimal spiral ganglion damage (sensoripresbycusis).

Figure 6-5 depicts results consistent with the classification of striapresbycusis or metabolic presbycusis: minimum hair cell damage and spiral ganglion pathology but diffuse striavascularis abnormality. Note the excellent PB score (100%), which is consistent with this diagnostic classification.

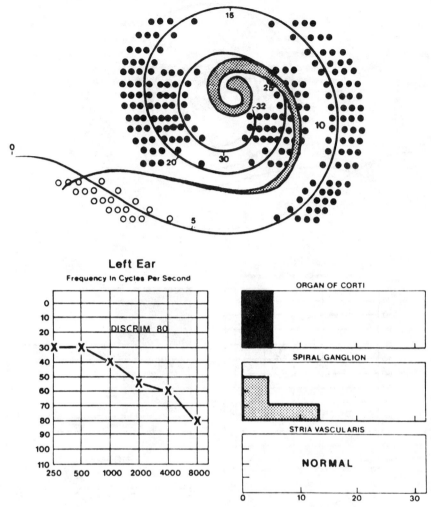

FIGURE 6–2. Pathology consistent with sensoripresbycusis. Open circles indicate areas of damage in the cochlea.

Figure 6–6 depicts the results obtained from a patient with diffuse damage of the organ of Corti, spiral ganglia, and stria vascularis (a combination of types of presbycusis). Note the very poor word identification score. Of all the patients described, certainly this individual would have the poorest prognosis for benefit from the use of hearing amplification.

Of significance, when one reviews Figures 6–1 through 6–6, is that conventional pure-tone audiometry, in terms of signal detection, most comfortable listening level, and tolerance discomfort thresholds, may

not provide enough information to predict the benefit to be expected in understanding intended verbal messages when hearing aid amplification is provided.

Although conventional word identification tests are suspect in ferreting out the best hearing aid device from among several choices, it is readily apparent that some form of speech or speech-like assessment is critical to the successful management of the aging patient. For example, the relatively low identification score show in Figure 6–4 may suggest that appreciable improvement in speech understanding over

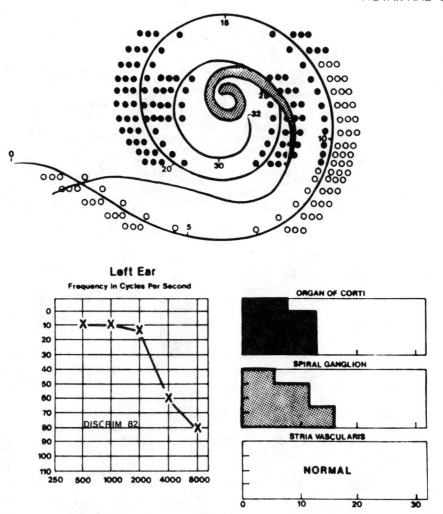

FIGURE 6–3. Pathology found in a patient with basal cochlear damage and marked changes in the spiral ganglion. Open circles show areas of cochlear damage.

time will not differ greatly from the measures obtained initially. Such an observation would have a profound effect on the counseling strategy devised to deal effectively with this patient as a result of the limitations imposed not only by the hearing aid but also by the auditory system itself.

Vasodilation is a common medical treatment for various inner ear diseases, including Meniere's, sudden hearing loss, tinnitus, and presbycusis. The dependence of the inner ear on a single-ended artery without cross circulation has led to speculation that vascular insufficiency may, in part, be

the cause of these inner ear disorders.

Further understanding of pathologic processes in the internal auditory canal that are responsible for inner ear vascular degeneration and neural loss was contributed by the excellent observations of Krmpotic-Nemanic (1971). She studied 2600 temporal bones of all ages and demonstrated an apposition of fibrous osteoid and bony material in the fundus of the internal auditory canal in the region of the spiral tract, beginning at the basal coil. This process reduced the diameter of the hole in the spiral tract through which nerve bundles

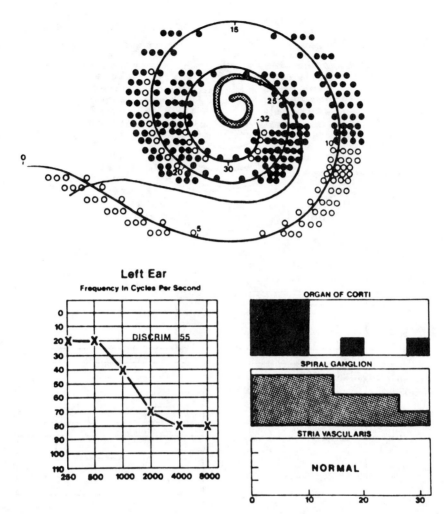

FIGURE 6–4. Pathologic findings for the patient shown indicate significant hair cell loss as well as spiral ganglion damage. Such findings are consistent with neuropresbycusis. Open circles indicate areas of damage in the cochlea.

cross from the inner ear to the internal auditory canal. For patients who exhibit severe cochlear-vascular changes, the hearing health care professional should be aware of the pronounced limitations imposed on the probable contributions of the hearing aid.

Extrinsic Etiologic Factors

Hearing loss in the aging ear is believed to be the end result of the cumu-

lative effects of various extrinsic factors in addition to genetically determined patterns of aging. There is a growing interest in environmental factors known to cause hearing loss that can be attenuated or eliminated as part of the overall efforts of hearing conservation.

Glorig and Nixon (1962) used the term *socioacusis* to describe the inevitable effects of daily, nonoccupational noise exposure. The hearing loss of aging, therefore, is the combined result of presbycusis (physio-

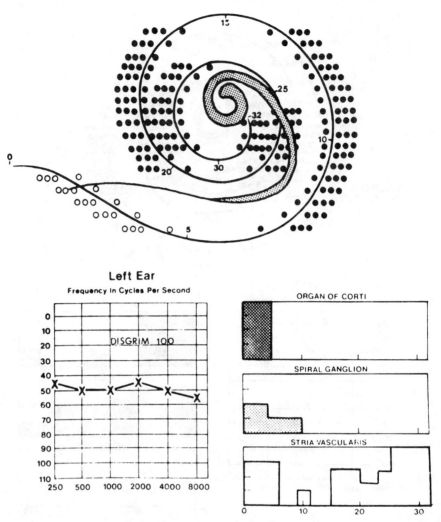

FIGURE 6–5. Hair cell loss consistent with striapresbycusis or metabolic presbycusis. Note the excellent word identification score. Open circles indicate areas of damage in the cochlea.

logic aging), socioacusis, and occupational noise.

Relation to Amplification

The end result of the many factors that cause hearing loss in the aged individual is multifaceted and highly complex. Some of these factors affect the application of amplification more than others. The primary biologic factor that limits adapting amplification to the aged ear is related to the pathol-

ogy in the inner ear. Pathology that affects the spiral ganglion causes the most difficulty in applying successful amplification. In general, in the absence of causes directly affecting the hair cells, such as noise and ototoxicity, the pathology of aging lies principally in the changes in the spiral ganglion and the neural elements that leave the calyces of the hair cells and proceed through the auditory nerve to the various stations in the midbrain and cortex.

The cochlea serves as (1) a coding mechanism in which the hair cells are the

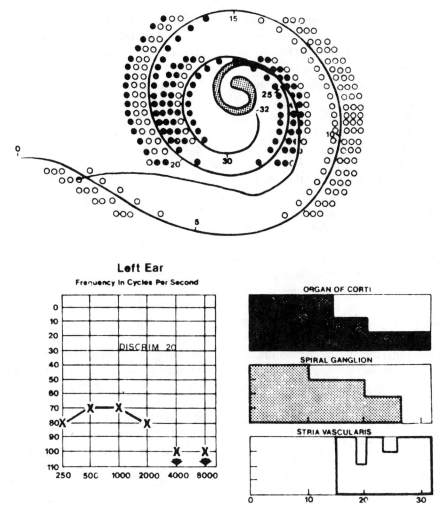

FIGURE 6-6. Pathology found in a patient with widely diffused damage of the organ of Corti, spiral ganglion, and stria vascularis. Note the poor word identification score for this patient. Cochlear hair cell loss is indicated by the open circles.

center of the coding system and (2) a processor of information, which is garnered by the hair cells and then transferred to the central nervous system by way of the neural elements.

In the case of abnormal first-order auditory neurons, the neural elements leaving the cochlea are reduced in their ability to process information. The decoding system, the central nervous system, thus receives sparse, poorly coded auditory information. In other words, the principal site of auditory processing is the neural system of

the cochlea. If this is faulty, it is difficult to build an extrinsic signal processor (hearing aid device) to correct it. The success of extrinsic signal processing is highly dependent on the degree of pathology in the spiral ganglion and the neural elements that transmit auditory information to the cortex. Differences in amplification results found in patients with similar test data may be explained by differences in cochlear pathology that are not apparent in the test data. In these cases, amplification can be compared to trying to use a public address system with a defective microphone by tailoring the input to the microphone so that the output of the system will be understandable. This has never been done successfully. Good public address systems depend on good microphones or transducers. Successful use of traditional hearing aids depends on a functioning cochlea, which is present in varying degrees in persons with various types of presbycusis.

In spite of this fact, hearing health professionals should not give up trying to apply amplification to older persons with hearing losses because, to date, there is no other alternative. Minimal improvement in speech understanding skills is better than no improvement. The challenge for clinicians is to develop assessment procedures that allow the most specific application of amplification to each older hearing-impaired client. To fully appreciate the magnitude of the problems related to the geriatric population and hearing aid use, practitioners should also be aware of the sociological and psychological factors peculiar to this population of individuals.

SOCIOLOGICAL AND PSYCHOLOGICAL PERSPECTIVES

In addition to changes in sensory and neural processes, aging may be accompanied by modifications in adjustment strategies, problem solving capacities, emotional states, perception, and memory (Mauldin, 1976). These changes are not consistent across the elderly population and may also vary as a function of race and culture. The focus of this portion of the chapter is on the relationship these modifications have to the rehabilitation of hearing loss and specifically to the successful fitting of amplification devices in elderly populations.

Successful utilization of amplification by the geriatric population is dependent on a number of factors including the magnitude of loss in threshold sensitivity, reduced tolerance for loud sounds, and the subsequent reduction in word identification skills. Although a large percentage of hearing aid candidates have these problems, many hearing health professionals are not fully aware of other age-related factors that contribute to acceptance and use of amplification systems. Therefore, some of the behaviors manifested by the elderly are reviewed here and their importance in the consideration of hearing aid use is assessed.

Cultural influences, coupled with the aging process and the changes that accompany it, are often major determinants of the elderly adult's behavior. Social, physical, and economic conditions also may affect attitudes, assessment of need, and ability to afford hearing aid use and care in the face of other, sometimes more pressing, economic realities. The need for hearing amplification is a physical reality. The use and acceptance of any amplification system, however, is tempered by a number of other concerns.

The stereotype of the elderly as physically feeble, severely hearing impaired, partially sighted, and demented fits less than three percent of the aged population. This stereotype would be true if survival to the maximum life span of 110 years was typical (Eisenberg, 1985). Aging can be viewed as both positive and negative, as growth and decline (Birren, Imus, & Windle, 1959; Gottlieb, 1983).

Higher neurologic functions are often largely preserved in normal aging (Posner, 1982). For example, self-esteem scores of older persons living independently in the community have been found to be nearly double those of high school students (Atchley, 1983). However, older individuals admitted to retirement homes have been found to have more latent pathology than elderly subjects who remain in the community (Busse, 1965).

Seeking help for hearing loss is influenced by economic constraints. The U.S.

Department of Commerce (1975) reported that one in six persons over 65 years of age lives in poverty versus one in 10 under the age of 65 years. Maulding (1976) observed that certain consequences of aging present problems because they directly impact on the older person's consumer needs. Digestive and metabolic changes may require changed diets. Changes in sensory processes, such as eyesight and hearing, may require eyeglasses and hearing aids; physical disabilities may require medical services, medical products, and institutionalization. The hearing health care professional must determine whether the hearing loss is considered a problem by the aged individual and, if it is a problem, where the remediation of hearing loss fits into the older person's priorities of consumer needs. Elderly hearing aid candidates may be ill, poor, without resources, and surrounded by people who avoid them. They are often described as rigid, conservative, cautious, and uncertain. However, as Gelfand (1982) has stated, these characteristics may be cohort effects related to how individuals were parented and their struggle to achieve security as first- or second-generation Americans. Subsequent generations of elderly individuals may have improved quality of health care, better nutrition, higher long-term socioeconomic status, and better educational level thus influencing these characteristics.

Cultural Considerations

In American culture, if one can generalize, the aged often have not been given, or allowed to assume the esteemed role given to elders in some other societies (e.g., China). Rather, they are often treated with impatience and patronization. Approximately 6 percent reside in extended care facilities. For a significant subset of the older Americans, as their life expectancy increases, they are given less reason to live (Parenti, 1978). Chinese psychiatrist Wer

Chen-1 contended that depression in the elderly is found more often in western cultures because "the west extrudes older citizens, they lose place in the family, industry, community, their sphere of influence collapses as does their morale, leaving them vulnerable to disability and disease" (Greenblat & Chien, 1983). When hearing loss exists in the older American client, great potential for depression and low morale must be assessed as possible etiologies of a lack of desire to communicate and to pursue use of amplification and aural rehabilitation.

It is very difficult to make generalizations about older Americans due to the ethnic diversity of the population in the United States and the existence of relatively pure ethnic and cultural subgroups, such as Asians, native Americans, and "neighborhood" Hispanics and blacks. The sociological ramifications of group membership, sexual differences, and educational and economic levels in each of these subcultures relative to hearing help-seeking behaviors of their older members are complex and should be assessed. For example, Cheng (1988, interview) described three subgroups of Asians in America: new immigrants; refugees, including those from Indochina, Vietnam, Laos, and Cambodia; and second-generation Asian-Americans.

New immigrants are defined as people who came to the United States as young people after 1950. If they have hearing problems, they are the most likely to seek help. Refugees may rely on remedies from nontraditional health care providers for various ailments, including hearing loss. There are many sheltered, protected, and isolated older people in this subgroup who do not speak English and who live with their extended families. Barriers to the pursuit of hearing health care and hearing aid use in this group include:

- Fear of American culture
- Illiteracy in their own language and lack of knowledge of English
- Lack of knowledge of available help

■ Psychological maladjustment to life in the United States

The third subgroup is American-born Asians. Cheng described two subgroups within this group. The "Chinatown ghetto" group whose members are born, raised, and never leave the Chinatown area is limited in its understanding of hearing problems and in access to audiologic services. On the other hand, individuals who left Chinatown early and established their own life-styles typically have their own English-speaking physicians and may seek help if they have a hearing problem.

For all groups, Asian cultural themes affect behavior in response to significant hearing loss. A general Asian belief that aging is a natural process that does not require intervention is common. In Asian cultures, for example, the young show respect for hearing-impaired aged by either speaking loudly or nodding to the elder during conversation, even when they cannot hear or understand the speech. In this case the elders may not feel a need to improve communication because they are consistently acknowledged during family conversations. If they purchase a hearing aid and it does not work satisfactorily, they will simply not wear it rather than seek confrontation. When asked if a problem exists, they will deny it ("How can the audiologist or the dispenser be wrong? It must be me"). Cheng (1988) asserted that these problems will not subside through acculturation in the forseeable future because increasing numbers of immigrants from Hong Kong and mainland China are expected in the coming decades. Culturally specific issues related to hearing help-seeking behaviors and application of amplification devices in all ethnic subgroups of the American population demand further investigation.

Demographics

Hearing impairment ranks second only to arthritis (Maurer & Rupp, 1979) as a chronic disability affecting the aged. In 1971 the American Speech and Hearing Association reported that at least 2.5 million U.S. citizens over the age of 65 years had significant bilateral hearing loss (Alpiner, 1982). Of persons 65 years and over with bilateral hearing loss, 7.2 percent had onset of loss before 21 years of age. Of that 7.2 percent, 10.2 percent could at best hear shouted speech unaided, and 4.8 percent could hear normal conversational speech. The remainder had varying degrees of difficulty understanding speech (Gentile, 1971). Persons over 70 years of age represent only 5.2 percent of the hearing population, but 30.2 percent of the population with hearing loss. Forty-nine percent of the total population with serious hearing loss (able to hear only shouted speech unaided) are over 70 years of age (Feller, 1981). Ries (1982) examined the hearing ability of older persons as a function of the sociodemographic characteristics of sex, race, family income, and level of education. Table 6–1 summarizes his findings for persons over the age of 64 years.

McCartney (1977) found that 84 percent of nursing home residents in a Sacramento study had significant bilateral hearing loss. In 126 older residents in nursing homes in San Diego, Novak (1980) found mean pure tone thresholds in the best ear were 47 dB HL (re: ANSI, 1969) at 500 Hz, 46 dB at 1000 Hz, 51 dB at 2000 Hz, 61 dB at 4000 Hz, and 69 DB at 8000 Hz. Ries (1982) found that of persons with serious hearing loss who lived independently, 49 percent of those 30 to 44 years old cited hearing loss as the main cause of limited activity, whereas only 6 percent of the same age group with normal hearing said they were limited in activity. In contrast, only 6 percent of those over 64 years old with severe hearing loss said that hearing loss was the main cause of limitation in activity. Ries concluded that younger, severely hearing-impaired people have few other limitations of activity and therefore view hearing loss, when it is serious, as a primary deficit.

TABLE 6-1. Hearing ability of persons over 64 years of age as a function of sex, race, family income, and level of education.

Hearing Ability	Sex		Race		Family Income			Years of Education		
	M	F	White	Black	<7K	7K-14.9K	>15K	<12	12	>12
No trouble hearing	38*	62	90	10	53	30	17	60	22	18
All levels of loss	49	51	94	6	60	26	14	68	18	14
At best hears shouted speech (71–91 dB HL)	50	50	95	5	61	24	15	76	14	10

* All data in percent of total population over 64 years.
Adapted from Ries (1982) with permission.

Older people, however, have a greater array of causes for limited activity and view even severe hearing loss as minimally responsible for limitations of activity. Ries (1985) concluded that hearing impairment is generally overrepresented in the elderly population, with highest incidence occurring in individuals who are low income, poorly educated, and ill. These groups may view even a serious hearing loss as insignificant.

Novak and Ybarra (1988) found that perception of handicap can vary across ethnic subgroups. In correlating perceived hearing handicap with objective measures of hearing loss, they found that, although the relative prevalence of varying degrees of hearing loss was similar for their non-audiology clinic samples of older urban black and native American subjects, the native Americans, regardless of degree of hearing loss, tended to perceive greater hearing handicap. In fact, several native Americans with clinically normal hearing (audiometric thresholds better than 25 dB HL for 500–3000 Hz) perceived significant hearing handicap. A possible explanation for this is that the older native Americans were hunters and gatherers and thus relied on a keen sense of hearing for their success and safety. In this study, the older blacks had less cultural emphasis on the importance of hearing as an isolated sense.

The Nursing Home Population

Of elderly individuals living in the United States at any one time, only 5 to 6 percent live in extended care facilities. The nursing home subpopulation consists of four subgroups:

1. Residents who are in nursing homes for rehabilitation with the realistic expectation of again living independently in the community, depending to various degrees on community-based services and their own resources
2. Residents who have physical limitations that prevent them from living independently but otherwise are mentally intact
3. Residents who, like group 2, are limited physically and are also mentally impaired
4. Residents who are critically and terminally ill

Nursing home residents, like all older people, have an increased desire for privacy. The paradox, however, is that institutional living reduces the ability to maintain privacy. For a significant subset of hearing-impaired, long-term nursing home residents, hearing loss may be their source of privacy, their insulation from the ever-present intrusions on their personal space. Ulatowska (1985) cited gestures, degree of eye contact, gaze, and orientation of body parts as methods used by nonambulatory nursing home residents to declare their territory and desire for solitude. Even a slight movement of the body or chair away from a fellow resident or staff member can indicate the termination of a conversation (Lipman, 1968). With this in mind, the hearing health care professional must ask what maintenance-of-privacy function the hearing loss serves for each of the subgroups of residents, and how truly motivated each group is to improve hearing for purposes of communication.

Specific hearing-aid related services that the hearing health care professional might provide for each of these subgroups include the following:

GROUP 1. Maximization of electroacoustic function of existing hearing aids and assurance of proper use and application of the hearing aids by the patient and nursing home staff, respectively. Electroacoustically appropriate loaner hearing aids or new hearing aids should be provided in cases where patients need amplification and do not have their own hearing aids.

Maximum use of residual hearing by members of this group is of paramount importance if they are to have optimum receptive and expressive communication during the rehabilitation process.

GROUP 2. Maximization of long-term life quality in the nursing home by allowing the hearing-impaired resident the option of using appropriate amplification when they desire to communicate. The ability to succeed in communicating when they desire to and when others must "get through" is imperative to the quality of life for this population of nursing home residents. The hearing health care professional, therefore, must ensure that the residents have optimum access to and use of:

- Appropriate amplification
- Ongoing staff inservice instruction in

the use of amplification systems including personal hearing aids and assistive listening devices
- Regular follow-up with residents using hearing aids on site
- Hearing aid assessment and fitting procedures that ensure valid application of amplification
- An in-house loaner hearing aid bank to ensure access to amplification for new and experienced hearing aid users

The hearing aids in the loaner bank can be donated by former residents, their families, and staff members, and electroacoustically analyzed and catalogued for appropriate use. Supportive aural rehabilitation programs and the availability of trained resident peer support and hearing-impaired patient advocate groups are also important for the optimum use of hearing aids by this subgroup.

GROUP 3. Maximization of functional mentation through the enhancement of meaningful sensory stimulation. The questions the hearing health care professional must answer for this group are: To what degree is inadequate and inconsistent sensory input responsible for the resident's impaired mental health? Are the symptoms displayed by this subgroup indicative of true chronic brain degeneration (dementia) or can the symptoms in part be described as signs of pseudodementia with the etiology of those symptoms being reduced meaning of sensory input (e.g., remediable auditory dysfunction)? To the extent that the latter is true, the hearing health professional is challenged to determine and fit appropriate amplification and optimize successful use through effective staff involvement and support. The availability of portable auditory brainstem evoked potential equipment for assessing hearing loss and probe tube microphone systems for assessing the insertion gain provided by hearing aids can be very helpful in working with this subgroup.

One in five persons over 65 years of age exhibits dementia at varying stages of severity; 25 percent are severely demented, and 75 percent have mild or moderate intellectual impairment (Mortimer, Schuman, & French, 1981). "Dementia must be greeted as a diagnostic challenge, not as an inevitable harbinger of death or a cause for nihilistic despair" (Cummings, 1985, p. 55).

GROUP 4. Maximization of receptive and expressive communication through the final stages of the terminally ill resident's life. The hearing health care professional may be critical in facilitating meaningful communication of the terminally ill hearing-impaired resident with his or her family physician, clergy, nursing staff, and friends. If hearing-impaired members of this subgroup are not currently hearing aid users, they are logical candidates for use of hearing aids provided from the facility's loaner hearing aid bank or use of institutionally owned assistive listening devices.

The hearing health care professional often must act as a vocal advocate for access of this patient subgroup to hearing aids and associated improved receptive communication function. Access to the hearing-impaired nursing home resident, in most cases, is determined by requests for services by the patient, nursing home staff, patient's physician, or family. Extended care facilities should have nonexclusive contracts with appropriate health care professionals to whom referrals for medical and audiologic intervention can be made. In most states, however, it is only with the consent of the resident's physician that these referrals can be consummated. Therefore, it is imperative for the nursing staff and personal physicians of extended care facility residents to be educated as to the potential benefit of appropriate intervention (e.g., hearing aids, assistive listening devices, aural rehabilitation therapy, otologic medical and surgical treatment) by hearing health care professionals.

Physically Impaired Adults Living at Home

Ten percent of the elderly individuals who live at home are as functionally impaired as individuals who live in nursing homes. Mutual access of this subgroup of the aged population to the variety of hearing health care services is limited by the individual's motivation to seek help for hearing problems either because of low priority in the list of more fundamental human needs or because of minimal demands for communicative efficacy (i.e., few visitors, no televison or radio, no telephone use, or use of communication devices at high volume to compensate for the individual's hearing loss). Access is also limited by the person's ability to get hearing health care services for initial and necessary follow-up appointments. The logistical problems of follow-up may be so overwhelming to the individual that it may seem impossible to overcome them; therefore, the person does not try. If services are to be provided to this group they must be more accessible to them than they typically are to the more flexible ambulatory hearing-impaired consumer.

Independent Ambulatory Adults

Eighty-five percent of the older population live independently in varying stages of wellness and well-being. This group by far contains the majority of aged hearing-impaired persons. The total population of aged hearing-impaired individuals constitutes 55 percent of adults with hearing losses severe enough to interfere with receptive communication (Berkowitz, 1975). Of this hearing-impaired population, Maurer and Rupp (1979) asserted that four out of five individuals are probably experiencing some communication problems in listening. Less than 25 percent of the hearing-impaired persons over age 65 who need and could benefit from amplification have purchased hearing aids (Skafte, 1986). The reasons for this, surmised from clinical experience, include:

■ Lack of acknowledgment of hearing loss as a problem

■ Lack of desire to rehabilitate acknowledged hearing loss

■ Lack of knowlege of available services and technology

■ Lack of appropriate support system and ability to manage use of hearing aids

■ Financial inability to purchase hearing aids

■ Erroneous understanding of what hearing aids can do and dissatisfied testimony from other hearing aid users or their own dissatisfaction with previous hearing aid use

■ Inadequate audiometric and psychosocial assessment of the residual auditory function and communication needs of the hearing-impaired aged

■ Amplification that was inappropriately applied because of electroacoustic and personal style preference inappropriateness

■ Lack of or poor supportive aural rehabilitation services for the first-time hearing aid user

Psychology of Adult Onset Hearing Loss

The emphasis of this chapter is on the application of amplification systems to the post-lingually hearing-impaired older adult, particularly adults who experience progressive hearing loss through middle and into old age. For this population, psychological adjustment to hearing loss and the ability to accept responsibility in the rehabilitation process are of profound importance in attaining maximum aural rehabilitation.

Becker (1980) stated that prelingually deafened adults have created a society in which group membership allows them a nonstigmatized personal identity and normalized social relationships. "These factors stand them in good stead throughout the life cycle. It is when they become old however that these factors are especially useful in coping" (p. 98). For this population,

hearing loss, which can be so catastrophic to the socialization of the aged post-lingually hearing impaired, is of no concern.

Glass (1985) suggested that there are two distinct older populations, the deaf who are growing old and the old who are growing deaf. She asserted that each group is affected similarly by the physical changes of aging but that the two populations undergo very different social, emotional, and behavioral effects related to hearing loss.

Factors important to the assessment of the effects of adventitious hearing loss include age at onset of loss, degree of impairment, rapidity of onset, and audiometric configuration. The earlier in adult life the loss is acquired, the more abnormal and catastrophic it is perceived as being. Hearing health professsionals typically assess severity of loss through tests of pure tone sensitivity, word identification, and binaural auditory integration. Weinstein and Ventry (1983), however, concluded that hearing handicaps in the elderly are more appropriately measured by a self-report format than audiometric test data. This is discussed further in a later section of this chapter.

Sudden adult-onset hearing loss is most traumatic. Mulrooney (1973) described grief as an overwhelming response to sudden deafness. Ashley (1985) used adjectives such as "thunderbolt," "devastating," "shattering," "desolating sense of loss," and "life-long burden" to describe his reaction to adventitious hearing loss.

Depression and withdrawal with resultant isolation are the most prevalent responses to significant hearing loss (Myklebust, 1964). Although Myklebust found this to be more true of "deafened" adults who are of employment age than older adults and equally true of the moderately and severely hearing impaired, it is a common clinical finding in the hearing-impaired elderly population. They assess themselves as withdrawing unwillingly from the mainstream of their social lives. Other symptoms found in adventitiously hearing-impaired adults are nervousness, anxiety, heightened fearfulness, irritability, embarrassment, and fatigue from trying to communicate (Meadow-Orlans, 1985; Oyer & Oyer, 1979).

Myklebust (1964) reported that hearing-impaired men were less well adjusted than hearing-impaired women; however, this may be a cohort effect reflective of the work status of men versus women, relative demands on communication, and the concomitant effects of retirement and accompanying isolation. Although paranoia is frequently ascribed to the adventitiously hearing-impaired adult, this has not been empirically substantiated (Myklebust, 1964; Thomas & Gilhome-Herbst, 1980).

Severe social effects of adult onset hearing loss have also been reported. There may be loss of some old friends who will not struggle with labored communication or who are threatened by the intensity of the hearing-impaired person's feelings (Luey, 1980). In a group of newly severely hearing-impaired adults, Hunter (1978) found that 86 percent made new friends, 50 percent divorced, and 68 percent changed career objectives. In spite of the seeming advisability of socialization with people with similar problems, elderly hearing-impaired individuals are not likely to join organizations for the hearing impaired, especially if they lose their hearing late in life (Miller, 1975). As a result, hearing loss can render the elderly "prime candidates for needless senility" (Maurer & Rupp, 1979). Hearing loss accentuates social isolation, dependency, and loss of status (Beattie, 1981). Group aural rehabilitation sessions run by hearing health care professionals and Self-Help for the Hard of Hearing (SHHH) organizations, available in many cities nationally and internationally, can be critical factors in determining successful use of amplification systems and optimum aural rehabilitation of elderly individuals.

Although there is abundant evidence, particularly when hearing-impaired adults are asked to discuss the concept in aural re-

habilitation settings, that older hearing-impaired adults believe that they are stigmatized by hearing persons, the nature and degree of the stigma is imprecise (Meadow & Orlans, 1985). It seems to be related to hearing-impaired persons' negative projections of what others think when they see a person wearing a hearing aid and normal hearing people's inability to understand the variability in the hearing ability of hearing-impaired persons in different listening situations.

Some adult clients believe that wearing a hearing aid elicits negative reactions in others, who consider a hearing aid a sign of old age and lack of intelligence. The negative stigma attached to hearing aid use, called the "hearing aid effect," has been demonstrated for normal hearing and speaking adolescent boys rated by college students (Blood, Blood, & Danhauer, 1978), geriatric patients rated by nursing home personnel (Knoll, 1979), and normal hearing and speaking preschool-age boys rated by audiologists, speech language pathologists, and college students (Danhauer, Blood, Blood, & Gomez, 1980). Iler, Danhauer, and Mulac (1982), however, found no differences in peer ratings of elders either wearing or not wearing hearing aids, using factors such as achievement, personality, or appearance. More recently, the wearing of hearing aids by the former president of the United States, Ronald Reagan, has served to reduce the self-perceived stigma of hearing aid use by the elderly.

Adjustment to Adult Hearing Loss

Kyle, Jones, and Wood (1985) presented a model that described the phases of acquisition and adjustment to adventitious hearing loss in adults. It is important to assess which stage an individual is in when hearing aid assessment and fitting is being attempted. Phase 1, acquisition of hearing loss, is described as the period when the loss is not acknowleged. It may last less than a month or go on for 20 years or more. It is the time period between initial onset of loss and the first visit to a hearing health care provider. Up to 75 percent of the population with acquired hearing loss may be in this phase at any time (Medical Research Council, 1981). During this phase the unaided person receives feedback from the environment that he or she is talking too loud, the television or radio is too loud, he or she has misheard important information, and so on. During the initial stages of this phase, the hearing-impaired person ascribes the inability to hear to the faulty speech of others and other problems external to him- or herself. The initial visit to a hearing health care professional for evaluation may be made only in aquiescence to the demands of family members. Since realization of the existence of the loss is fundamental to initiation of help-seeking behavior. Kyle and colleagues suggested that when persons are forced to be in situations where they cannot control the volume of speech (e.g., lectures, church), they are apt to more quickly realize the extent of their impairment than if their time is spent in listening activities where they can control the volume of speech (e.g., watching television) or ascribe their inability to understand to faulty connections (e.g., using the telephone).

Phase 2 is described as the time between first contact with a professional and diagnosis of permanent hearing loss and the receipt of a hearing aid. Kyle and colleagues found that in England, where hearing aids are provided at no charge, this phase lasted a few months. In the United States, where the cost of hearing aids represents a significant financial investment, this phase may last a year or more. It is marked by uncertainty as to the ramifications of the newly identified hearing loss, and the resolution of this phase in large part is dependent on the accommodation and support of the person's family and friends. The resolution of this phase is also dependent on the person's willingness to accept responsibility for his or her own successful use of assertive communication techniques and speechreading skills taught in supportive aural rehabilitation sessions.

Phase 3 is the period of subsequent accommodation to the hearing loss. This phase is characterized by the individual's realization of the level of control he or she can expect to have in various communication settings. The ultimate goal of hearing aid fitting and supportive rehabilitation is to maximize the independence and control of the hearing-impaired individual in all desired communication environments. Kyle and colleagues cited maladaptive behaviors in this phase as behavioral changes resulting in (1) excessive introversion and control of conversations with minimal listening and (2) withdrawal from communication situations that threaten control and independence.

An acceptable resolution of Phase 3 is dependent on how the individual adjusts to the hearing aid, to personal and social situations, vocational and avocational demands, and the dynamics of family life. Fundamental to adjustment to the hearing aid is acceptance of its physical appearance, optimum electroacoustic compatibility with and compensation for the hearing loss, independence in the use of the amplification system, acknowledgment of the use of a less than perfect amplification system to others with whom communication is initiated, and realistic expectations of others regarding the aided benefit the new hearing aid user can derive in a variety of listening environments. Kyle and Wood (1983) found that, although 89 percent of their aided respondents had difficulty with street conversations, 79 percent would not tell people that they had a hearing problem. This is also typical of the reactions of new hearing aid users in the United States. If audiologists and dispensers were able to perfectly match the hearing aid configuration to the psychophysical needs of the client, there would be no need for public acknowledgment of the loss and the use of hearing aids.

However, given the as yet imperfect match of electroacoustic hearing aid parameters to clients' psychophysical needs and our incomplete understanding of the optimum psychophysical measures needed to adequately define the aidable parameters of the hearing loss, acknowledgment of the hearing loss and use of hearing aids remains critical to the successful resolution of the aural rehabilitation process.

The remainder of this chapter deals with assessment and intervention strategies.

AUDITORY ASSESSMENT FINDINGS IN THE AGED POPULATION

This section concentrates on threshold and suprathreshold auditory function in the aged listener. This information is, of course, most important when considering appropriate assessment and intervention strategies to amplify the older hearing-impaired client.

Marshall (1981) suggested the following hypotheses in the clinical evaluation of the older hearing-impaired listener: (1) Aging listeners are no different than young listeners with equal degrees of hearing loss and (2) Aging listeners will show auditory function problems in addition to those shown by younger listeners with similar hearing losses, possibly due to peripheral problems associated with presbycusis, which are not adequately assessed by the pure tone audiogram, central auditory nervous system degeneration, cognitive differences, or a combination of all of the above.

Assessment Problems Related to Age

The incidence of excessive impacted cerumen is higher in the older versus younger population (Fisch, 1978; Schow, Christensen, Hutchinson, & Nerbonne, 1978). Otoscopy must be performed prior to auditory and hearing aid evaluation.

Collapsing ear canals with the application of earphones has also been found to occur more frequently in older listeners (Zucker & Williams, 1977; Schow & Goldbaum, 1980) and may explain the high frequency conductive loss cited in several studies (Rosen, Plester, El Mofty, & Rosen, 1964). The implication is to assess the anterior posterior relationship of the tragus to the cavum of the concha and the relative collapsibility of the tragus and cartilagenous portion of the external auditory meatus. If circumaural earphones or canal inserts are used to eliminate this problem, calibration of the audiometer must be completed with the modifications in place. As described earlier, collapsing ear canals also present a challenge for the fabrication of earmolds and ITE hearing aids.

It has been suggested that aged listeners are more conservative in their threshold criterion than younger listeners when they are asked to respond yes or no to the presence of an auditory signal (Rees & Botwinick, 1979; Potash & Jones, 1977). Clinical observations indicate that aged listeners may be less willing to guess in their discrimination of suprathreshold auditory signals if only a portion of the signal is heard (as with a suprathreshold single-word identification task). This symptom may be representative of older listeners or it may be endemic only to the current aged population as a consequence of low self-esteem and the low value generally placed on the aged by our society. In either case, the implication for the hearing health care professional is to reduce auditory test anxiety and reinstruct the older client regarding the clinician's expectation that errors in signal identification are expected, and in fact necessary, if an accurate evaluation is to be obtained. Implications for the test procedures include changing the threshold response to a two-interval forced choice task (eliminating the possibility of a nonresponse) and using closed-set, forced choice suprathreshold speech identification tests, such as a Modified Rhyme type test, the

Synthetic Sentence Identification Index, or a comparison of closed set (high redundancy) to open set (low redundancy) word identification performance using a tool such as the Speech in Noise test (SPIN).

Loudness and Adaptation

Because of the bilateral symmetry of most hearing losses in the aged population and the difficulty of comparing loudness levels of very different frequencies in the same ear, it is not possible to use the alternate binaural loudness balance test (ABLB) or the monaural loundess balance (MLB) test to behaviorally assess loudness recruitment. Short Increment Sensitivity Index (SISI) results are equivocal (Jerger, Shedd, & Harford, 1959) or similar to those shown with cochlear hearing losses of non-age related etiologies. Since this test is typically done in a yes or no paradigm, given the potential for conservative response, it may also be inappropriate as a measure of recruitment in the older client. "Other than using uncomfortable loudness thresholds as a recruitment measure, there is currently no behavioral test of recruitment for elderly listeners" (Marshall, 1981). It has been suggested by clinical audiologists that uncomfortable loudness measures using speech and pure tones lack validity as representations of the levels of sound a person will truly accommodate when they are motivated to do so (i.e., in social or vocational situations).

In spite of this perception it is important to assess frequency specific tolerance limits, known by various names such as uncomfortable loudness levels (UCLs), upper limits of comfortable loudness (ULCL), loudness discomfort levels (LDLs), and most comfortable listening levels (MCLs), in each ear for each subject in order to make the most appropriate initial decisions regarding the appropriate frequency-specific gain and saturation sound pressure level (SSPL) characteristics of hearing aids.

Adaptation, or reduction in the loudness percept of suprathreshold continuous pure tones, has been assessed in older individuals using Bekesy and conventional tone decay tests. Bekesy tracings are usually consistent with normal hearing or a cochlear site of lesion (type I or II tracings, respectively) (Jerger, 1960; Harbert, Young, & Menduke, 1966), and tone decay is typically less than 30 dB, also consistent with cochlear site of lesion (Olsen & Noffsinger, 1974; Ganz, 1976).

Implications for Amplification

The primary behavioral assessment of recruitment for the aging listener is loudness tolerance for pure tones, warble tones, or speech. The dynamic range from threshold to these levels is reduced in all persons with sensorineural hearing loss. Although the usable auditory dynamic range is not inordinately reduced for aged hearing-impaired listeners, they often have a decreased ability to ignore the presence of loud environmental noise, which interferes with their understanding of important auditory input.

The aided listener with sensorineural hearing loss requires a comparatively wide range of input signal intensities to be amplified to suprathreshold levels and maintained within the compressed suprathreshold dynamic range of the individual. These findings suggest that, if maximum hearing aid benefit is to be achieved for the elderly and all persons with sensorineural hearing loss, SSPL90 values that closely correspond to obtained frequency-specific UCLs must be utilized, while at the same time providing enough gain to boost important auditory stimuli to the person's MCLs. Depending on the separation in dB between the person's MCL and UCL at each frequency, these criteria may be met without the use of a compression circuit in the aid. However, as MCLs approach the levels of the UCLs, reducing the dynamic range, it may be possible only to provide adequate gain for lower level input signals in order to keep all amplified signals below the UCLs. This situation would necessitate the use of a compression circuit. If compression is utilized, it is therefore important to keep the "knee" or threshold of compression as high as possible in order to maximize gain for speech input (particularly for frequencies at and above 1000 Hz). The audiologist or the dispenser who uses frequency-specific stimuli to determine MCLs and UCLs should also evaluate whether MCLs and UCLs for more complex signals (e.g., speech and environmental noise) might be somewhat lower due to loudness summation resulting from the simultaneous presentation of the multiple frequency components contained in these stimuli.

Frequency Discrimination

Reduced frequency selectivity in persons with sensorineural hearing loss has been shown using difference limens for frequency (DLF) (Zurek & Formby, 1979). DLFs have been shown to increase with increased magnitude of loss and for low frequencies as well as high frequencies in persons with only high frequency pure tone loss. It has not been established whether aged hearing-impaired listeners have inordinately greater DLFs than their younger counterparts when learning effects and potential age-related criterion effects are controlled (Marshall, 1981).

Psychophysical tuning curves for listeners with sensorineural hearing loss, obtained by fixing the level and frequency of a probe tone and measuring the level of a second tone at various frequencies required to mask the probe, have shown abnormal broadening, abnormal shape, and loss of the tip in regions of hearing loss (Zwicker & Shorn, 1978; Tyler, Fernandes, & Wood, 1984) and abnormality in regions of normal hearing sensitivity (Mills, Gilbert, & Adkins, 1979), especially in the presence of significant high frequency loss (Nelson, 1979). It is not clear whether these results differ in older versus younger persons with similar audiograms (Marshall, 1981).

It has been suggested that each frequency is surrounded by its own critical bandwidth of frequencies and that all frequencies within the critical band of a probe frequency are processed equally. Thus, formants in the speech signal that are separated by a critical bandwidth are perceived as different frequencies; however, environmental noise located within the critical band of each formant frequency is processed along with the speech signal. A widening of critical bandwidths, or loss of frequency selectivity, has been found with the advent of sensorineural hearing loss (deBoer & Bowmeester, 1974, 1976). The widening of critical bands may be due to cochlear changes (efferent olivocochlear neuron degeneration) not related to afferent input, and frequency discrimination may be independent of loss of pure tone hearing threshold sensitivity (Bienvenue & Michael, 1979). It has not been definitively shown, however, that the widening of critical bandwidths in aged listeners with sensorineural loss is in excess of that for young hearing-impaired listeners. Bienvenue and Michael (1979) listed four functions of critical bands: (1) to band limit the effect of background noise on the target signal serving to enhance the signal-to-noise ratio; (2) to determine ability to perceive harmonic content and formant content (in the case of speech) of complex signals; (3) to determine ability to perceive phase relationships among tone complexes; and (4) to sharpen frequency discrimination beyond that which can be described by basilar membrane mechanics.

Critical ratios (signal-to-noise ratio at masked threshold) and upward spread of masking have been assessed in aged listeners and are a reflection of critical bandwidth. Critical ratios have been demonstrated to increase for higher frequencies in both normal hearing (Reed & Bilger, 1973) and high frequency noise-induced hearing-impaired listeners (Tyler, Fernandes, & Wood, 1984). Margolis and Goldberg (1980) concluded that critical ratios are not a simple reflection of auditory filter bandwidth in aged listeners. Upward spread of masking in aged hearing-impaired listeners has not been shown to be any greater than for younger cochlear hearing-impaired counterparts. Although upward spread of masking has been found to be detrimental to speech discrimination of normal hearing listeners at high signal intensities (95–100 dB SPL) (Danaher, Osberger, & Pickett, 1973), it has not been shown to be abnormally broad in all listeners with sensorineural hearing loss (Jerger et al., 1960; Leshowitz & Lindstrom, 1979).

Implications for Amplification

It is quite possible that peripheral deterioration of the frequency selectivity of the cochlea accounts in large part for the reduced understanding of speech in noise in the aged hearing-impaired listener. It is also possible that aged persons with different audiometric configurations and etiologies of hearing loss have varying degrees of alteration in critical bandwidths and cochlear-based frequency specificity.

Once a reliable data base is established regarding the frequency discrimination of older versus younger hearing-impaired listeners with controls for loss configuration, etiology, and task response criterion effects, it seems imperative that tasks that assess frequency discrimination be included in the hearing aid assessment process. The information obtained would make it possible to severely band limit the amplified signal, based not only on the audiometric configuration of the pure tone loss, but also on the extent of abnormality of frequency selectivity across the frequency range, even in the presence of what appear to be normal pure tone thresholds. This would be quite possible with the use of digital filtering which, unfortunately, is not currently available in the majority of hearing aids.

Speech Discrimination

From the previous discussion of the importance of peripheral frequency selec-

tivity to the discrimination of complex signals (speech) in noise, it can be argued that if population-specific information was available, much of the responsibility for reduction in speech discrimination in noise demonstrated by significant numbers of aged hearing-impaired listeners could be described on the basis of impaired frequency selectivity at the level of the cochlea. If this were true, particularly with the advent of digital processing technology, algorithms could be designed into the hearing aid to compensate specifically for abnormal cochlear function. An additional portion of the reduction in speech understanding in aged listeners can be explained on the basis of inadequate sensation levels, particularly of high frequency speech sounds and high formant frequencies within those speech sounds.

To determine age-only related changes in auditory temporal processing, Blackington, Novak, and Kramer (1988) examined NU-6 word identification in normal hearing young and elderly subjects with 0 and 60 percent temporal compression of the speech signals. The authors compared these data to forward masking threshold results using 500 and 2000 Hz as the target stimuli with wide band noise as the masker. The older subjects, ages 60 to 79 years, obtained 70 percent correct identification on the compressed speech presented at 40 dB HL compared to 82 percent correct identification for the young controls. There was no difference in word identification scores between the two groups for non-compressed speech stimuli (97–99% for all subjects). Blackington, Novak, and Kramer also found that, for separations between the masker and target stimuli of 0 to 250 ms, the older subjects required higher tone sensation levels in order to achieve the same 70 percent correct detection level as their younger counterparts. This was particularly true for the 2000 Hz stimuli.

A common clinical observation from aged hearing-impaired listeners is that their understanding of speech improves with a mildly reduced rate of speech. The results of many of the altered speech studies have showed excessively reduced performance in aged hearing-impaired listeners. The results of Blackington, Novak, and Kramer (1988), which showed the same reduction of performance in normal hearing aged listeners, suggest that the critical causal factors are age-related central factors that are not dependent on changes in pure tone sensitivity.

Binaural Integration

Binaural auditory fusion and release from masking tasks have been used to assess central auditory nervous system integrity. Binaural auditory fusion compares word identification when high and low frequency information is presented monaurally versus when high-pass filtered speech is presented to one ear and low-pass filtered speech to the other. Breakdown in the former task can be attributed solely to abnormal cochlear filter effects, whereas breakdown in the dichotic high pass–low pass task can also be impaired by brainstem pathology and bilateral and diffuse cerebral pathology (Lynn & Gilroy, 1976). Investigators have found that the aged listener's binaural fusion ability is not significantly poorer than younger listeners with similar pure tone thresholds (Harbert et al., 1966; Palva & Jokenen, 1970). In fact, older listeners often perform more poorly on the monaural task than on the dichotic speech fusion task, which is consistent with peripheral auditory system pathology. Franklin (1975) also found this to be true with young (13–23 years) listeners with sensorineural hearing loss.

The binaural masking level difference (MLD) is a psychophysical task which also relies on intact lower brainstem function for maximum MLD results. Many studies that have reported MLD results for presbycusic listeners have concluded that MLDs are generally smaller for the presbycusic population (Olsen, Noffsinger, & Carhart, 1976; Warren, Wagener, & Herman, 1978),

in spite of considerable overlap of MLD values between young normal hearing and older hearing-impaired groups. Novak and Anderson (1982) were the first to attempt to systematically control for age, degree of hearing loss, bilateral symmetry of loss, shape of loss, and central auditory integrity in the evaluation of the MLD in older hearing-impaired listeners. They found that, for older listeners, MLD magnitudes for 500 Hz were significantly reduced only for the neural presbycusic (Schuknecht, 1964, 1974) group. The authors concluded that central auditory system function as measured by the MLD task was significantly different only for the neural presbycusic group with high frequency sloping sensorineural hearing loss and single-word identification scores less than 70 percent. These binaural speech fusion and MLD studies support the contention that binaural integration is intact for many aged hearing-impaired listeners.

Implications for Amplification

From the results of the studies cited in the previous two sections, it must be concluded that, although problems of speech understanding in the aged hearing-impaired listener can be attributed in large part to cochlear filtering effects due to pathology at the level of the cochlea, even older normal hearing listeners show poorer performance than their younger counterparts on temporal masking tasks (compressed speech identification, forward masking signal detection). In this case, age appears to be a critical factor in determining the ability to understand rapid speech. On the basis of the recent forward masking data of Blackington, Novak, and Kramer (1988), even normal hearing older listeners may benefit from mild high frequency emphasis amplification in order to improve their detection and processing of rapidly presented auditory information.

In the case of bilaterally symmetrical hearing loss and PB word discrimination scores in excess of 80 percent, binaural fitting of aids must not be ruled out solely on the basis of concern for inability to binaurally integrate dichotically presented information (typical sound-field listening). Age, in and of itself, does not appear to be a significant factor in reduction of binaural auditory fusion or binaural release from masking abilities in older persons with cochlear-based hearing loss.

The implications of all of the psychoacoustic findings with aged hearing-impaired listeners are that:

■ The population is indeed composed of subgroups as defined by different peripheral and central auditory system function.
■ The pure tone audiogram, in and of itself, is not an adequate descriptor of important auditory psychophysical abilities.
■ The onus is on the audiologist to develop a valid, reliable, and efficient test battery that will delineate cochlear versus retrocochlear function as it relates specifically to the specification of hearing-aid parameters.

This test battery must differentiate between improved auditory function that can be expected based solely on differential hearing aid design and benefits from "appropriate" amplification predicted on the basis of psychosocial motivational parameters unique to each aged listener.

HEARING AID EVALUATION PROCEDURES SUGGESTED FOR USE WITH THE AGED LISTENER

The audiologist must apply hearing aids that (1) have the electroacoustic characteristics most appropriate for the client's residual auditory function and (2) are acceptable to the client. Satisfaction of the first requirement does not always ensure

satisfaction of the second. Barford (1979) stated that user satisfaction across clients, as measured by speech perception ability, can be high or low with similar sudden significant changes in aided versus unaided auditory sensitivity. High satisfaction results if the additional frequency information provided to the "recognition device" is indeed meaningful and useful. Low satisfaction results when enhanced aided sensitivity for high frequencies relative to low frequencies causes a "mismatch of the recognition device and the input code." A degradation in speech perception ability at the time of initial hearing aid use "will result if the latter effect dominates." Barford suggested that, "this mismatch will gradually decrease as a result of adaptation, if adaptation is possible." However, the length of the adaptation is not easily predicted (re: age of client, type of loss, and a variety of psychosocial variables) for each individual client and may last from a few days to 6 months or longer. Because of the potential existence of this very real paradox between self-assessed user benefit and objectively measured improvement in aided versus unaided sensitivity, recent investigations indicate that it is important to include client self-assessment of aided versus unaided hearing handicap (Alpiner, 1982; Weinstein & Ventry, 1983; Demorest & Erdman, 1984a; Hawkins, 1985) as well as objective measures of auditory ability in order to maximize appropriate application of hearing aids to the hearing-impaired older adult population.

The steps in the geriatric hearing aid evaluation can be divided into measurements required for:

■ Selection of client-specific optimum hearing system (hearing aid plus acoustic coupler) electroacoustic characteristics
■ Assessment of client's perception of the communication handicap imposed by the hearing loss
■ Assessment of the client's auditory, psychological, and physical ability to bene-

fit from amplification
■ Assessment of the reduction in handicap afforded by appropriate application of amplification as measured by objective and subjective procedures

Selection of Electroacoustic Parameters of Hearing Aids

Many articles have been written on procedures for determining appropriate gain, frequency response, and SSPL90 characteristics of hearing aids, as well as the need for directional microphones, compression amplification, binaural fitting, and acoustically modified earmolds or ITEs. It is not at all obvious, however, that the typical auditory measures of thresholds, MCLs, and LDLs for pure tones and speech measured under earphones versus the same measures made in the sound field for aided versus unaided assessment are sufficient to model the auditory needs that must be accomodated by the hearing aid. For example, might it not also be beneficial to assess critical bandwidths? This could be done for high as well as low frequencies and differential discrimination of frequency across the critical auditory spectrum (500–6000 Hz) in order to better identify the signal processing parameters that would maximize use of these auditory abilities in the hearing-impaired client. This information would tell us if the older client can discriminate between target frequencies in the hearing aid response curve, thereby helping the hearing aid provider to determine which frequency response curve modifications are most meaningful. For example, attempting to increase gain for frequencies above 3000 Hz would be unnecessary if the client is unable to discriminate differences between frequencies in the 4000 to 6000 Hz target range. These considerations are crucial to optimum design of future "speech processor" type hearing aids but are beyond the scope of this chapter.

Efficiency, speed, validity, and reliability of test procedures are critical when assessing auditory function in aged clients in order to select appropriate electroacoustic characteristics available in current hearing aids.

Auditory Evaluation

It is recommended that, at a minimum, the following parameters should be assessed:

1. Pure tone thresholds and MCLs under earphones in order to specify general frequency response characteristics and absolute gain requirements. Methods for calculation of desired frequency specific gain values on the basis of pure tone audiometric data (thresholds or MCLs relative to assumed frequency specific values for the long-term speech spectrum) have been desvribed by Berger, Hagenberg, and Rane (1977); Pascoe (1978); Skinner, Pascoe, Miller, and Popelka (1982); McCandless and Lyregaard (1983); Cox (1985, 1987); Byrne and Dillon (1986); Libby (1986); Byrne (1987); and Skinner (1988). In applying audiometric data to determinations of frequency response requirements and preselection of specific hearing aids, it is important to realize that 2 cc coupler values indicated on manufacturers' specification sheets may underrepresent desired functional gain (aided versus unaided thresholds for warble tones or narrow band noise) or insertion gain (aided versus unaided ear canal sound response level) (Hawkins & Schum, 1984). This difference will be greater for BTE than for ITE hearing aids, particularly for frequencies above 1000 Hz. Lower insertion and functional gain will also be seen in persons with large ear canal volumes medial to the tip of the hearing aid on the earmold and with very flaccid middle ear systems.

2. Immittance testing with special attention to the physical volume measure and the Peak Y amplitude value of the tympanogram.

3. Frequency specific LDLs for those frequencies for which amplification is desired in order to specify SSPL90 values to which the aid should first be adjusted. It is suggested that the client's own earmold coupled to an external hearing aid receiver, which is coupled to the output of the audiometer (Hawkins, 1984), be used in order to arrive at LDL values in dB SPL that correlate directly to hearing aid specification data. Etymotic insert earphones, available through the Etymotic Research Lab, calibrated in the 2 cc coupler are a less cumbersome alternative. LDLs should be obtained for both frequency specific and broad band stimuli (speech or speech noise) to determine the extent to which loudness summation may necessitate the lowering of the SSPL90 requirements.

4. Word identification scores using the receiver described by Hawkins (1984) on the etymotic earphones with speech presented at precalculated frequency specific gain levels (as afforded by a master hearing aid-type audiometer). This enables assessment of speech perception that is less contaminated by the upward spread of masking and distortion, which might be created by the overamplification of lower frequencies and underamplification of higher frequencies when using the typical flat spectrum speech audiometer set to the client's MCL.

5. DLFs for frequencies needing significant amplification in order to determine the individual's ability to discriminate between adjacent frequencies. This is particularly helpful in determining how important it really is to try to achieve significant target gain values for 3000, 4000, and 6000 Hz.

In a less than optimal testing environment, the effects of background noise are reduced for persons with thresholds ≥ 40 dB HL at or above 500 Hz. Methods utilized include assessment of pure tone thresholds, UCLs, and MCLs under earphones using a portable audiometer, and identification of recorded words under earphones using a tape recorder with dB HL settings marked on the dial, as determined by previous 6 or 2 cc (depending on the earphones used) coupler calibration of the speech levels. Probe microphone measures are invaluable in allowing a quick and reliable comparison of aided versus unaided ear canal sound pressure levels (insertion gain) to assess adequacy of hearing aid gain without requiring subjective judgments from the client. Aided versus unaided speech identification can be assessed in the sound field at a pragmatic distance of 3 feet with the clinician's speech being monitored at 55 to 60 dBA at the patient's location using a sound level meter. The speech stimuli used will vary with the abilities of the client (standard word lists for more intact clients or abbreviated word lists emphasizing high frequency words, the Ling 5 sounds test incorporated into real words [e.g., shaw, she, shoe, saw, see, sue], and more meaningful questions about the client and his or her environment for less intact clients). Speech testing, aided versus unaided, should also be done with and without the use of lip cues in order to show the older client the importance of enhancing hearing aid use by watching the speaker's face.

Assessment of Self-Perceived Handicap Imposed by the Hearing Loss

There are a variety of self-assessment inventories designed to allow clients to rate the psychological, social, vocational, and emotional handicaps imposed by their hearing losses. These include the Hearing Handicap Scale (High, Fairbanks, & Glorig, 1964), Hearing Measurement Scale (Noble & Atherley, 1970), Social Hearing Handicap Index (Ewertson & Birk-Nielsen, 1973), Denver Scale of Communication Function (Alpiner, Chevrette, Glascoe, Metz, & Olsen, 1974), Hearing Performance

Inventory (Giolas, Owens, Lamb, & Schubert, 1979), Revised Hearing Performance Inventory (Lamb, Owens, & Schubert, 1983), Hearing Problem Inventory (Hutton, 1980), Hearing Handicap Inventory for the Elderly (Ventry & Weinstein, 1982), McCarthy-Alpiner Scale of Hearing Handicap (McCarthy & Alpiner, 1983), Communication Profile for the Hearing Impaired (Demorest & Erdman, 1984).

Use of the Hearing Handicap for the Elderly (Weinstein & Ventry, 1983) is recommended because it has been used and validated with hearing-impaired older persons typically seen in speech and hearing clinics. It is relatively short and assesses the critical concerns of the emotional and social and situational effects of the hearing loss. Weinstein and Ventry found that older clients with pure tone averages of 0 to 25 dB HL (500, 1000, 2000 Hz) almost never described their hearing losses as handicapping. Half of the clients with pure tone averages of 26 to 40 dB HL perceived the hearing loss as a handicap and half did not. Older clients with hearing losses greater than 41 dB HL very often (88–92%) perceived their hearing loss as handicapping. There was, however, considerable variability even for the greater-than-40-dB loss group in the degree (mild to significant) of perceived handicap. Results for older persons were very similar to the results for younger persons, and audiometric data (e.g., pure tone averages, speech reception thresholds, and speech discrimination scores) accounted for less than 50 percent of the variance in self-assessed hearing handicap. These results are consistent with the recommendation that, although pure tone thresholds are important for the description of the desired hearing aid electroacoustic parameters, they do not adequately describe the functional deficits imposed by a given hearing loss, particularly for losses less than 40 dB HL for the three-frequency pure tone average.

The Demorest and Erdman (1984) Communication Profile for the Hearing Impaired is also recommended for use in problematic cases that require very specific aural rehabilitation procedures. The test battery allows assessment of adequacy of communication in the individual's social environment. Problem awareness, communication need, physical environment, attitudes and behaviors of others, maladaptive behaviors, verbal and nonverbal communication strategies, self-acceptance, acceptance of loss, anger, defensiveness, guilt, discouragement, stress, withdrawal, and denial are also assessed. Some items from this tool are not appropriate for retired adults and would therefore have to be deleted.

Most aged clients who admit that they are having communication difficulties secondary to hearing loss complain that with previous hearing aids sounds were often too loud, and speech was difficult to understand when background noise was present (e.g., informal group gatherings). If bilaterally impaired, sounds originating on the unaided ear were often difficult to initially detect and process if relocation was not easy (e.g., when seated in a car). Mueller, Hawkins, and Sedge (1984) suggest that, for the majority of the hearing-impaired population, who have potential for bilateral amplification, it is preferable to use compression, directional microphones, and binaural fitting. If the client is over 70 years of age and a first-time hearing aid user, the recommendation for binaural fitting might be qualified, based on the person's ability to physically and mentally cope with, at first, just one new hearing aid and then, at a later time, possibily a second hearing aid.

Prediction of Ability to Successfully Use Amplification

The Rupp Feasibility Scale for Predicting Hearing Aid Use (Rupp, Higgins, & Maurer, 1977) differentially weights factors of motivation, fault, initial impression, age, vision, significant others, self assessment, functional gain for speech, adaptability, manual dexterity, and financial resources and, accordingly, allows for scoring of each client from poor (0) to excellent (100) prognosis for successful use of hearing aids Hosford-Dunn and Baxter (1985) found that in a group of 95 clients ranging in age from 20 to 29 years old (mean age, 65 years) with mild to severe hearing losses at 1000 to 4000 Hz, clinician-assessed "motivation" and "initial subjective impressions of amplification" to be the two best predictors of long-term (first 3 months of aid use) satisfaction. As Hosford-Dunn and Baxter suggested, for clients older than 70 years of age, other factors of this instrument may have predictive value as well and should not be eliminated for that population. Hosford-Dunn and Baxter also examined the predictive value of standard audiometric measures relative to the successful use of amplification. Only aided versus unaided single-syllable word identification scores in quiet were found to be of predictive value. Although predictive studies with aged hearing aid users have not been reported using data from the Communication Profile for the Hearing Impaired, the completeness of the range of parameters assessed by this test battery would make it very useful in identifying problems that could interfere with an otherwise seemingly good prognosis for successful hearing aid use. The length of the test battery and scoring time may preclude its use in some clinical settings.

Assessment of Reduction of Handicap Afforded by Amplification

Audiometric indications of a successful hearing aid fitting are aided versus unaided functional gain for warble tones and narrow band noises, allowing for aided thresholds from 1000 to 6000 Hz of 30 to 35 dB HL with aided speech in quiet for words presented at 50 dB HL in excess of 88 percent, and aided conversational to loud speech levels reported by the listener to be comfortable and within their tolerance limits, respectively. Coupled with discrimination scores greater than 88 percent for speech in environmental noise with +10 dB or poorer signal-to-noise ratios and tolerance of all ranges of aided environmental noise levels, these results should assure most hearing aid dispensers that their fitting of the aid was successful. However, it is rare for all of these conditions to be met in more typical cases of aged hearing aid users. As stated earlier, even with optimum electroacoustic matching of the hearing aid to the hearing loss with near normalization of aided auditory sensitivity for important speech frequencies, aged hearing aid users may reject hearing aids. Rejection may occur because the aided auditory signals are too different from the internal auditory code they have used to previously encode the auditory speech signal (Barford, 1979). With the aged client, therefore, it is advisable to include pre- and post-aided self-assessment inventories of handicap, as discussed earlier, to validate audiometric suggestions of a successful hearing aid fitting. This might be accomplished through pre- and post-administration of the Hearing Handicap Inventory for the Elderly (Weinstein & Ventry, 1982) or, as Hosford-Dunn and Baxter (1985) have done, pre-and post-fitting administration of the Hearing Performance Inventory (Lamb, Owens, & Shubert, 1983) using only the 38 items (HPI$_{38}$) related to speech understanding. Lamb and colleagues measured HPI$_{38}$ scores of clients in their sixties and seventies with primarily moderate losses prior to hearing aid fitting and 3 months post-fitting. They concluded that if the difference score was in excess of 10 percent, there was "no chance of dissatisfaction" with the aid. It would be ideal if this type of assessment could be done within the currently mandated 30-day trial period. However, since adjustment to the hearing aid may take in excess of 6 months for an older first-time user, it might be argued that this type of pre–post assessment within the current 30-day trial period would not give a valid reflection of the client's ability to benefit from hearing aid use. This period may be dramatically affected by intensive aural rehabilitation counseling immediately post hearing aid fitting. The critical question, however is: How do age when first amplified, degree and slope of hearing loss, amount of change in unaided versus aided sensitivity, and nonauditory psychosocial and cultural factors interact with the amount and type of counseling necessary to optimize adjustment within the 30-day trial period? Even with daily rehabilitation sessions, 30 days may not be long enough for some aged hearing aid users to adapt to hearing aid use.

The aged hearing-impaired population presents infinitely complex diagnostic and rehabilitative challenges to hearing health care professionals. Older hearing aid candidates may have a variety of physical changes in addition to hearing loss, which provide a complicated backdrop to problems created by hearing loss, or hearing loss may be their only significant disorder. Aged clients may present themselves alone with no one to assist in the aural rehabilitation process, or they may be warmly supported by a child, a spouse, or a friend in their adaptation to the use of hearing aids and new assertive communication skills. They may have predominantly cochlear-based sensorineural hearing loss and seem no different than their younger counterparts, or they may have more difficulty understanding aided speech than would be predicted on the basis of their pure tone audiograms. They may present themselves at hearing aid clinics because they truly realize the extent of their disability and desire rehabilitation or may come only to appease a significant other with no acknowledgment of responsibility for the communication problems they are having.

Knowledge of appropriate psychophysical data necessary to discretely describe the auditory function of presbycusic sub-groups is incomplete. Our ability to model "normal" auditory function in each aged hearing-impaired client with uniquely appropriate amplification is, therefore, also imperfect. The procedures that are used in the assessment of the aged client for use of amplification should specifically define unique cochlear versus retrocochlear function in presbycusic subgroups. The resultant data should be adaptable to a prescriptive approach for the recommendation of hearing aids to minimize the time spent in hearing aid evaluation and fitting.

In the final analysis, the clinician is best advised to listen to elderly clients and to understand, as much as possible, the orientation (cultural, social, psychological) of the client with respect to the hearing aid and aural rehabilitation process. Successful aural rehabilitation of the older client is possible only if there is mutual respect and honesty between the client and the hearing health care professional. The onus is on the individual professional to recommend the most appropriate hearing aid, or aids, to provide supportive aural rehabilitation counseling to the aged client, and to involve the client in a manner that will maximize independent use of all of the equipment and communication strategies offered.

REFERENCES

Alpiner, J. G. (1982). *Handbook of adult rehabilitative audiology.* Baltimore: Williams & Wilkins.

Alpiner, J. G., Chevrette, W., Glascoe, G., Metz, M., & Olsen, B. (1974). *The Denver Scale of Communication Function.* Denver, CO: University of Denver.

Ashley, J. (1985). A personal account. In H. Orlans (Ed.), *Adjustment to adult hearing loss.* Boston: College-Hill Press.

Atchley, R. C. (1983). *Aging: Continuity and change.* Belmont, CA: Wadsworth.

Barford, J. (1979). Speech perception processes and fitting of hearing aids. *Audiology, 18,* 430–441.

Beattie, J. A. (1981). *Social aspects of acquired hearing loss in adults.* Report on research project, 1978-1981 (summary of contents and findings). Bradford, England: Post Graduate School of Applied Social Studies, University of Bradford.

Becker, G. (1980). *Growing old in silence.* Berkeley: University of California Press.

Berger, K., Hagenberg, N., & Rane, R. (1977). *Prescription of hearing aids.* Kent, OH: Herald Publishing.

Berkowitz, A. (1975). Audiologic rehabilitation of the geriatric patient. *Hearing Aid Journal, 8,* 30-34.

Bienvenue, G., & Michael, P. (1979). Digital processing techniques in speech discrimination testing (critical bandwidth measurements for use in hearing aid testing). In P. Yaneck (Ed.), *Rehabilitative strategies for sensorineural hearing loss.* New York: Grune & Stratton.

Birren, J. E., Imus, H. A., & Windle, W. F. (1959). *The process of aging in the central nervous system.* Springfield, IL: Charles C. Thomas.

Blackington, B., Novak, R. E., & Kramer, S. A. (1988). Temporal masking effects for speech and pure tone stimuli in normal hearing aged subjects. Unpublished masters thesis, San Diego State University, California.

Blood, G. W., Blood, I. M., & Danhauer, J. L. (1978). Listeners' impressions of normal hearing and hearing impaired children. *Journal of Communicative Disorders, 11,* 573-578.

Busse, E. W. (1965). Research on aging: Some methods and findings. In M. A. Barezin & S. H. Cath (Eds.), *Geriatric psychiatry.* New York: International University Press.

Byrne, D. (1987). Hearing aid selection formulae: Same or different. *Hearing Instruments, 38,* 5-13.

Byrne, D., & Dillon, H. (1986). The National Acoustic Labs (NAL) new procedure for selecting gain and frequency response of a hearing aid. *Ear and Hearing, 7,* 257-265.

Cheng, L. R. (1988). *Personal interview with R. E. Novak.* San Diego, CA.

Corso, J. F. (1963). Age and sex differences in pure tone thresholds. *Archives of Otolaryngology, 77,* 53-73.

Cox, R. (1985). A structured approach to hearing aid selection. *Ear and Hearing, 6,* 226-239.

Cox, R. (1987). The MSU hearing instrument prescription procedures. *Hearing Instruments, 39,* 6-10.

Crowe, S. J., & Guild, S. R. (1934). Observation of the pathology of high tone deafness. *Johns Hopkins Hospital Bulletin, 54,* 315-380.

Danhauer, J. L., Blood, G. W., Blood, I. M., & Gomez, N. (1980). Professional and lay observations of preschoolers wearing hearing aids. *Journal of Speech and Hearing Disorders, 45*(3), 64-71.

Danaher, E. N., Osberger, M., & Pickett, J. (1973). Discrimination of formant frequency transitions in synthetic vowels. *Journal of Speech and Hearing Research, 16,* 439-451.

deBoer, E., & Bowmeester, J. (1974). Critical bands and sensorineural hearing loss. *Audiology, 13,* 236-259.

deBower, E., & Bowmeester, J. (1975). Clinical psychophysics. *Audiology, 14,* 274-299.

Demorest, M., & Erdman, S. (1984a). Applications of self assessment inventories. *Hearing Instruments, 35,* 32-40.

Demorest, M., & Erdman, S. (1985b). A database management system for the communication profile for the hearing impaired. *Journal of the Academy of Rehabilitative Audiology, 17,* 87-96.

Eisenberg, S. (1985). Communication with elderly patients: The effects of illness and medication on mentation, memory, and communication. In H. K. Ulatowska (Ed.), *The aging brain and communication in the elderly.* Boston: College-Hill Press.

Ewertson, H., & Birk-Nielsen, H. (1973). Social hearing handicap index: Social handicap in relation to hearing impairment. *Audiology, 12,* 180-187.

Fabini, G. (1931). Regarding morphological and functional changes in the internal ear arteriosclerosis. *Laryngoscope, 4,* 663-670.

Feller, B. (1981). Prevalence of selected impairments. *United States, 1977* (Series 10, No. 134) National Center for Health Statistics. Washington, DC: U.S. Government Printing Office.

Fisch, L. (1978). Special senses: The aging auditory system. In J. C. Brocklehurst (Ed.), *Textbook of geriatric medicine and gerontology.* New York: Churchill Livingstone.

Fisch, U. (1972). Degenerative changes of the arterial vessels of the internal auditory meatus during the process of aging. *Acta Otolaryngologica, 73,* 259-260.

Franklin, B. (1975). The effects of combining low- and high-frequency pass bands on consonant recognition in the hearing impaired. *Journal of Speech and Hearing Re-*

search, 18, 719–727.

Ganz, R. P. (1976). The effects of aging on the diagnostic utility of the roll over phenomenon. *Journal of Speech and Hearing Disorders, 41,* 63–69.

Gelfand, D. (1982). *Aging: The ethnic factor.* Boston: Little, Brown.

Gentile, A. (1971). Persons with impaired hearing. *United States, 1971* (Series 10, No. 134). Washington, DC: U.S. Government Printing Office.

Giolas, T. G., Owens, E., Lamb, S., & Schubert, E. (1979). Hearing Performance Inventory. *Journal of Speech and Hearing Research, 44,* 169–195.

Glass, L. (1985). Psychosocial aspects of hearing loss in adulthood. In H. Orlans (Ed.), *Adjustment to adult hearing loss.* Boston: College-Hill Press.

Glorig, A., & Davis, H. (1961). Age, noise and hearing loss. *Annals of Otology, 70,* 556–571.

Glorig, A., & Nixon, H. L. (1962). Hearing loss as a function of age. *Laryngoscope, 27,* 1596–1610.

Goldman, R. (1971). Decline in organ function with aging. In I. Rossman (Ed.), *Clinical geriatrics,* Philadelphia: Lippencott.

Gottlieb, B. H. (1983). *Social support strategies.* Beverly Hills, CA: Sage.

Greenblat, N., & Chien, C. (1983). Depression in the elderly. In L. Breslau & M. Haug (Eds.), *Depression and aging: Causes, care and consequences.* New York: Springer-Verlag.

Harbert, R., Young, J., & Menduke, H. (1966). Audiological findings in presbycusis. *Journal of Auditory Research, 6,* 297–312.

Hawkins, D. B. (1984). Selection of a critical electroacoustic characteristic: SSPL-90. *Hearing Instruments, 35,* 28–32.

Hawkins, D. B. (1985). Reflections of amplification: Validation of performance. *Journal of the Academy of Rehabilitative Audiology, 17,* 87–96.

Hawkins, D. B., & Schum, D. J. (1984). Relationship among various measures of hearing aid gain. *Journal of Speech and Hearing Disorders, 49,* 94–97.

High, W. S., Fairbanks, G., & Glorig, A. (1964). Scale for self assessment of hearing handicap. *Journal of Speech and Hearing Disorders, 29,* 215–230.

Hosford-Dunn, H., & Baxter, J. H. (1985). Prediction and validation of hearing aid wearer benefit: Preliminary findings. *Hearing*

Instruments, 36, 34–41.

Hunter, C. C. (1978). *A pilot study of late deafened adults.* Unpublished master's thesis, California State University, Northridge.

Hutton, C. (1980). Responses to a hearing problem inventory. *Journal of the Academy of Rehabilitative Audiology, 12,* 133–154.

Iler, K., Danhauer, J. L., & Mulac, A. (1982). Peer perceptions of geriatrics wearing hearing aids. *Journal of Speech and Hearing Disorders, 47,* 433–438.

Jerger, J. (1960). Bekesy audiometry in analysis of auditory disorders. *Journal of Speech and Hearing Research, 3,* 275–287.

Jerger, J., Shedd, J., & Harford, E. (1959). On the detection of extremely small changes in sound intensity. *Archives of Otolaryngology, 69,* 200–211.

Knoll, C. (1979). *The influence of the hearing aid on the attitudes of nursing home personnel.* Master's thesis, Wichita State University, Kansas.

Krmpotic-Nemanic, J. (1971). A new concept of the pathogenesis of presbycusis. *Archives of Otolaryngology, 93,* 161–166.

Kyle, J. G., Jones, L. G., & Wood, P. L. (1985). Adjustment to acquired hearing loss: A working model. In H. Orlans (Ed.), *Adjustment to adult hearing loss.* Boston: College-Hill Press.

Kyle, J. G., & Wood, P. L. (1983). Social and vocational aspects of acquired hearing loss. Final report to MSC School of Education, Bristol. (Reported in Kyle, J. G., Jones, L. G., & Wood, P. L. [1985]. Adjustment to acquired hearing loss: A working model. In H. Orlans [Ed.], *Adjustment ot adult hearing loss.* Boston: College-Hill Press.)

Lamb, S. H., Owens, E., & Schubert, E. D. (1983). The revised form of the Hearing Handicap Inventory. *Ear and Hearing, 4,* 152–157.

Leshowitz, B., & Lindstrom, R. (1979). Masking and speech-to-noise ratio. *Audiology and Deaf Education, 6,* 5–8.

Libby, E. R. (1986). The ⅓–⅔ insertion gain hearing aid selection guide. *Hearing Instruments, 3,* 27–28.

Lipman, A. (1968). A socio-architectural view of life in three homes for older people. *Gerontologica Clinica, 10,* 88–101.

Luey, H. S. (1980). Between worlds: The problems of deafened adults. *Social Work in Health Care, 5,* 253–265.

Lynn, G. E., & Gilroy, J. (1976). Central aspects

of audition. In J. Northern (Ed.), *Hearing disorders.* Boston: Little, Brown.

Margolis, R., & Goldberg, S. (1980). Auditory frequency selectivity in normal and presbycusic subjects. *Journal of Speech and Hearing Research, 23,* 603-613.

Marshall, L. (1981). Auditory processing in aging listeners. *Journal of Speech and Hearing Disorders, 46,* 226-236.

Mauldin, C. R. (1976). Communication and the aging consumer. In H. J. Oyer & E. J. Oyer (Eds.), *Aging and communication.* Baltimore: University Park Press.

Maurer, J. F., & Rupp, R. R. (1979). *Hearing and aging: Tactics for intervention.* New York: Grune & Stratton.

Mayer, O. (1970). Das Anatomische Substrat der Altersschwerhovigkeit. *Arch. Ohren-Nasen-u-Kehlkopfh., 105,* 1313.

McCandless, G., & Lyregaard, P. (1983). Prescription of gain/output (POGO) for hearing aids. *Hearing Instruments, 1,* 16-21.

McCarthy, P. A., & Alpiner, J. G. (1983). An assessment scale of hearing handicap for use in family counseling. *Journal of the Academy of Rehabilitative Audiology, 16,* 256-270.

McCartney, J. (1977, November/December). A look at hearing loss. *Perspectives on Aging,* 10-11.

Meadow-Orlans, K. P. (1985). Social and psychological effects of hearing loss in adulthood: A literature review. In H. Orlans (Ed.), *Adjustment to adult hearing loss.* Boston: College-Hill Press.

Medical Research Council Institute of Hearing Research. (1981). Population study of hearing disorders in adults. *Journal of the Royal Society of Medicine, 74,* 819-827.

Merluzzi, F., & Hinchcliffe, R. (1973). Threshold of subjective auditory handicap. *Audiology, 12,* 65-69.

Miller, L. V. (1975). The adult and the elderly: Health care and hearing loss. *Volta Review, 77,* 57-63.

Mills, J. H., Gilbert, R. M., & Adkins, W. V. (1979). *Some effects of noise on auditory sensitivity, temporal integration and psychophysical tuning curves.* Paper presented at Second Midwinter Research Meeting of the Association for Research in Otolaryngology, St. Petersburg, FL.

Mueller, H. G., Hawkins, D., & Sedge, R. K. (1984). Three important variables in hearing aid selection. *Hearing Instruments, 35,* 14-17.

Mulrooney, J. (1973, October). The newly-deafened adult. In *Proceedings, National Conference on Program Development for and with Deaf People* (pp. 40-43). Sponsored by Office of Public Service, Gallaudet College and Cooperative Extension. Washington, DC: University of Maryland.

Myklebust, H. R. (1964). *The psychology of deafness.* New York: Grune & Stratton.

Nelson, D. A. (1979). *Frequency selectivity in listeners with sensori-neural hearing loss.* Paper presented at Second Midwinter Research Meeting of the Association for Research in Otolaryngology, St. Petersburg, FL.

Nixon, J. C., & Glorig, A. (1962). Changes in air and bone conduction thresholds as a function of age. *Journal of Laryngology, 76,* 288-292.

Noble, W. G., & Atherley, G. R. (1970). The Hearing Measurement Scale: A questionnaire for the assessment of auditory disability. *Journal of Auditory Research, 10,* 229-250.

Novak, R. E. (1980). *Demographics of hearing loss and staff awareness of hearing loss in primary and secondary care nursing homes in San Diego.* Unpublished study.

Novak, R. E., & Anderson, C. V. (1982). The differentiation of types of presbycusis using the masking level difference. *Journal of Speech and Hearing Research, 25,* 504-508.

Novak, R. E., & Ybarra, S. (1988). Hearing loss. Hearing handicap and help seeking behaviors in American Indians and Black elders. Unpublished master's thesis, San Diego State University, California.

Olsen, W. O., & Noffsinger, D. (1974). Comparison of one new and three old tests of auditory adaptation. *Archives of Otolaryngology, 99,* 94.

Olsen, W., Noffsinger, D., & Carhart, R. (1976). Masking level difference encountered in clinical populations. *Audiology, 15,* 287-301.

Oyer, H. J., & Oyer, E. J. (1979). Social consequences of hearing loss for the elderly. *Allied Health and Behavioral Sciences, 2,* 123-137.

Palva, A., & Jokenen, H. (1970). Presbycusis V. Filtered speech test. *Acta Otolaryngologica, 70,* 232-241.

Parenti, M. (1978). *Power and powerlessness.* New York: St. Martin's Press.

Pascoe, D. (1978). An approach to hearing aid selection. *Hearing Instruments, 6,* 12-16, 26-27.

Posner, J. D. (1982). Particular problems of antibiotic use in the elderly. *Geriatrics, 37,* 49–54.

Potash, M., & Jones, B. (1977). Aging and decision criteria for the detection of tones in noise. *Journal of Gerontology, 32,* 436–440.

Reed, C. M., & Bilger, R. C. (1973). A comparative study of S/NO and E/NO. *Journal of the Acoustical Society of America, 53,* 1039–1044.

Rees, J. N., & Botwinick, J. (1971). Detection and decision factors in auditory behavior of the elderly. *Journal of Gerontology, 26,* 133–136.

Ries, P. W. (1982). Hearing ability of persons by sociodemographic and health characteristics. *United States* (Series No. 10, No. 140). National Center for Health Statistics. Washington, DC: U.S. Government Printing Office.

Ries, P. W. (1985). The demography of hearing loss. In H. Orlans (Ed.), *Adjustment to adult hearing loss.* Boston: College-Hill Press.

Rosen, S., Bergman, M., Plester, D., El Mofty, A., & Sotti, M. (1962). Presbycuses study of a relatively noise free population in the Sudan. *Annals of Otolaryngology, 71,* 727–743.

Rosen, S., Plester, D., El Mofty, A., & Rosen, H. High frequency audiometry in presbycusis. *Annals of Otolaryngology, 79,* 18–32.

Rupp, R., Higgins, J., & Maurer, J. F. (1977). A feasibility scale for predicting hearing aid use (FSPHAU) with older individuals. *Journal of the Auditory Rehabilitation Association, 10,* 81–194.

Schow, R. L., Christensen, J. M., Hutchinson, J. M., & Nerbonne, M. A. (1978). *Communicative disorders of the aged.* Baltimore: University Park Press.

Schow, R. L., & Goldbaum, D. E. (1980). Collapsed ear canals in the elderly nursing home population. *Journal of Speech and Hearing Disorders, 45,* 259–267.

Schuknecht, H. F. (1951). Lesions of the organ Corti. *Transactions of the American Academy of Ophthalmology and Otolaryngology, 57,* 366.

Schuknecht, H. F. (1955). Presbycusis. *Laryngoscope, 65,* 42.

Schuknecht, H. F. (1964). Further observations on the pathology of presbycusis. *Archives of Otolaryngology, 80,* 369–382.

Schuknecht, H. F. (1974). *Pathology of the ear.* Cambridge, MA: Harvard University Press.

Skafte, M. (1986). Communicate for a longer life.

Hearing Instruments, 37, 4.

Skinner, M. (1988). *Hearing aid evaluation.* Englewood Cliffs, NJ: Prentice-Hall.

Skinner, M., Pascoe, D., Miller, J., & Popelka, G. (1982). Measurements to determine the optimal placement of speech energy within the listener's auditory area: A basis for selecting amplification characteristics. In G. Studebaker & F. Bess, *The Vanderbilt hearing aid report: Monographs in contemporary audiology.* Upper Darby, PA.

Thomas, A., & Gilhome-Herbst, K. (1980). Social or psychological implications of acquired deafness for adults of employment age. *British Journal of Audiology, 14,* 76–85.

Tyler, R. S., Fernandes, M., & Wood, E. J. (1984). Masking temporal integration and speech intelligibility in individuals with noise induced hearing loss. In G. Taylor (Ed.), *Disorders of auditory function III.* New York: Academic Press.

Ulatowska, H. K. (1985). *The aging brain: Communication in the elderly.* Boston: College-Hill Press.

U.S. Department of Commerce. (1975, February 10). Reported in *U.S. News and World Report.*

Ventry, I. M., & Weinstein, B. E. (1982). The Hearing Handicap Inventory for the Elderly: A new tool. *Ear and Hearing, 3,* 128–134.

Warren, L. R., Wagener, J., & Herman, G. (1978). Binaural analysis in the aging auditory system. *Journal of Gerontology, 33,* 731–736.

Weinstein, B. E., & Ventry, I. M. (1983). Audiometric correlates of the Hearing Handicap Inventory for the Elderly. *Journal of Speech and Hearing Disorders, 84,* 379–383.

Zucker, K., & Williams, P. S. (1977). *Audiological services in extended care facilities.* Paper presented at the American Speech and Hearing Convention, Chicago, IL.

Zurek, P., & Formby, C. (1977). *Frequency discriminability of sensorineural listeners.* Paper presented at the Second Midwinter Research Meeting of the American Speech and Hearing Association, Chicago, IL.

Zwaardemaker, H. (1891). Der Verlust an Horen Tonen Mit Zunehemendum Alter: Ein Neues Gesetz. *Arch Ohr Nas.-Kehlk-Heilk, 32,* 53.

Zwicker, E., & Shorn, K. (1978). Psychoacoustical tuning curves in audiology. *Audiology, 17,* 120–140.

7

THE APPLICATION OF SPEECH STIMULI IN HEARING AID SELECTION AND EVALUATION

DAN F. KONKLE ■

JILL M. MOLLOY ■

Amplification represents the single most important rehabilitative tool available to the hearing-impaired population (Ross, 1975; Ross & Giolas, 1978; Bess & McConnell, 1981). When used appropriately, amplification devices provide a valuable communicative link between the acoustic environment and the hearing-impaired listener. Conversely, malfunctioning, inappropriate, or misused amplification can substantially degrade communication ability; and under certain conditions, can cause additional damage to the auditory system (Rintelmann & Bess, 1977; Humes & Bess, 1981). Therefore, it is important to give special consideration to procedures used for assessing amplification parameters that are known to interact with communication and auditory function, especially those that relate to electroacoustic output and listener performance.

The majority of procedures currently advocated to assess amplification were developed for use with personal wearable hearing aids. The American National Standards Institute (ANSI), for example, has published measurement standards (ANSI, 1982) for defining the electroacoustic performance of hearing aids. Moreover, various methods and procedures have been proposed to assess listener performance while wearing personal hearing aids. Although the ANSI standard has been widely accepted by American manufacturers, health care providers, and consumers, acceptable procedures for evaluating "as worn" hearing aid performance have not emerged despite clinical and research efforts that span more than 50 years (Studebaker, 1980).

Nonetheless, a need exists for procedures that can be used to evaluate the performance of a listener when wearing an amplification system. The purpose of this chapter is to discuss the use of speech stimuli to examine the variables associated with defining listener performance when using a hearing aid. First, several important variables associated with listener performance, hearing loss, and specific amplification criteria are considered. Next, various speech-based behavioral methods for selecting amplification are reviewed; and finally, potential applications for speech stimuli related to the selection and evaluation of hearing aids in current clinical practice are presented.

LISTENER PERFORMANCE AND ELECTROACOUSTIC CHARACTERISTICS OF HEARING AIDS

The assessment and subsequent selection of an appropriate amplification system for a specific hearing-impaired individual is based, in part, on assumptions related to the electroacoustic parameters of the device and the auditory characteristics of the impaired ear. For the past several years, the prevailing view has been that the optimal amplification system: (1) compensates in some way for the particular characteristics of an individual's hearing loss, (2) provides greatest amplification in the high frequencies (i.e., above 1000 Hz) to enhance speech perception and at least some low frequency extension to retain sound quality, and (3) minimizes the disruption of ear canal resonance effects produced when the external ear canal is occluded by an earmold, (Libby, 1982).

Electroacoustic parameters associated with the amplification device that typically are considered important include gain, saturation sound pressure output, and frequency response. These parameters have received extensive study in terms of their interactions with types and magnitudes of hearing loss, preferred listening and loudness detection levels, and the audiometric configuration of hearing impairment.

Gain Requirements

Gain represents the amount of amplification the instrument produces at a speci-

fied volume control setting, (i.e., the dB difference between input and output intensities). Although intuitively it seems reasonable to assume that one can compensate for an auditory deficit by selecting an overall gain equal to the degree of hearing loss, in practice this notion is fallacious because increases in hearing loss are not necessarily accompanied by similar increases in preferred listening level (i.e., the intensity level, or range of levels, preferred by a particular individual for everyday listening). Indeed, preferred listening levels increase at a slower rate than hearing loss. Hence, if gain is selected to equal an individual's hearing level, then everyday sounds, particularly speech, are amplified excessively.

In general, research has shown that the gain needed to amplify speech to a preferred listening level increases linearly with hearing level (HL), but at about one-half the rate, the so-called half-gain principal (Lybarger, 1944; Brooks, 1973; Martin, Grover, Worral, et al., 1973; Millin, 1973; Boorsma & Courtoy, 1974; Byrne & Fifield, 1974; McCandless, 1976; Byrne & Tonisson, 1976; Schwartz & Larson, 1977). An examination of the slope data for the gain-HL relationship, derived from the majority of available research, suggests that the best estimate of the overall gain-HL function ranges from 0.45 to 0.49 (Byrne, 1983). Stated differently, about 4.5 to 4.9 dB of gain is required for every 10 dB of hearing loss. In clinical practice, however, this rule is used to select the "operating gain" that should be otained at a volume control setting 10 to 15 dB below the system's maximum gain. This allows for a gain reserve that should be adequate for the user under most listening conditions.

While there is general agreement about the gain-HL relationship for ears with sensorineural loss, additional gain is needed to overcome a conductive or mixed type disorder. The amount of extra gain required for these types of hearing loss, however, is controversial. Most individuals involved in the practice of fitting amplification tend to support the recommendation of Lybarger (1944) that conductive or mixed hearing losses require additional gain equal to one-fourth of the difference between the air and bone conduction thresholds. Brooks (1973), on the other hand, calculated a slope of 0.57 for conductive losses, whereas Berger (1980) increased gain by one-fifth of the air-bone gap. Regardless of which value is selected for use, the concept that individuals with conductive or mixed hearing loss require more gain than their sensorineural counterparts holds.

Saturation Sound Pressure Level (SSPL) Requirements

The SSPL of an amplification device refers to the maximum output intensity that the instrument can produce, regardless of the intensity of the input signal. For the purpose of optimal amplification the SSPL should be sufficiently high to permit delivery of relatively undistorted amplified speech above the wearer's audibility threshold and below the loudness discomfort level (LDL). Failure to limit the output, however, may lead to overamplification and hence result in either temporary or permanent deleterious shifts in auditory thresholds. For excellent detailed reviews of the area of overamplification, see Rintelmann and Bess (1977), Markides (1980), and Humes and Bess (1981).

Another variable associated with the concept of SSPL is that the intensity output of the amplification device should not exceed the user's LDL. As a general clinical guide to ensure user preference, the maximum output from the device when adjusted to "operating gain" should not exceed the user's measured LDL at any point across the effective amplification bandwidth of the particular system. That is, the maximum output for an amplification device, determined for a given level of "operating gain" under an input intensity characteris-

tic of everyday listening conditions, should not be specified as an average figure selected according to average LDL because the latter will vary as a function of frequency. If, for example, output is set according to an average value derived from computations involving several frequencies, it is possible for the output to exceed the listener's actual LDL at some frequencies with resultant discomfort, while at the same time being inadequate at other frequencies and thereby reducing the level of the signal delivered above the individual's threshold of audibility. Averaged output data cannot be applied to averaged LDL because intersubject variability among sensorineural listeners and actual LDL measures is too large (Hood & Poole, 1966; Kamm, Dirks, & Mickey, 1983; Kamm, Morgan, & Dirks, 1983). Thus, it is best to determine that the amplification system is not providing too much output by directly measuring LDL under use conditions while the system is being worn by the listener.

Frequency Response Requirements

The importance of selecting an amplification system having a frequency range and relative gain-by-frequency response appropriate for a given hearing loss can be understood best by relating these concepts to factors that are important to amplification acceptance. As indicated in the previous discussion of gain and SSPL, the primary goal in selecting amplification is to provide an amplified signal that is maximally useful (i.e., improves speech communication) and comfortable for long-term listening to everyday acoustic signals. The following observations serve to summarize the current trends in frequency response requirements applied by most professionals who are involved in the process of selecting appropriate amplification.

The basic function of any amplification system is to make audible as many of the phonemic elements of speech needed to improve speech intelligibility. The findings from a variety of investigations designed to establish the optimum frequency-gain characteristics of personal hearing aids, summarized by Braida, Durlach, Lippman, et al. (1979), have rejected the long-held view of Davis, Stevens, and Nichols (1947) that, "As a practical matter, the best choice for all ears" (p. 6) is an amplification system that permits selection of a frequency response that is either flat or offers a high frequency emphasis of about 6 dB per octave.

In recent years many audiologists have subscribed to the notion that the optimal frequency response is one characterized by high frequency emphasis extending beyond 4000 Hz and low frequency suppression with little amplification below 750 Hz (Bess & Bratt, 1979; Harford & Fox, 1980; Schwartz, 1982). The high frequency emphasis, of course, is to enhance the perception of the relatively low intensity consonant sounds critical to speech intelligibility. The reason for minimizing the low frequencies is based on the observation that amplification of low frequency speech sounds and noise has been shown to interfere with the perception of high frequency consonants by the upward spread of masking phenomenon (Danaher, Osberger, & Pickett, 1973).

There is a growing trend in amplification research toward preserving a balance between the high frequency amplification needed to enhance speech intelligibility and the low frequency amplification needed to maximize sound quality (Pascoe, 1975; Punch & Beck, 1980; Skinner, 1980; Lippmann, Braida, & Durlach, 1981; Skinner, Karstaedt, & Miller, 1982). Specific to audiometric configuration, these researchers contended that listeners with gradually sloping audiometric contours require frequency-gain characteristics that provide 15 dB more "real ear" gain at 2000 Hz as compared to 500 Hz in order to maintain maximum speech intelligibility in combination with acceptable sound quality. Conversely

listeners with steeply sloping audiograms need 20 to 30 dB less gain at 500 Hz than at 2000 Hz (Skinner & Miller, 1983).

Current thought related to matching the electroacoustic characteristics of an amplification system to the physical characteristics of the impaired ear was summarized by Libby (1982) who stated that the optimal amplification system of today is one that:

1. Eliminates the peak at 1000 Hz and provides relative smoothness in the response curve at other frequencies.
2. Compensates for the insertion loss at 2700 Hz caused by the occlusion effects of an earmold.
3. Increases the bandwidth up to 8000 Hz to ensure greater fidelity for speech and music.
4. Preserves a balance between high and low frequency amplification to enhance both speech intelligibility and sound quality.

STRATEGIES FOR SELECTING AMPLIFICATION

The underlying premise of hearing aid selection (HAS) and hearing aid evaluation (HAE) is to select an instrument that will maximize an individual's communicative abilities under everyday listening conditions. While the previous section on electroacoustic characteristics briefly dealt with parameters important for understanding the relationships between hearing loss and amplification, the HAS and HAE attempt to use various data to select the best amplification system for a given hearing-impaired listener. The myriad of procedures that have been advocated to accomplish this goal over the past 50 years can be divided into two broad categories: comparative strategies and prescriptive or theoretical selection methods. Other chapters in this book detail the specifics associated with the use of prescriptive methodology for HAS and HAE. The following section, therefore, is concerned with the use of the comparative approach to HAS and HAE since this strategy typically has employed speech stimuli as a measure of hearing aid performance. Conversely, only a brief review is provided of the prescriptive or theoretical selection methods.

Comparative Strategies

Historically, comparative strategies for hearing aid evaluation have enjoyed the most popularity in the audiologic community. This approach incorporates some form of criterion measure, either objective or subjective, to assess which of several amplification systems is potentially best suited for a given individual. The most time-honored of these methods is the speech-test-based procedure advocated by Carhart (1946) and subjective judgments of hearing aid sound quality or speech intelligibility. In recent years, however, measures of real ear functional and insertion gain have received considerable clinical and research attention.

Speech Test Methods

Using this approach to hearing aid evaluation, the selection of a specific hearing aid is made on the basis of composite performance results on each of several speech tests obtained in an unaided condition and then again while the individual is wearing one of several hearing aids. Speech tests are administered in a sound field rather than under earphones. The hearing aid selected is the one that permits the greatest improvement in the individual's speech recognition in the presence of quiet and noise from the unaided condition. (For a detailed review of the Carhart [1946] method, see Schwartz and Walden [1983].)

While the speech-based comparative HAE approach continues to be widely used, it is plagued by serious pitfalls related to the variability of listener responses on speech recognition tests. Shore, Bilger, and Hirsch (1960), for example, demonstrated

that speech recognition tests could not reliably differentiate among hearing aids, especially using Carhart's (1946) original criteria of an 8 percent difference between scores. Schwartz and Walden (1983) investigated the results of word recognition scores for eight patients over a five-day period and reported day-to-day variability as great as 30 percent. Beattie and Edgerton (1976) examined test-retest reliability of word recognition in the presence of noise and concluded that a 14 percent criterion should be used in comparison of different hearing aids. In addition to the use of monosyllabic words to assess recognition scores between hearing aids, nonsense syllables (e.g., the Nonsense Syllable Test [NST] of Levitt and Resnick, 1978) and sentence stimuli (e.g., the Synthetic Sentence Identification [SSI] developed by Speaks and Jerger, 1965, and the Speech Perception in Noise [SPIN] test proffered by Kalikow, Stevens, and Elliott, 1977) have been suggested to improve measurement reliability and validity. Regardless of the type of stimuli, however, it must be stressed that the reliability of a given speech recognition score depends on the number of items in the test as well as the performance of the listener (Thornton & Raffin, 1978).

Subjective Methods

In view of the questionable power of most speech recognition tests to distinguish among hearing aids, professionals involved in hearing aid fitting have sought alternative methods for selecting the "best" amplification system. The most commonly used alternative method is the paired-comparison subjective approach in which the listener makes some form of preference judgment based on the perception of either sound quality or the relative intelligibility of hearing-aid-processed speech. The advantage of this method is that the response is a simple binary decision as to which hearing aid in a given pair produces the best sound quality or the more intelligible speech. Through a process of elimination, or sequential rankings, the hearing aid consistently judged as providing superior quality and intelligibility is selected as the most suitable instrument. Unfortunately, listeners appear to depend on a different set of electroacoustic parameters to rate quality as compared to intelligibility (Schwartz & Walden, 1983). Thus, a common outcome with this method is that one hearing aid is preferred for quality, whereas a different system is judged better for intelligibility.

Real Ear Methods

The *real ear gain* of a hearing aid represents the decibel difference between aided and unaided sound pressure as measured either by the listener's response (e.g., functional gain) or by a miniature microphone or probe tube placed directly in the external ear canal (e.g., insertion gain). The functional gain method is based on the dB difference between a listener's sound field threshold determined with and without a hearing aid. The unaided condition is used as a control with the hearing aid that provides the greatest amount of gain or most closely matches a predetermined criterion considered most appropriate. The insertion gain method utilizes a subminiature probe microphone seated in the ear canal of the listener or, more commonly, a flexible probe tube that serves as a sound channel between the listener's ear canal and an external microphone. Using pure tone, warbled tone, or various noise type stimuli, including speech spectrum noise, a real ear gain-by-frequency curve is measured in both the unaided (real-ear response) and aided (in situ response) conditions. The difference between the in situ response and real-ear response is termed the insertion gain. Here again, the aid of choice is the one that provides the greatest gain relative to the unaided values across frequencies commensurate with the individual's hearing loss or best satisfies a preselected frequency response based on one of the available prescriptive-theoretical strategies. Since these strategies are discussed in detail elsewhere in this book, the following discussion is limited to a brief consideration of several concepts considered to be important for understanding the relationship and general limitations associated with real-ear measures as applied to the hearing aid selection process.

Prescriptive-Theoretical Strategies

Due to the work of Byrne and Tonisson (1976) and Berger, Hagberg, and Rane (1977), there is a growing trend toward using prescriptive methodology for hearing aid selection. This strategy postulates that specific amplification parameters relate to the auditory characteristics of the impaired ear. Thus, in lieu of attempting to select the optimal hearing aid on the basis of patient performance on a series of tests as in comparative methods, this approach presupposes some general principals regarding the gain-by-frequency response required to optimize the reception of amplified speech at a comfortable listening level, as discussed previously under electroacoustic considerations. Most prescriptive methods involve the use of simple mathematical formulae to determine effective operating gain across frequencies for a given hearing-impaired individual. Moreover, some of these procedures are based on listener threshold data, while others not only require threshold responses but also depend on listener judgments of comfortable and uncomfortable listening levels.

To avoid mathematical computations of the gain-by-frequency response formula, the majority of currently advocated prescriptive procedures use a series of reference tables to determine the maximum gain requirements necessary to provide optimal amplification for a specific hearing loss at each frequency. In many cases, the tabled data are adjusted to account for the average difference between real ear and 2 cc coupler measured gain, although the specific correction factors used by each method are often different. This application also lends itself well to the use of personal computer software whereby the necessary threshold data (or comfort or loudness discomfort measurements) are entered into a computer program that calculates a defined prescriptive insertion gain. Regardless of the method used, after computing the required gain-by-frequency specifications, a series of trial hearing aids that have electroacoustic characteristics consistent with the predicted criteria are selected for evaluation. The objective is to prescribe the instrument that will result in aided sound field thresholds (functional gain) or microphone/probe tube measurements (insertion gain) that most closely approximate the values predicted from the tabled data.

Functional and insertion gain have been used most commonly to verify that an individual hearing aid meets the specifications of a given prescription. Either method is appropriate, and accurate predictions of gain can be made from either measure. From a practical standpoint, however, functional gain measures require listener cooperation and are limited by the noise floor in the test environment and the maximum intensity output of the audiometric instrumentation. Thus, verification of a prescription to be used with a difficult-to-test patient, or with a listener who has a mild or profound hearing loss, is best accomplished by using insertion gain methodology. Finally, it is important to stress that the prescriptive theoretical strategies do not represent a comparative evaluation of potential amplification systems. The use of either functional or insertion gain comprises the comparative aspect of determining if a hearing aid system meets a particular prescription. Indeed, when specific criteria for a prescription are met, it remains equally important to ensure that the prescription is appropriate for the listener.

SPEECH STIMULI AND SELECTION/EVALUATION STRATEGIES

In his discussion on the enigma of the hearing aid evaluation, Schwartz (1982) concluded that research findings raised serious questions as to whether any of the selection strategies was effective. Resnick and Becker (1963) and Walden and colleagues (1983) identified and evaluated several of the underlying assumptions of comparative hearing aid assessment. The findings from these investigations make it clear that the speech-based comparative evaluation, at least as applied to the use of monosyllabic stimuli, is an unreliable and invalid method to distinguish reliably between hearing aids that have similar amplification outputs.

Conversely, since it appears that most professionals are interested in matching the electroacoustic characteristics of the device to the auditory characteristics of the user's impaired ear, the theoretical-prescriptive methodology seems to have the greatest merit (Byrne, 1983). In general, regardless of the specific prescriptive procedure used, this technique is simple to apply because it requires only consultation of prepared tables, most conveniently via a computer program, to predict the gain needed at each frequency to optimize the reception of speech at a preferred listening level. No instrumentation or behavioral assessment is required to specify which set of electroacoustic response characteristics is appropriate for a given user if — and only if — the individual fitting the device has prior knowledge about the potential user's hearing loss and audiometric configuration. The electroacoustic output of the particular amplification system also must be known in order to match the system's electroacoustic parameters to the criteria determined best for the specific individual listener.

The recommendation that prescriptive theoretical methodology is preferred over the comparative approach in HAS and HAE does not imply that speech stimuli are unimportant in assessing hearing aid performance. Rather, the shift from comparative to prescriptive-theoretical methods reflects a change in clinical philosophy. With the comparative approach, for example, much clinical time is spent on evaluating different hearing aids by repeating various speech tests with each aid. As stated previously, the information obtained from this sequential testing cannot differentiate the "best" hearing aid; thus, spending significant amounts of clinical time in the comparative approach is simply not justified. Prescriptive-theoretical methods, on the other hand, require minimal time to obtain the prescribed insertion gain. The majority of clinical time then can be spent in direct interaction with the listener, either in fine-tuning the amplification system or in counseling sessions concerning hearing aid use or listening expectations.

Regardless of the methodology used to select or evaluate a hearing aid (i.e., comparative or prescriptive-theoretical), the specific method used must have a defined goal and employ procedures that permit a valid prediction of how well a particular hearing aid actually meets the defined goal. Since the fundamental purpose of amplification is to assist the communicative ability of hearing-impaired individuals, it follows that the amplification system recommended by any HAS and HAE method should improve speech recognition ability compared to unaided listening. While it may not be possible to obtain normal speech intelligibility under aided conditions, the listener must achieve some degree of improved communicative ability in order to justify use of the recommended hearing aid. Therefore, the reader is cautioned to pay careful attention to the rationales that support the various prescriptive-theoretical strategies.

While it is clear that speech-based comparative strategies for HAS and HAE are not justified in terms of reliability and validity, it is equally clear that most prescriptive-theoretical procedures are limited if a hearing aid is recommended solely on the basis of matching electroacoustic information to the results of audiometry. Several authors have recommended that prescriptive-theoretical methods be used in conjunction with measures of speech intelligibility or word recognition. The prescriptive electroacoustic output, usually in the form of a functional or insertion gain frequency response, is either confirmed as appropriate or is modified based on the results of speech testing.

Cox (1985) suggested that the HAS and HAE procedure should be based on the concept of using all available data from a given listener. This approach uses a series of sequential data collection, interpretation of data, and logical decisions to derive the recommended hearing aid. If, for example, the listener is only able to provide reliable pure tone threshold data (e.g., a young child), a prescriptive method that uses threshold measurements is appropriate rather than a technique that requires suprathreshold loudness data. Conversely, if the listener is able to respond reliably to a variety of psychoacoustic measures, the clinician must decide how much unaided and aided audiologic data are necessary in order to make a confident hearing aid recommendation. Given an appropriate listener, Cox (1985) outlined the use of speech intelligibility comparisons to select an appropriate hearing aid. This procedure requires the listener to rate speech intelligibility on a scale of 0 to 10 for each of the selected hearing aids. The speech stimuli consist of a 35 s passage of connected discourse presented in a background of speech babble at a predetermined signal-to-babble ratio. According to Cox (1985), this procedure may identify an aid that is clearly superior to the other systems being assesed, or it may indicate a clearly inferior aid. Regardless, in situations where two systems produce the same intelligibility rankings, the listener will typically express a preference based on a quality judgment of the reproduced speech.

For additional information concerning this procedure, the reader is referred to Cox and McDaniel (1984).

Another approach to the use of speech stimuli in combination with a prescriptive-theoretical strategy incorporates acoustical indices such as the Articulation Index (AI) (ANSI, 1969), the Speech Transmission Index (STI) (Houtgast & Steeneken, 1985), or the modified STI (mSTI) described by Humes and associates (1986). The AI and STI or mSTI are algorithms used to predict speech recognition performance.

Conceptually, these indices have several common features. Each divides the speech spectrum into various bands, derives a speech-to-noise ratio (SNR) for each band, applies weighting factors to equate the relative contribution of the various bands to overall speech intelligibility, and sums the individual contributions in the form of a ratio ranging from 0.0 to 1.0. There are substantial differences between the articulation and speech transmission indices in the way these factors are applied to derive various predictions. The AT, for example, divides the speech spectrum into 20 bands, although ANSI also expresses weighting for one-third octave bands with centered frequencies from 200 through 6300 Hz; whereas the STI and mSTI divide the speech spectrum into seven octave bands centered at 125 through 8000 Hz. Moreover, the SNR for the AI is computed as the difference between the rms intensity of the speech signal in each band plus 12 dB compared to the rms noise level in the same band. For the STIs, however, the SNR for each band is obtained by comparing the percent of intensity modulation present in the output signal of a system when the input signal is long-term average rms speech intensity modulated at 100 percent for rates of 0.63 to 12.5 Hz. The result is a modulation transfer function (MFT) that is converted to an SNR for each of the seven octave bands. Another difference between the AI and STI or mSTI is that the weighting factors used for the latter indices are

similar for all octave bands compared to the former index in which weighting factors for one-third octaves between 1000 and 4000 Hz are significantly greater than for other frequencies. Finally, since the STIs are based on MFTs, they are sensitive to both frequency and temporal characteristics of acoustic stimuli and essentially reflect system (i.e., hearing aid) performance.

The use of acoustical indices in conjunction with prescriptive-theoretical methods appears valuable for the following reasons. First, the theories, rationales, objectives, and validation procedures that support various prescriptive approaches vary widely among the different methods. Despite this variation, however, Humes (1986) has demonstrated in a theoretical study that many of the prescriptive techniques are able to optimize speech recognition performance equally, given adjustments in overall hearing aid gain (i.e., volume control rotation). This does not suggest a change in the hearing aid's frequency response to maximize speech perception, rather, acoustical indices are excellent tools that can be used to predict the amount of gain adjustment necessary to optimize speech recognition performance. Second, the patient's performance on a word recognition task while wearing the prescribed amplification system, as determined by real-ear insertion gain and frequency response, can be compared to performance predicted by the acoustical index. If the patient's aided word recognition score is comparable to the predicted performance, plus or minus 95 percent confidence intervals recommended by Thornton and Raffin (1978), it is logical to assume that the overall goal of maximizing speech recognition has been accomplished. This strategy appears particularly useful when word recognition performance is measured with speech stimuli presented in both quiet and in a background of competing noise. Conversely, if the patient's aided speech recognition performance is significantly poorer than predicted, appropriate counseling and follow-up aural rehabilitation strategies are warranted. Finally, the patient's unaided speech recognition performance can be predicted and compared to measured performance in quiet and competing noise conditions. These values, when contrasted to measured and predicted aided performance, yield an indication of the derived benefit to be expected from the use of amplification. Such information is often useful when making judgments about hearing aid candidacy or when counseling patients during pre- and post-selection sessions.

Additional research is needed concerning the relationship between the use of acoustical indices, prescriptive-theoretical procedures, and measures of real-ear aided and unaided insertion gain. Nonetheless, the AI, STI, or mSTI allow the clinician to fine tune the amplification system based on the prescribed insertion gain and predicted speech recognition performance for individual listeners. These predictions can then be verified using word recognition tests, such as the NST or SPIN, presented under unaided and aided conditions. The intensity of the NST or SPIN materials should be presented at a level consistent with the individual patient's listening environment. For average everyday listening, an intensity of 70 dB SPL is recommended. Likewise, the intensity of the background noise should also reflect the patient's listening environment. For everyday average conditions, the SNR should be adjusted to +7 dB. In some cases, sampling predicted and actual speech recognition performance in several SNR conditions may be appropriate, especially if the hearing aid wearer typically experiences varied listening environments (e.g., those characterized by different intensity levels of background noise).

Although the computations associated with acoustical indices are somewhat complex, the use of personal computers is ideally suited for this application. Currently, there are several commercially available software programs that compute these indices in combination with various pre-scriptive theoretical methods. The majority of time devoted to HAS is spent in non-patient contact activity, leaving additional time for patient interaction or fine tuning the system. As noted previously, Cox (1985) proposed a philosophy for prescriptive HAS and HAE based on obtaining as much information from the patient as possible, whereas Byrne and Dillon (1985) have advocated a prescriptive approach based on limited patient data. Regardless of the philosophical approach, however, the application of speech audiometric measures to the HAS and HAE is most appropriate and efficient when restricted either to obtaining information for prescriptive judgments or validating an already prescribed amplification system.

REFERENCES

American National Standards Institute. (1966). *Methods for the calculation of the Articulation Index.* New York: Author.

American National Standards Institute. (1982). *Specification of hearing aid characteristics* (ANSI S3.22). New York: Author.

Beattie, R., & Edgerton, R. (1976). Reliability of monosyllabic discrimination tests in white noise for differentiating among hearing aids. *Journal of Speech and Hearing Disorders, 41,* 464–476.

Berger, K. (1980). Gain requirements of conductive hearing loss. *British Journal of Audiology, 14,* 137–141.

Berger, K., Hagberg, N., & Rane, R. (1977). *Prescription of hearing aids.* Kent: Herald Publishing.

Bess, F., & Bratt, G. (1979). Spectral alterations of hearing aids and their effects on speech intelligibility. In V. Larson, D. Egolf, R. Kirlin, & S. Stiles (Eds.), *Auditory and hearing prosthetics research.* New York: Grune & Stratton.

Bess, F., & McConnell, F. (1981). *Audiology, education, and the hearing impaired child* (pp. 152–183). St. Louis: C.V. Mosby.

Boorsma, A., & Courtoy, M. (1974). Hearing evaluation with hearing impaired children. *British Journal of Audiology, 8,* 44–46.

Braida, L., Durlach, N., Lippman, R., et al. (1979). Hearing aids: A review of past research on linear amplification, amplitude compression and frequency lowering. *ASHA Monographs* (No. 19). Rockville, MD: American Speech-Language-Hearing Assn.

Brooks, B. (1973). Gain requirements of hearing aid users. *Scandinavian Audiology, 2,* 199–205.

Byrne, D. (1983). Theoretical prescriptive approaches to selecting the gain and frequency response of a hearing aid. In D. Schwartz, F. Bess, & R. Libby (Eds.), *Monographs in Contemporary Audiology, 4,* 1.

Byrne, D., & Dillon, H. (1986). The National Acoustics Laboratories' (NAL) new procedure for selecting the gain and frequency response of a hearing aid. *Ear and Hearing, 7,* 257–265.

Byrne, D., & Fifield, D. (1974). Evaluation of hearing aid fittings for infants. *British Journal of Audiology, 8,* 47–54.

Byrne, D., & Tonisson, W. (1976). Selecting the gain of hearing aids for persons with sensorineural hearing impairment. *Scandinavian Audiology, 5,* 51–59.

Carhart, R. (1946). Selection of hearing aids. *Archives of Otolaryngology, 44,* .1–8.

Cox, R. (1985). A structured approach to hearing aid selection. *Ear and Hearing, 6,* 226–239.

Cox, R., & McDaniel, D. (1984). Intelligibility ratings of continuous discourse: Application to hearing aid selection. *Journal of the Acoustical Society of America, 76,* 758–766.

Danaher, E., Osberger, J., & Pickett, J. (1973). Discrimination of formant frequency transitions in synthetic vowels. *Journal of Speech and Hearing Research, 16,* 439–451.

Davis, H., Stevens, F., & Nichols, R. (1947). Hearing aids. *An experimental study of design objectives.* Cambridge: Harvard University Press.

Harford, E., & Fox, J. (1980). The use of high-pass amplification for broad frequency sensorineural hearing loss. *Audiology, 17,* 10–26.

Hood, J., & Poole, J. (1966). Tolerable limits of loudness: Its clinical and physiological significance. *Journal of the Acoustical Society of America, 40,* 47–53.

Houtgast, T., & Steeneken, H. (1980). A review of the MTF concept in room acoustics and its use for estimating speech intelligibility in auditoria. *Journal of the Acoustical Society of America, 77,* 1069–1077.

Humes, L. (1986). An evaluation of several rationales for selecting hearing aid gain. *Journal of Speech and Hearing Disorders, 51,* 272–281.

Humes, L., & Bess, F. (1981). On the potential deterioration in hearing due to hearing aid usage. *Journal of Speech and Hearing Disorders, 24,* 3–15.

Humes, L., Dirks, D., Bell, T., et al. (1986). Application of the Articulation Index and the Speech Transmission Index to the recognition of speech by normal-hearing and hearing-impaired listeners. *Journal of Speech and Hearing Research, 29,* 447–462.

Kalikow, D., Stevens, K., & Elliott, L. (1977). Development of a test of speech intelligibility in noise using sentence materials with controlled word predictability. *Journal of the Acoustical Society of America, 61,* 1337–1351.

Kamm, C., Dirks, D., & Mickey, M. (1983). Effect of sensorineural hearing loss on loudness discomfort level and most comfortable loudness measurements. *Journal of Speech and Hearing Research, 21,* 668–682.

Kamm, C., Morgan, D., & Dirks, D. (1983). Accuracy of adaptive procedure estimates of PB-max level. *Journal of Speech and Hearing Disorders, 48,* 202–209.

Levitt, H., & Resnick, S. (1978). Speech reception by the hearing impaired: Methods of testing and the development of new tests. *Scandinavian Audiology, 6*(Suppl.), 207–230.

Libby, R. (1982). In search of transparent insertion gain hearing aid responses. In G. Studebaker & F. Bess (Eds.), *The Vanderbilt hearing aid report: Monographs in contemporary audiology* (pp. 112–123). Upper Darby, PA.

Lippmann, R., Braida, L., & Durlach, N. (1981). Study of multichannel amplitude compression and linear amplification for persons with sensorineural hearing loss. *Journal of the Acoustical Society of America, 69,* 524–534.

Lybarger, S. (1944, July 3). United States patent application No. FN 543, 278.

Markides, A. (1980). The effect of hearing aid amplification on the user's residual hearing. In R. Libby (Ed.), *Binaural hearing and amplification* (pp. 341–356). Chicago: Zenetron.

Martin, M., Grover, B., Worral, J., et al. (1973). The effectiveness of hearing aids in a school population. *British Journal of Audiology, 10,* 33–40.

McCandless, G. (1976). Special considerations in evaluating children and the aging for hearing aids. In M. Rubin (Ed.), *Hearing aids.* Baltimore: University Park Press.

Millin, J. (1973, October). The relationship between electroacoustic response of hearing aid and pure tone audiometric configuration. *Hearing Aid Journal,* 14–17.

Pascoe, D. (1975). Frequency responses of hearing aids and their effects on the speech perception of hearing-impaired subjects. *Annals of Otology, Rhinology, and Laryngology, 84*(Suppl. 23), 1–40.

Punch, J., & Beck, E. (1980). Low-frequency response of hearing aids and judgments of aided speech quality. *Journal of Speech and Hearing Disorders, 45,* 325–335.

Resnick, D., & Becker, M. (1963). Hearing aid evaluations: A new approach. *ASHA, 5,* 695–699.

Rintelmann, W., & Bess, F. (1977). High-level amplification and potential hearing loss in children. In F. Bess (Ed.), *Childhood deafness: Causation, assessment and management* (pp. 267–294). New York: Grune & Stratton.

Ross, M. (1975). Hearing aids for young children. *The Otologic Clinics of North America, 8,* 125–142.

Ross, M., & Giolas, T. (1978). Introduction. In M. Ross & T. Giolas (Eds.), *Auditory management of hearing impaired children: Principles and prerequisites for intervention* (pp. 1–14). Baltimore: University Park Press.

Schwartz, D. (1982). Hearing aid selection methods: An enigma. In G. Studebaker & F. Bess (Eds.), *The Vanderbilt hearing aid report: State of the art — research needs. Monographs in contemporary audiology* (pp. 180–187). Upper Darby, PA.

Schwartz, D., & Larson, V. A. (1977). A comparison of three hearing aid evaluation procedures for young children. *Archives of Otolaryngology, 103,* 401–406.

Schwartz, D., & Walden, B. (1980). Current status of the clinical hearing aid evaluation. In *Studies in the use of amplification for the hearing impaired* (pp. 15–28). Munich: Excerpta Medica.

Schwartz, D., & Walden, B. (1983). Current status of the clinical hearing aid assessment: A reappraisal of an old philosophy. In D. Konkle & W. Rintelmann (Eds.), *Principles of speech audiometry* (pp. 321–352). Baltimore: University Park Press.

Shore, I., Bilger, R., & Hirsh, I. (1960). Hearing aid evaluation: Reliability of repeated measurements. *Journal of Speech and Hearing Research, 25,* 152–170.

Skinner, M. (1980). Speech intelligibility in noise-induced hearing loss: Effects of high-frequency compensation. *Journal of the Acoustical Society of America, 67,* 306–317.

Skinner, M., Karstaedt, M., & Miller, J. (1982). Amplification bandwidth and speech intelligibility for two listeners with sensorineural hearing loss. *Audiology, 21,* 521–568.

Skinner, M., & Miller, J. (1983). Amplification bandwidth and intelligibility of speech in quiet and noise for listeners with sensorineural hearing loss. *Audiology, 22,* 235–279.

Speaks, C., & Jerger, J. (1965). Method for measurement of speech identification. *Journal of Speech and Hearing Research, 8,* 185–194.

Studebaker, G. (1980). Fifty years of hearing aid research: An evaluation of progress. *Ear and Hearing, 1,* 57–62.

Thornton, A., & Raffin, M. (1978). Speech discrimination scores modeled as a binomial variable. *Journal of Speech and Hearing Research, 21,* 263–273.

Walden, B., Schwartz, D., Williams, D., et al. (1983). Test of the assumptions underlying comparative hearing aid evaluations. *Journal of Speech and Hearing Disorders, 48,* 264–273.

8

COCHLEAR IMPLANTS AND REHABILITATIVE PRACTICES

DIANNE J. MECKLENBURG ■

*I*t is estimated that 90,000 to 200,000 individuals in the United States are profoundly hearing impaired and cannot benefit from amplification through a hearing aid (Ries, 1982). This population consists of individuals who are unable to effectively transform an acoustic stimulus to auditory sensation through the normal mechanical processes that take place within the cochlea due to hair cell loss.

The unimpaired cochlea allows acoustic signals to be transformed by mechanical shearing of the hair cells, which causes chemical changes within the cell body and results in synapse to dendrites projecting from the auditory nerve. In the case of the pathological cochlea where hair cells — or other cochlear structures — are nonfunctional, the hydromechanical shearing effects cannot occur and transmission to the auditory nerve cannot take place (Figure 8-1).

Communication for these profoundly deaf individuals can be augmented with speechreading as well as by learning a signed language. Alternative devices that attempt to utilize the pathological cochlea, such as air conduction hearing aids or temporal bone oscillating units, are ineffective in overcoming the impairment because these amplifying and mechanical transmission devices stimulate only the remaining hair cells and are thus limited by the impaired sensory system. In people with profound deafness, the auditory sense can be stimulated only if the nonfunctioning sense organ (cochlea) is by-passed and the auditory nerve is excited directly by electrical stimulation. This is accomplished through the application of cochlear implants (see Luxford & Brackmann, 1985).

COMPONENTS OF COCHLEAR IMPLANTS

A cochlear implant is an electronic device designed to simulate an acoustic signal with an electrical analog and to excite auditory neural fibers directly through elec-

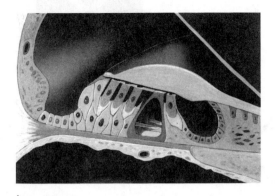 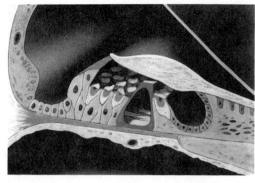

A   B

FIGURE 8-1. A. Normal cochlea with full complement of hair cells. B. Pathological cochlea showing loss of hair cells and the inability to provide mechanical transduction of the acoustically elicited signal.

trical stimulation. Although more than 29 different cochlear prostheses have been designed throughout the world, most systems consist of similar component parts: a receiving microphone, a speech processing unit, a transmitting coil or wire, a receiving coil, an implanted electronics package, an electrode array, and batteries (Figure 8–2).

Receiving Microphone

A receiving (pick-up) microphone similar to those used in hearing aids is placed at ear level, within an earmold, in the speech processing unit, or attached separately to the clothing with a clip. A directional, electret microphone is most commonly used. The directionality of the microphone allows an enhanced signal-to-noise ratio.

Speech Processing Unit

The acoustic signal received through the microphone is directed to an electronics box that converts the acoustic signal into a processed electrical signal. The method by which a signal sent to the implant recipient is derived is called the *coding strategy* (Moore, 1985; Mecklenburg & Lee, 1986). Most cochlear implant systems uti-

lize either a filter bank or a feature extraction procedure for coding. In the first instance, the signal is separated into a number of different frequency bands and transmitted as the analog of the input (Eddington, Dobelle, Brackmann, Mladejovsky, & Parkin, 1978; Merzenich, 1983). The feature extraction procedure focuses on the aspects of a signal that theoretically provide the greatest degree of speech recognition. These features have been described by Clark and Tong (1985); Liberman, Harris, Hofman, and Griffith (1957); and Tong, Blamey, Dowell, and Clark (1983).

Transmitting Coil or Wire

The externally processed signal is sent to the internal (implanted) components of the cochlear prosthesis directly by connecting the signal through percutaneous wires (Figure 8–3a) or transcutaneously (Figure 8–3b) by using a transmitting coil with either a radiofrequency link or passive magnetic induction.

Receiving Coil

Cochlear implant designs that incorporate transcutaneous transmission require a subcutaneous coil situated to allow for its alignment with the external transmit-

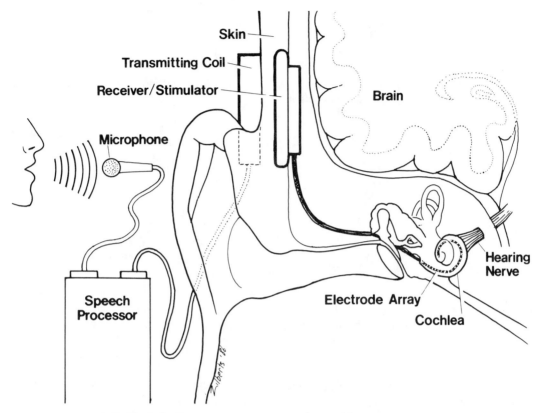

Skin

Transmitting Coil

Receiver/Stimulator

Brain

Microphone

Hearing Nerve

Speech Processor

Electrode Array

Cochlea

FIGURE 8-2. Common components of a cochlear implant system.

ting coil for effective transfer of information (Clark, Tong, Patrick, Seligman, Crosby, Kuzma, & Money, 1984; Rebscher, 1985). Both speech data and power are received by electromagnetic coupling. The receiver coil is usually located outside the implanted electronics package.

Implanted Electronics Package (Receiver)

The function of the receiver package is to decode the transmitted signal into electrical stimuli to be presented to the electrode array. This package can be referred to as the *receiver-stimulator* because it receives the signal from the internal receiver coil, decodes the transmitted signal, and directs the electrical signals to cochlear electrodes, which stimulate the auditory nerves.

Electrode Array

The function of an electrode in a cochlear implant is to transmit an electrical signal that initiates a physiological event by stimulating the auditory nerve. Electrode arrays vary in shape, size, stimulation configuration, and number of active electrodes. In most cases, the number of electrodes is synonymous with the number of channels of the device. However, the number of *active* electrodes defines the channels in a cochlear implant. Multichannel is best described as multi-sited stimulation. Thus, an array that has multiple electrodes but chooses only one set for stimulation is considered a single channel system. Any implant with only one active electrode and a reference is a single channel device.

Generally, cochlear implant electrodes are made of pure platinum or a combina-

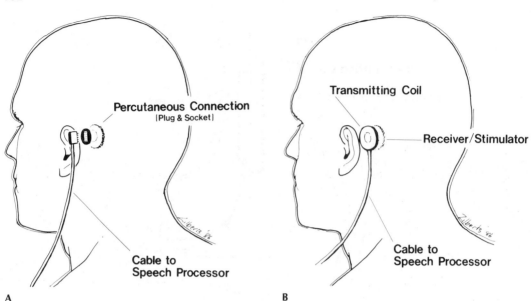

FIGURE 8-3. A. Percutaneous link where transmission is through the skin via a plug and socket. B. Transcutaneous link where transmission is across the skin via magnetic induction from a transmitting coil to a receiving coil.

tion of platinum and iridium (Rebscher, 1985). Although not yet implanted in human subjects, research continues toward the design of thin-film electrodes using photolithographic technology as described by White, Roberts, Cotter, and Kwon (1983).

Since postmortem histological studies showed that a relatively stiff, long wire, as used with the early House/3M designs, caused damage to cochlear structures during insertion (Burgio, 1986), electrodes have been redesigned. Electrode length has been shortened (Figure 8–4a).

Bundled array electrodes are characterized by a set of independent leads and electrodes that can be inserted individually into or onto the cochlear (Figure 8–4k). An array designed by Chouard (1980) and his colleagues allowed each electrode to be inserted separately into the scala tympani through different sites along the bony labyrinth. The array was later redesigned to be inserted through the round window with the electrode located in a carrier (Figure 8–4c). Another bundled array (Eddington, 1982), which was studied histologically and shown

to have caused extensive insult to cochlear structures (Galey, 1984), was redesigned with all electrodes housed in a silastic carrier. The extracochlear bundle (Banfai, Kubik, & Hortmann, 1984), in which individual electrodes could be placed on the promontory of the middle ear and into (but not through) the bony labyrinth, was adapted to a carrier plate (Figure 8–4f). Generally, the use of these electrode styles has been abandoned.

Several other shapes of electrodes have been clinically implanted in humans. Ball electrode designs (Figure 8–4a, e, i, and j) are the most common. Variations in single electrode designs include length of the lead wire, diameter of the ball, and stiffness of the lead wire. Multiple ball electrodes can be used as a multielectrode array. The ball electrodes may be partially embedded in silastic (Hochmair-Desoyer et al., 1983), gathered in silastic (Parkin, Eddington, Orth, & Brackmann, 1985), or extended from an earmold (Douek et al., 1983).

Banded electrodes have evolved from an early wrapped design by House-Urban (Johnsson, House, & Linthicum, 1982) to a

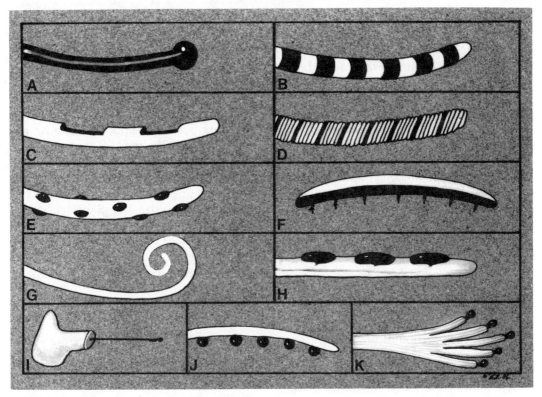

FIGURE 8–4. Electrode designs: A. ball, B. banded, C. recessed, D. wrapped band (discontinued), E. imbedded, F. plate, G. coiled memory, H. mushroom, I. earmold, J. gathered, and K. bundled.

series of tapered pure platinum bands (Figure 8–4b) on a silastic carrier (Clark et al., 1984).

Mushroom-shaped electrodes (Figure 8–4h) integrated into a silicone rubber carrier that is molded into a spiral have also been used. This particular multielectrode array (Figure 8–4g) is designed to maintain a degree of elastic memory (Rebscher, 1985).

The plate-electrode array is an example of an extracochlear design. This unit evolved from spring-loaded electrodes to the pointed-tip array shown in Figure 8–4k. The plate array is designed to be placed on the medial wall of the middle ear (Banfai, Kubik, & Hortmann, 1984; Hortmann, 1986).

Insertion depth varies from 0 mm (outside the cochlear) to 25 mm. Typically, the longer arrays are associated with multielectrode designs. Electrode arrays are either free-fit (nonspace filling) or space-filling.

The latter type must be carefully designed to avoid occluding the flow of perilymph within the scala tympani, which may result in localized neural degeneration (Leake-Jones & Rebscher, 1983).

Batteries

In percutaneous systems, power is supplied directly to the implant from batteries in the speech processing unit. Transcutaneous systems also rely on external batteries located in the speech processing unit. Listings of the different battery types and battery life for the various devices are described in Wilson and Finley (1985).

More complete descriptions of the various systems most widely in use are discussed in Eddington (1983); Banfai, Kubik, and Hortmann (1984); Clark and colleagues

(1984); Hochmair-Desoyer (1984); Millar, Tong, and Clark (1984); White, Merzenich and Gardi (1984); Fretz and Fravel (1985); Rebscher (1985); Staller (1985); and Hopkinson (1986).

An analogy between a cochlear implant and a normal auditory system can be made from a description of sound reception and perception (Chermak, 1981). In effect, the cochlear implant, in combination with the pathological auditory system, serves as a translator in much the same way as the mechanical functioning of the outer, middle, and inner ear serve to transfer acoustic energy. Figure 8–5 describes the similarities:

1. Acoustic signals are collected (through the microphone).
2. Preliminary signal processing is performed (the function of the speech processor).
3. The signal is distributed to the sensory system (decoded and transmitted to the receiver-stimulator).
4. The signal energy is transduced into electrochemical energy (electrode array).
5. The electrochemical energy is transmitted to the central nervous system (CNS) for further processing (residual neural population).

DESIGN CONSIDERATIONS

Cosmetic considerations, including size, weight, and color, are important for all of the external components. Ease of operation, power consumption, durability, reliability, cost of replacement parts, and repair charges should also be considered.

Receiving Microphone

The directional characteristics of the microphone play an important part in pro-

viding a more intelligible signal in noise. Directional microphones allow the processor to receive a better signal when it is embedded in noise. If this is not possible, the signal transmitted to the patient will also be noisy, and speech recognition will be more difficult. Enhancement of the signal is particularly important because patients are usually implanted monaurally and normal binaural squelch cannot take effect. This results in less effective cortical processing of speech in noise. Another consideration is the size and placement of the microphone. It is important to consider the different placements of the microphone and the impact of these sites on frequency response and directionality (Clark & Tong, 1985).

Speech Processing Unit

It is particularly important that the processing unit be lightweight, as small as possible, and durable. Controls should be large enough and simple to manipulate to accommodate the needs of both children and older cochlear implant wearers.

Controversy surrounds the selection of coding strategies. To date, clear evidence supporting the superiority of one strategy over another has not been demonstrated. Several factors have influenced the selection; however, the major element appears to be a theoretical consideration. It can be argued that the auditory system has always received a complete signal representing the original source-acoustic signal. The auditory system selects the most important elements from that complete signal. Thus, theoretically, the best model should be the one that most closely approximates normal cochlear reception. The auditory system, whether normal or pathologic, will select the features necessary for understanding.

The alternative coding strategy, which uses feature extraction, suggests that a com-

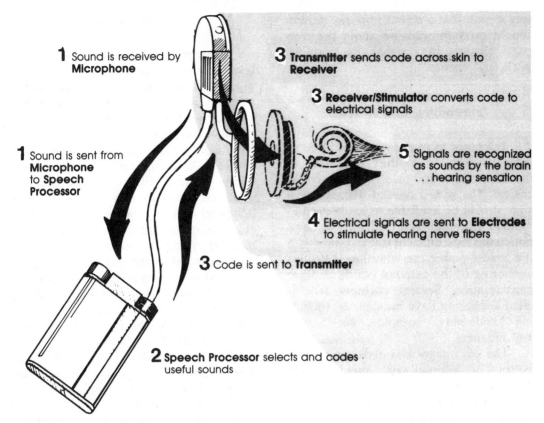

1 Sound is received by **Microphone**

1 Sound is sent from **Microphone** to **Speech Processor**

3 **Transmitter** sends code across skin to **Receiver**

3 **Receiver/Stimulator** converts code to electrical signals

5 Signals are recognized as sounds by the brain . . . hearing sensation

4 Electrical signals are sent to **Electrodes** to stimulate hearing nerve fibers

3 Code is sent to **Transmitter**

2 **Speech Processor** selects and codes useful sounds

FIGURE 8–5. Process through which a cochlear implant produces sound sensation. Reprinted with permission of Cochlear Corporation.

plete signal may be too noisy for a pathologic cochlea. Evidence to support this theory was presented by Wilson and Finley (1986), who suggested that a cochlea with poor neural reserve may not be capable of processing a complete signal. Current research by these investigators is aimed toward modifying the signal by limiting the amount of information transmitted to the cochlea. The goal of feature extraction systems is to present only the speech features that provide important information for speech recognition, such as fundamental frequency, maximum spectral energy peaks within different formant frequencies, and amplitudes of different formants (Patrick, Seligman, Dowell, & Blamey, 1986).

In a comparative study of four different cochlear implant systems with 17 patients, Ganz, McCabe, Tyler, and Preece (1985) concluded that all four devices (two single channel and two multichannel systems) enhanced speechreading ability but that "multichannel cochlear implant systems that provide spectral information in addition to temporal and intensity cues are consistently allowing profoundly deafened postlingual adults to recognize some words without visual cues." Such perceptual abilities were not reported for users of single channel devices. These findings support the theoretical considerations purported by Uttal (1973), who suggested in his discussion of sensory coding of auditory stimuli that a neural response pattern should carry information about the temporal changes in a signal, its loudness, pitch, and timbre.

Transmitting Coil or Wire

Tolerance to movement should be as great as possible so that alignment of the transmitting and receiving coils is less critical. The widest coaxial distance possible should be available to easily accommodate different skin thicknesses and obtain the most efficient transmission with the lowest power consumption. Effective anchoring of the external coil is another consideration. Several attempts at efficient anchoring have been made, including headbands, earmolds, ear hooks, and magnets.

The advantages and disadvantages of external to internal component linkage should be considered. Due to the absence of a direct feedthrough, transcutaneous transmission can be affected by skin thickness and hair and does not provide direct access to electrode measurements and direct control of electrical stimulation. Transcutaneous links require an equal number of transmitting and receiving coils.

Percutaneous linkage allows direct access; however, it may be confounded by the risk of postoperative infection. Parkin (1985) reported that percutaneous linkage presented only minimal risk of infection since the surrounding tissue forms a seal with the pedestal. Mild problems, reported by Parkin to occur in less than 20 percent of the patients with percutaneous linkage, were skin sagging around the pedestal, ingrown hairs surrounding the pedestal, mild infections resolved with the application of topical antibiotics, and the development of granuloma. Other considerations include the patient's ability to plug and unplug the pins into the pedestal and the age of the patient.

Receiving Coil

Currently, the number of coils for transcutaneous transmission is determined by the number of independent transmission links required. If more than one electrode is to be stimulated at exactly the same time (simultaneously), there must be a separate transmission link for each electrode. An example of a multiple coil system is shown in Figure 8-6. To overcome this need, other systems that present multichannel information multiplex the input so that the signals are carefully timed to occur rapidly in succession (sequentially). Continued research is needed to determine whether one method is more effective than the other in providing speech recognition without lipreading. To date, significant differences have not been demonstrated clinically.

The most important requirements are that the coil be effectively sealed from the ingress of body fluids to prevent failures and that the transmission characteristics of the coil allow the most efficient reception of magnetically induced signals.

Implanted Electronics Package

The electronics package should be as small as possible and thin enough so that it can be placed in the mastoid bone of both children and adults. It should be sealed against the invasion of body fluids. The most reliable method has been hermetic sealing, which is welding the package with either an electron or laser beam in a vacuum or inert atmosphere (Rebscher, 1985).

The Electrode Array

Several requirements may be imposed on electrode design such as biocompatibil-

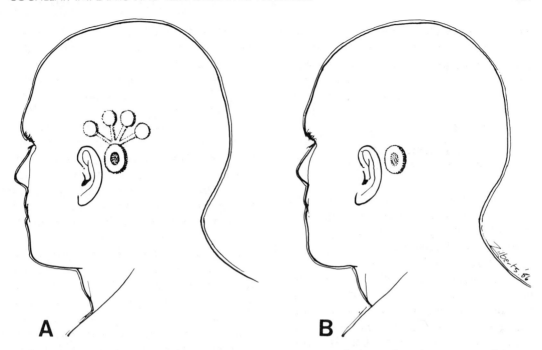

FIGURE 8-6. Illustration of multiple subcutaneous receiver coils (A) and single receiver coil (B).

ity, mechanical stability, practical fabrication, localized current control, and atraumatic insertion characteristics. Considerations related to atraumatic insertion include size, insertion distance, and the stiffness of the wire or carrier.

Control of stimulation is related to the amount of current flowing between an active and an indifferent, or reference, electrode. If current flows between two points (electrodes) that are very close together, the narrow region between the electrodes will be stimulated electrically. The greater the distance between the two electrodes, the wider the current spread. In a monopolar stimulus configuration, current flows between an active electrode and a remote ground. The active electrode is located within the cochlea or at the round window or promontory. The reference (ground) electrode is located away from the active electrode, typically in the temporalis muscle. Thus, a wide, undefined population of neural fibers is stimulated.

Bipolar stimulation, which utilizes closely spaced electrode pairs, results in a narrow distribution of current. The close physical proximity of the two electrodes, in part, determines the selective stimulation of discrete bundles of auditory nerves. Michaelson, Merzenich, and Pettit (1973) suggested that the fine discriminations needed for speech require stimulation of small groups of fibers. Keidel, Kallert, and Korth (1983) and Parkins and Houde (1983) agreed that there is a relationship between pitch sensation and the site of excitation in the cochlea. In multichannel devices, bipolar stimulation provides the ability to direct stimulation to specific regions within the cochlea, taking advantage of normal tonotopic organization.

Batteries

Size, life, and cost are important factors in battery design. Rechargeable batteries can be used in most systems; however their life per day is not as long as alkaline batteries. The fact that nicad batteries should be completely discharged to achieve the best recharging has not discouraged the use of this type of battery.

CLINICAL APPLICATION OF COCHLEAR IMPLANTS

Since 1976, any product that is to be injected, ingested, connected, or implanted in a human being is under the regulation of the Federal Food and Drug Administration (FDA), which requires that the product demonstrate safety, effectiveness, and performance of its designed function. In the case of cochlear implants, national clinical trials have been undertaken by several manufacturers to satisfy these requirements and to show that stimulation of the auditory nerve is both a safe and an effective means of treating deafness. As of 1989, three devices had received approval from the FDA for application in adults: the single channel 3M/House, the percutaneous 4 channel Symbion, and the transcutaneous Nucleus 22 channel devices. Other cochlear implants continue to be classified as investigational.

Patient Selection

A careful review of patients who have received a cochlear implant suggests that selection of candidates for implantation with the goal of predicting performance is confounded by several interacting variables (Mecklenburg & Brimacombe, 1986). Demographic and pre- and postsurgical audiologic data were gathered from 65 subjects, all of whom received the Nucleus 22-channel multielectrode system (Figure 8–7, Table 8–1). Data were collected 3 months postoperatively. The mean age at implantation was 49 years (range 20–78), and all patients were postlinguistically deafened adults who could obtain no benefit from a hearing aid or tactile device as defined by inability to score on a series of speech recognition measures.

Table 8–2 summarizes the findings of the study. Patients with progressive hearing loss demonstrated a trend to score higher on a selected test battery (recorded CID sentences, NU-6 word and phoneme scores, live-voice vowel recognition, consonant recognition, and speech tracking difference scores). This is in agreement with Punch, McConkey, Myres, Pope, and Miyamoto (1985) who studied the performance of subjects who had single channel devices. Interestingly, women scored higher on all measures than men. For the Nucleus system, patients who had 15 or more channels were more likely to score higher on the test battery than patients who had fewer channels, thus patency of the scala tympani was a factor. Consistent with reports by Eisenberg (1986) and McCandless (1986), years of deafness and age at implantation also were found to be significantly related to post-implantation performance.

Pre- and Postoperative Evaluations

Pre- and postoperative evaluation protocols for cochlear implant candidates should be consistent to document changes in performance as a result of cochlear implantation. Each patient should act as his or her own control with preoperative test results compared to the same battery of tests administered postoperatively. The test battery should be selected from standard test materials according to the needs of a particular clinic. The test battery should aid in the selection of individuals for candidacy and document relative performance between pre- and post-implant conditions.

The type of implant, single or multichannel, will affect the composition of the test battery. Since open-set speech recognition is limited for single channel users (Gantz et al., 1985), it is important to include tests that demonstrate effects related

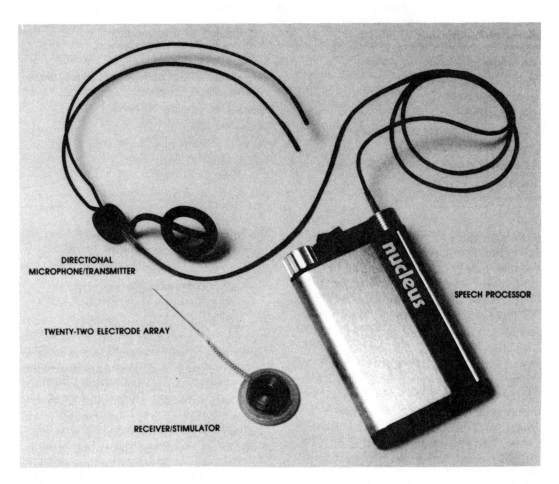

FIGURE 8–7. Component parts of the Nucleus 22-channel cochlear implant. Reprinted with permission of Cochlear Corporation.

TABLE 8–1. Design features of the Nucleus 22-channel cochlear implant.

Intracochlear placement
Bipolar stimulation
Feature extraction coding (F0, F1, F2)
22 electrodes (21 bipolar pairs)
Multiplexed, sequential signal processing
Transcutaneous linkage
Individually programmable stimulation

TABLE 8-2. Relationship of patient characteristics to post-implantation performance of profoundly deaf adults fitted with cochlear implants.

Related to Performance	Not Related to Performance
Type of loss (progressive vs. sudden)	Etiology of hearing loss
Sex	Preoperative aided threshold data (aided residual
Age at implantation	vs. no aided response)
Years of deafness	Absence or presence of tinnitus
Linguistic ability (pre- vs. postlingual)	Lipreading ability
Appropriate expectations	Years of sensorineural hearing loss
Desire to communicate in a hearing society	Age at onset of hearing loss
Patency of scala tympani	

to prosodic cues. Clinics evaluating multichannel subjects have often eliminated tests that rely mainly on the perception of time and intensity cues. This, of course, depends on the needs of the evaluating facility.

Typically, a complete test battery consists of audiometric and impedance measurements, a hearing aid evaluation, recorded speech tests, live-voice speech tests, a measure of speechreading, speech tracking, speech production evaluation, an environmental sounds test, and electrophysiologic measures (Mecklenburg & Brimacombe, 1985). Commonly used speech intelligiblity tests include the Minimal Auditory Capabilities (MAC) Battery (Owens, Kessler, & Schubert, 1981), the Iowa Cochlear Implant Test (Tyler, Preece, & Lowder, 1983), the Monosyllabic, Trochee, Spondee (MTS) Test (Erber & Alencewicz, 1976), and Discrimination after Training (DAT) Test (Thielemeier, 1982).

All cochlear implants are designed to provide, at a minimum, a sensation of sound that is neither too loud nor too soft for comfortable recognition. Thus, all systems require dynamic range measurements to allow determination of the output parameters of the speech processing unit. Some implant devices also require psychophysical testing to estimate loudness growth, frequency discrimination, loudness balancing, and sensitivity to stimulated electrode pairs. The amount and preciseness of

the testing required is dependent on the particular cochlear implant system.

REHABILITATION PROGRAM

The deaf population represents an extremely heterogeneous group. Even within the broad categories of mild to moderate to severel hearing impairment, performance varies greatly depending on a host of factors that influence all human behavior. Therefore, the structure of rehabilitation necessarily will be modeled to accommodate the needs of the individual patient.

Elements of a rehabilitation program for adult cochlear implant recipients include sound orientation, auditory training (including speechreading enhancement), speech production training (including voice and articulation monitoring), counseling, and ongoing assessment. Children require more intensive training, which should include therapy to assist educators in encouraging language development. The rehabilitation concepts discussed in this chapter deal with elements specifically related to reception and perception of sound.

Sound Reception

Understanding hearing aids, speech reception, the implementation of speech acoustics related to frequency specific perception, and an entire body of knowledge that hearing health professionals take for granted has been altered by the advent of cochlear implants. The most pervasive change is in the concept that speech intelligibility is predictable from measurements of the reception of frequency information, that is, the pure-tone or warble-tone audiogram. Depending on its coding strategy and filtering characteristics, each cochlear implant provides different information to a particular listener. In evaluating the frequency information received by an individual with a cochlear implant, an audiogram represents what the speech processing unit transmits, not what the pathologic cochlea receives. For example, if the microphone picks up a 3000 Hz signal, it will allow that frequency to be transmitted to the speech processing unit. If the speech processor's filtering capacity accepts 3000 Hz, a signal will be sent to the electrodes. It is virtually impossible to suggest that the 3000 Hz signal will stimulate the cochlea in the tonotopic (place-pitch) region where neural fibers sensitive to that frequency will fire or that the stimulation will elicit a 3000 Hz percept. However, in most cases, a sound sensation will be elicited. What the audiogram describes, post-implant, is the range of inputs that have been transmitted to the electrodes. It does not describe what the eighth nerve responds to.

This lack of specificity can be illustrated by comparing monopolar to bipolar stimulation. Each time current is applied between an active and a remote electrode pair, the distribution of current is wide and the stimulation of neural fibers nonspecific. Frequency specific cues (not related to neural firing rates) that are part of the tonotopic organization of the cochlea are not differentiated. This is true whether the speech processor receives a 1000 Hz signal or a 4000 Hz signal. The stimulation from either signal probably activates the same population of neural fibers between the active and reference electrodes. The listener may detect differences between signals due to other auditory cues, such as amplitude and temporality.

In bipolar stimulation, the situation is somewhat different. Greater control of the stimulating current allows specific bundles of nerves to be activated. However, it is not possible to suggest that a specific region in the cochlea, which is sensitive to a specific frequency, is activated. Consider that an electrode array is not situated in the same place in every cochlea. The lowest perceivable frequency for one person may be different for another person simply due to the length of insertion. One patient may have 10 mm of insertion length, another patient, 25 mm. It is clear that the lowest frequency (place-pitch) stimulated by closely placed bipolar pairs of electrodes will be different for the two patients, yet both individuals will "respond" to a warble tone of 500 Hz if the speech processor receives the signal and transmits it. The speech processor simply causes an electrode pair to be activated.

Further, audiometric threshold levels measured for cochlear implant users describe the sensitivity of the speech processor, rather than the receptive capabilities of the implant wearer. An implant, like a hearing aid, does not restore hearing. It artificially restores the possibility of the auditory system to respond to sound sensation. The speech processor determines the level at which hearing is activated. Post-implant audiometric thresholds suggest the softest sound that will cause the speech processor to send a signal to the electrodes in the cochlea. The output of the speech processor is adjusted to fit the needs of the patient. Therefore, even if a particular patient needs more output to recognize the sound at a soft level, the speech processor is the actual acoustic sound detector.

Therefore, assumptions that have been made in the past regarding what a person should or should not perceive on the basis of the audiogram must be different. What should concern the rehabilitationist of cochlear implant users is *pattern perception* (amplitude, timing, or pitch). The implication is broad, (re)habilitation for cochlear implant patients should be based on materials and exercises that progress from gross to specific differences in speech patterning. There are differences between training pre- and postlinguistically deafened adults. Although the progression holds true for both types of patients for the postlinguistically deafened adult, it is necessary to introduce the percept only in order to allow for comparison to remembered percepts.

SOUND ORIENTATION

The need for some directed familiarization with sound after implantation lies in the fact that, for postlinguistics at least, the perception of sound through a cochlear implant is different from that perceived through a normal auditory system or an auditory system that has been augmented by hearing aids (McFarland, 1986). Essentially, it is necessary to teach the cochlear implant subject to "hear" again and to adjust to the somewhat unnatural and new sounds transmitted by the speech processor.

The sound orientation phase of cochlear implant rehabilitation may be sufficient for the postlinguistically deafened individual to associate the new electrically elicited sound patterns with remembered receptive patterns that correspond to earlier sound sensations that were meaningful. It can include techniques that enhance listening skills and focus attention on relevant (and to the relevance of) sound stimuli.

Prelinguistically deaf patients require more than an introduction to sound. Nevertheless, this phase is an important element in their rehabilitation because this population first must learn to identify sound stimuli as meaningful. At this early stage, it is not important for the patient to understand speech, but rather to understand that speech elicits a perceivable sensation that carries meaning. Once this is established, it is possible to proceed with auditory training.

Training in the discrimination of environmental sounds has been recommended for people who receive single channel implants (Norton & Berliner, 1977). This type of training was introduced by Carhart for hearing aids in the late 1940s because it was believed that it provided a sense of being a part of a sound environment. However, more recent research has demonstrated that different cognitive strategies are used to process speech and nonspeech stimuli (Paterson, 1982; Raphael, 1986). More specifically, speech and environmental sounds have vastly different temporal characteristics. Thus, the choice of whether to directly train the recognition of environmental sounds rests in the determination of whether the rehabilitationist believes that speech recognition is possible for a given person. "Certainly, learning to discriminate environmental sounds may have some importance in itself, but there is no evidence that it will promote improvement in speech discrimination." (Paterson, 1982, p. 264).

Auditory Training

As early as 1961, Carhart defined auditory training as a process of teaching the hearing-impaired person to take full advantage of sound cues. Durity (1982) defined it as, "an instructional program ... designed to maximize use of residual hearing for the purpose of greater participation in the auditory [communication] environment" (p. 296). More specific to cochlear implants, Boothroyd (1986) described auditory training as taking advantage of the newly acquired access to speech information with the aim of enhancing the ability of implant subjects to utilize this information to understand speech.

McFarland (1986) suggested that rehabilitation strategies be based on the performance capabilities of the implant system. Thus, if time and intensity cues are available, as with single channel devices, the focus should be on elements such as stress, syllabification, duration, and so forth. A multichannel system, on the other hand, provides some information about frequency, and therefore the focus should be on different elements, such as vowel distinctions, word identification, and sentence recognition.

Modality Training

Multisensory Approach

The most widely used multisensory approach is total communication (TC). The fundamental principle underlying the use of TC was summarized by Dr. McCay Vernon in his presentation to the Alexander Graham Bell Society's national convention in 1971: "Language development is the key to the deaf child's hope for education and communication .... Total communication provides the deaf child a language environment of symbols he can see and learn to understand" (Scouten, 1984, p. 349). The operative word is *see;* hearing is not discussed. By definition, the TC method utilizes all sensory input: visual (speechreading, fingerspelling, manual sign language, natural gestures, facial expression, and written text) and auditory (self-monitored speech production and amplified audition). It is clear, however, that the opportunity to make use of visual input in TC is far greater than auditory input. Essentially, then, TC must be considered a visually based program in which most information is conveyed through the visual system. Since the goal of auditory training for cochlear implant recipients is to take the greatest advantage of the auditory channel, this multisensory approach is not recommended and may, in fact, inhibit the successful integration of sound sensation as meaningful stimuli. This idea is supported by Ross and Calvert (1984) who consider the use of TC an inhibiting factor in providing children the opportunity to take full advantage of residual hearing. However, before the advent of cochlear implants, when communication was possible only through an auditory system that was highly nonfunctional, TC training appeared to be most

appropriate. Erber (1982) supported this when he remarked that the majority of hearing-impaired individuals live in a multisensory environment and "... regardless of hearing loss, [a multisensory approach] probably is the best condition for overall language learning" (p. 25). This has not proved to be the case. Even the primary goal of providing better language development has not been achieved according to Geers, Moog, and Schick (1983). They surveyed 15 TC schools and 13 oral schools in a study that revealed that the spoken language of children trained in oral programs was richer than that of children who had received their education through TC.

The committee on developmental issues chaired by Stark, Bowman, Busse, Hasenstab, House, and Oller (1986) suggested that it may be possible to combine tactile (electro- or vibrotactile) with electrically elicited sound sensations (cochlear implants) and vision to provide an individual with the greatest possibility of receiving speech and language. This suggestion was based on work by Sparks, Kuhl, Edmonds, and Gray (1978) in which they reported that aspects of speech that are not available through speechreading are effectively presented by spectrally oriented tactile arrays. De Fillipo (1982) believes that tactile input can be used to supplement training for hearing-impaired individuals by aiding them in focusing their attention on minimal cues received through the auditory system. The primary goal is to enhance the auditory signal. She cited Geldard's (1961) work in which he suggested that the tactile system is not ideally suited to receive acoustic energy because the skin's resolving power is limited for time, intensity, and frequency information related to speech. However, research with persons using multi-arrayed tactile stimulators suggests that the recognition of words and sentences may be possible without the aid of audition (Brooks & Frost, 1983; Oller, Eilers, Vengara, & LaVoie, 1986).

Further study is needed to carefully evaluate individuals who have received rehabilitation therapy wearing both a cochlear implant and a tactile device.

Bisensory Approach

Bisensory training is also a combined auditory and visual method but employs only visual cues that are specifically associated with speech, that is, speechreading. Erber (1982) suggested that the integration of vision and audition allows for more effective reception and discrimination of speech than either modality alone. Sims (1982) reported that when sound is added to speechreading, significant improvement in consonant, word, and sentence recognition can be demonstrated.

Cochlear implant recipients benefit from the combined approach. The most widely used technique is speech tracking, which was first introduced by De Filippo and Scott in 1978. Since the use of this technique is growing, it is appropriate to review it in more detail.

Speech tracking is a training and evaluation technique that uses continuous discourse or prose. In the tracking procedure, the clinician reads a passage from 2 to 10 words long. The listener attempts to repeat the passage verbatim. If a mistake is made, the clinician uses a variety of strategies to assist the patient in making a correct response. Speech tracking is best described as an interactive, adaptive procedure that closely mimics a true communication process. It differs from other methods of speech recognition evaluation in that it requires the patient to respond with 100 percent accuracy from the stimulus material. This requirement not only allows a quantitative measure of how many words can be transmitted and repeated in a selected period of time but also takes into consideration the ease or difficulty of conveying a message once it has been understood. The better the individual's speech understanding, the faster he or she is able to perform the task and the higher the words per minute (wpm) score. Speech tracking can be used at several levels, including phonemes, words, phrases, and sentences. It is a purely synthetic approach in which direct training of visual and auditory reception of segmental elements of speech is not emphasized.

A few words of caution regarding the use of this technique as an evaluation tool are necessary. Speech tracking is more variable and less well-defined than other tests, although it more closely approximates a conversational situation and better approximates the full speech communication system. Confounding factors should be taken into account when collecting comparative data between different conditions (e.g., speechreading only, speechreading combined with implant, and implant alone) or when comparing results from session to session, clinician to clinician, or patient to patient. Other considerations include the materials used, the speaker, the test environment, and the technique (Mecklenburg, Dowell, & De Filippo, 1984). Further, it is very important to keep in mind that the goal of speech tracking is to teach and assess speechreading ability and its enhancement when sound is added to visible speech. This inherently implies that signing, common gestures, spelling out words in the air, fingerspelling, and writing are not effective strategies for enhancing speechreading skills. They are inappropriate methods for transmitting speech when the emphasis is on a uni- or bisensory approach and should not be part of the tracking technique.

The scoring of speech tracking results also should be clearly understood so that the effects of rehabilitation and the enhancement of speechreading through the addition of sound sensation can be clearly demonstrated. Speechreading ability varies greatly among hearing-impaired individuals, thus absolute scores suggest little more than the efficiency of a person's speechreading skill. A more representative method for estimating enhancement of speechreading skills when sound is added is through a difference score. To calculate a difference score (or rate), obtain scores with speechreading when the cochlear implant is activated and with speechreading only. Subtract the speechreading-only score from the speechreading plus implant score to obtain a difference score. Absolute values are useful only when relating subject performance to rates obtained from normal listeners (90–115 wpm).

As a rehabilitation technique, speech tracking has obvious advantages: similarity to a natural communication environment, active participation by the person, three-dimensional interaction, and the potential to maintain the individual's interest over time. The technique is less formal than analytic training in speechreading and lip movements and can be aimed at achieving understanding of spoken material. Although it can be argued that speech tracking is an artificial process, in fact, it utilizes all of the dynamic aspects of intercommunication. Further research is needed to determine if the strategies learned are internalized and generalized for use in nonclinical settings (Owens & Telleen, 1981).

Unisensory Approach

This training technique emphasizes sound reception through the auditory sense alone; therefore, speechreading is not taught. It is also referred to as the auditory method or acoupedic method (Ferguson, Hicks, & Pfau, 1982). Materials for use with single channel implants have been developed at the House Ear Institute (Eisenberg, 1985). The exercises represent a range of tasks related to the prosodic features of speech and recognition of environmental sounds. A set of materials for training of adult, postlinguistically deafened recipients of multichannel cochlear implants was developed by Mecklenburg and Dowell (1986) and revised by Mecklenburg, Dowell, and Jenison (1987). They employ a variety of word and sentence stimuli that can be utilized in closed- or open-set paradigms. When using a unisensory approach, materials should be highly redundant, simple, and familiar. They also should be designed for a high probability of success to positively reinforce the use of hearing.

Some multichannel implant patients can perform the speech tracking task using audition alone. This technique excludes the use of visual cues. Because of this difference, use of special strategies and tactics in which the set of options is considerably reduced is necessary. Consistent reinforcement is also important. Again, since this technique is gaining popularity in demonstrating cochlear implant patients' ability to achieve useful information from electrically induced speech signals, it is appropriate to briefly review the adapted procedure for hearing-only conditions.

The tracking period should always begin with a familiar passage. It is usually necessary to allow patients several sentences to refamiliarize themselves with the speaker's voice as it sounds without the aid of speechreading. During this reading period, repeats are used, but a full repertoire of strategies is not as it can be time consuming. If a word is missed, the patient is tapped on the shoulder, allowed to lipread and hear the correct word, then returned to the no-lipreading condition in which the phrase is repeated. When using repeats during a timed segment, a maximum of three repetitions are used. More can be both time consuming and frustrating. It is more effective to repeat a phrase than a single word.

Comparative results for 10 patients between lipreading only, lipreading combined with cochlear implant, and implant alone conditions are shown in Figure 8–8. All patients used the Nucleus 22 device. Enhancement of lipreading is shown in the mean difference score of 45 wpm. It can also be demonstrated that these patients, as a group, performed the speech tracking task at a mean rate that was greater than in the lipreading condition alone (Mecklenburg, 1984). Such information is important when assessing the effectiveness of cochlear implantation and also suggests that

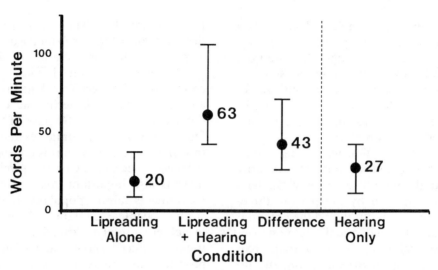

FIGURE 8-8. Means and ranges for speech tracking rates. Best score for three conditions (N = 12).

greater communication exchanges are possible through bisensory input.

Unisensory training should be used to direct and enhance listening skills rather than to achieve speech recognition without speechreading. The latter task is too difficult. It is easier to transfer from bisensory to unisensory discrimination than to receive auditory input only and be expected to integrate it with visual cues without training.

ANALYTIC VERSUS SYNTHETIC APPROACHES TO AUDITORY TRAINING

The committee on auditory training at the Durango meeting (Colloquium on Cochlear Implants in Children, 1986) recommended that both analytic and synthetic approaches be included in any auditory training program for children with cochlear implants but noted that the more structured approach was needed for patients who had no experience with sound (Osberger, 1986). Durity (1982) argued that it is artificial to isolate speech characteristics which, although perceptually important to speech recognition, are part of a dynamic, multidimensional process of conceptualization. It is one thing to receive and per-

ceive a stimulus, but the goal must be to attach meaning to that stimulus. Training simple differences or basic prosodics without attaching meaning leads to an ability to discriminate but not to cognate the sensations into an integrated signal-symbol. Ling (1976) amplified this thought, suggesting that analytic training is best used to familiarize subjects with elements such as rhythm, stress, intonation, and syllabification, but is not appropriate as a therapy technique. He stated: "Discrimination of sounds or sound sequences does not imply identification or the ability to recognize sounds or sound sequences." A commonly used analytic task requires the subject to distinguish between two stimuli in a same-different paradigm, such as recognizing whether two spondees are the same or different words, between male and female voices, or between noise and voice stimuli. Individuals who demonstrate the ability to score well above chance on such tests do not necessarily demonstrate the ability to obtain open-set speech recognition. Training on same-different tasks does not prepare the listener for linguistic discriminations needed to perceive ongoing speech. However, Erber (1982) supported the benefit of incorporating analytic training into (re)habilitation programs in order to aid the listener in recognizing general characteristics of speech patterns with the goal of enhancing speechreading as well as contributing to speech monitoring and control.

The method incorporated into the multichannel cochlear implant program (Mecklenburg, Dowell, & Jenison, 1987) employs both analytic and synthetic techniques. To acquaint the beginning implant user with the phonemic and syllabic elements of speech signals, initial sessions include repetition and contrast of a closed-set of vowels and consonants in three different conditions beginning with the easiest, speechreading combined with sound sensations from the implant, and progressing to the most difficult, implant alone. This drill work also is used to plot progress over time and to demonstrate the difference between conditions. All other training emphasizes a top-down approach in which materials systematically provide listening experiences in a realistic, meaningful language context. Related words and sentences, clue-word sentences, topic sentences and other similar materials adapted from speechreading exercises developed by Jeffers and Barley (1971) are used. Even prosodic elements of speech are embedded in contextual speech through a procedure called paragraph tracking in which the individual is required to follow (without the benefit of visual cues), but not necessarily understand, words in a paragraph as they are read aloud.

Generally, clinicians involved in auditory training agree that no single technique meets the needs of all individuals undergoing therapy. The aural rehabilitator should be conversant with a variety of strategies to provide the most effective training to the widest population.

Telephone Training

It is important to demonstrate, as early as possible, that the new sound sensa-tions are effective in providing individuals with usable hearing and allowing them to participate in a hearing community. For postlinguistically deafened adults, release from the dependence of relying on others to communicate is a strong motivating factor. One of the more frustrating effects of acquired deafness is the inability to contact friends, make appointments, make enquiries, and transmit information over the telephone. This is not surprising considering the extent to which the telephone is a part of most people's daily lives. Restoring the ability to communicate by telephone is an immediate reinforcer and encourages new listeners to use the cochlear implant for longer periods of time.

Erber (1985) suggested that nearly all hearing-impaired individuals are capable of using the telephone for the reception of acoustic speech, although people with profound hearing impairment demonstrate a range of telephone communication skills, which depend on the type of cues they use to understand speech. These range from cuing into very basic prosodic characteristics of the signal to recognizing words and sentences. This is also true of cochlear implant recipients. Several techniques, codes, and training methods have been suggested by Castle (1977, 1978) and Erber (1982, 1985).

Telephone communication should be encouraged for all cochlear implant wearers soon after they first have had their speech processing units set. It is essential that clinicians correctly estimate the level at which communication can take place. For instance, for most beginning listeners, a simple "yes yes" "no" code (Castle, 1977) suffices to introduce telephone use accompanied by familiarization with common telephone sounds, such as ringing, a dial tone, a busy signal, and the difference between a ringing sound and a person talking. Familiarization training is necessary for users of single channel implants but may also be needed by listeners with multichannel implants who lack experience in telephone use or who have lost confidence in their ability to make use of auditory cues. Users of multichannel devices are often able to recognize closed-set sentences of different lengths, selected numbers and colors, and the difference between yes and no within the first week. As listeners gain experience, more difficult tasks may be possible. In a group of 36 patients, who had completed 10 training sessions using the Nucleus multichannel cochlear implant, patients who achieved a speech tracking difference score of 30 wpm or greater were able to conduct interactive conversations over the telephone without the aid of a code (Mecklenburg, Brimacombe, & Dowell, 1985).

The most appropriate type of coupling between the telephone receiver and the speech processor must be made. Once this is accomplished, the person is shown how to answer the telephone, instruct the caller to wait while a microphone is attached, and hold the telephone receiver for best transmission and reception. Appropriate expectations should be taught so that the implant user understands that reception may be more difficult, depending on the distance between the callers, the weather, the type of telephone, and the fact that some speech sounds transmit more clearly across telephone lines than others.

Home exercises begin by requiring the person to simply answer the telephone in response to a ring and to pass the call on to someone else and progress to receiving known, simple messages spoken by a familiar speaker. Early therapy in the user's clinic should concentrate on activities in which the implant wearer experiences success and therefore gains greater confidence in using the telephone. If successful unisensory training is taking place, it is reasonable to assume that the listener will be able to do similar tasks over the telephone. It is important, however, to demonstrate that speech reception over the telephone is more difficult than a live-voice, auditory-only condition.

CONCLUSION

Rehabilitation for individuals who have received cochlear implants is a new frontier for hearing health professionals. A multifaceted, interdisciplinary team approach is required to provide emphasis on specific areas of development, yet it is important to maintain a unified goal. Ideally, that goal is to restore the possibility of receiving information similar to that received by normally functioning auditory systems. Realistically, the goal is to provide usable hearing sensations. Reasonable expectations gained through understanding how cochlear implant systems function help to encourage cooperation and communication between surgeons, speech pathologists, audiologists, educators, and family members.

REFERENCES

Banfai, P., Kubik, S., & Hortmann, G. (1984). Our extra-scalar operating method of cochlear implantation. *Acta Otolaryngologica* (Stockholm), *411,* 9–12.

Boothroyd, A. (1986, April 17–19). Effective rehabilitation techniques for the adult cochlear implant recipient. Paper presented at the conference on Speech Recognition with Cochlear Implant: Issues, Progress, and Trends. New York University Medical Center, New York.

Brooks, P., & Frost, B. (1986). Evaluation of a tactile vocoder for word recognition. *Journal of the Acoustical Society of America, 74,* 34–39.

Burgio, P. (1986, April 17–19). Safety considerations of cochlear implantation. Paper presented at the conference on Speech Recognition with Cochlear Implant: Issues, Progress, and Trends. New York University Medical Center, New York.

Carhart, R. (1961). Auditory training. In H. Davis & R. Silverman (Eds.), *Hearing and deafness* (p. 276). New York: Holt, Rinehart & Winston.

Castle, D. L. (1977). Telephone training for the deaf. *Volta Review, 79,* 373–378.

Castle, D. L. (1978). Telephone communication

for the hearing impaired: Methods and equipment. *Journal of the Academy of Rehabilitative Audiology, 11,* 91–104.

Chermak, G. D. (1981). *Handbook of audiological rehabilitation.* Springfield, IL: Charles C. Thomas.

Chouard, C. H. (1980). The surgical rehabilitation of total deafness with the multi-channel cochlear implant: Indications and results. *Audiology, 19,* 137–145.

Clark, G. M., & Tong, Y. C. (1985). The engineering of future cochlear implants. In R. F. Gray (Ed.), *Cochlear implants* (pp. 211–228). Boston: College-Hill Press.

Clark, G. M., Tong, Y. C., Patrick, J. F., Seligman, P. M., Crosby, P. A., Kuzma, J. A., & Money, D. K. (1984). A multi-channel cochlear prosthesis for profound-to-total hearing loss. *Journal of Electrical and Electronic Engineering* (Australia), *4*(2), 111–117.

De Filippo, C. E. (1982). Tactile perception. In D. G. Sims, G. G. Walter, & R. L. Whitehead (Eds.), *Deafness and communication — Assessment and training* (pp. 40–52). Baltimore: Williams & Wilkins.

De Filippo, C. L., & Scott, B. L. (1978). A method for training and evaluating the reception of ongoing speech. *Journal of the Acoustical Society of America, 63*(4), 1186–1192.

Douek, E., Fourcin, A. J., Moore, C. J., Rosen, S., Walliker, J. R., Frampton, S. L., Howard, D. M., & Abberton, E. (1983). Clinical aspects of extracochlear electrical stimulation. *Annals of the New York Academy of Science, 405,* 332–336.

Durity, R. P. (1982). Auditory training for severely hearing-impaired adults. In D. G. Sims, G. G. Walter, & R. L. Whitehead (Eds.), *Deafness and communication — Assessment and training* (pp. 296–311). Baltimore: Williams & Wilkins.

Eddington, D. K. (1982). Multiple channel intracochlear stimulation. In D. E. Brackmann (Ed.), *Neurological surgery in the ear and skull base* (pp. 199–205). New York: Raven Press.

Eddington, D. K. (1983). Speech recognition in deaf subjects with multichannel intracochlear electrodes. In C. W. Parkins & S. W. Anderson (Eds.), *Cochlear prostheses: An international symposium* (pp. 183–190). New York: New York Academy of Sciences.

Eddington, D. K., Dobelle, W. H., Brackmann, D. E., Mladejovsky, M. G., & Parkin, J. L. (1978). Auditory prosthesis research with multiple channel intracochlear stimulation in man. *Annals of Otology, 87*(53), 5–39.

Eisenberg, L. S. (1985). Training strategies for the post-implant patient. In R. A. Schindler & M. M. Merzenich (Eds.), *Cochlear implants* (pp. 511–520). New York: Raven Press.

Eisenberg, L. S. (1986, April 17–19). Rehabilitation strategies for children with a cochlear implant. Paper presented at the conference on Speech Recognition with Cochlear Implants: Issues, Progress, and Trends. New York University Medical Center, New York.

Erber, N. P. (1982). *Auditory training.* Washington, DC: Alexander Graham Bell Association for the Deaf.

Erber, N. P. (1985). *Telephone communication and hearing impairment.* Boston: College-Hill Press.

Erber, N. P., & Alencewicz, C. M. (1976). Audiologic evaluation of deaf children. *Journal of Speech and Hearing Disorders, 41,* 256–267.

Ferguson, D. G., Hicks, D. E., & Pfau, G. S. (1982). Education of hearing impaired learners. In N. J. Lass, L. V. McReynolds, J. L. Northern, & D. L. Yoder (Eds.), *Speech, language, and hearing: II. Hearing disorders* (pp. 1067–1069). Philadelphia: W. B. Saunders.

Fretz, R. J., & Fravel, R. P. (1985). Design and function: A physical and electrical description of the 3M House cochlear implant system. *Ear and Hearing, 6*(Suppl.), 14S–19S.

Galey, F. R. (1984). Initial observations of a human temporal bone with a multi-channel implant. *Acta Otolaryngologica* (Stockholm), *411,* 38–44.

Gantz, B. J., McCabe, B. F., Tyler, R. S., & Preece, J. P. (1985). Evaluation of four cochlear implant designs. *Annals of Otology, Rhinology, and Laryngology, 96*(1, Part 1) (Suppl. 128), 145–147.

Geers, A., Moog, J., & Schick, L. (1983, Fall). National results compare oral/"total" communication. *CID Bulletin.*

Geldard, F. A. (1961). Cutaneous channels of communication. In W. Rosenblith (Ed.), *Sensory communication* (pp. 73–87). Boston: MIT Press.

Hochmair-Desoyer, I. J., Hochmair, E. S., & Burian, K. (1983). Design and fabrication of multiwire scala tympani electrodes. In C.

W. Parkins & S. W. Anderson (Eds.), *Cochlear prostheses* (pp. 173–182). New York: New York Academy of Sciences.

Hopkinson, N. (1986). Report of the ad hoc committee on cochlear implants. *ASHA, 28,* 29–52.

Hortmann, G. (1986, February 10–11). Eight channel cochlear implant. Paper presented at Ear International Conference, Aspen, CO.

Jeffers, J., & Barley, M. (1971). *Speechreading.* Springfield, IL: Charles C. Thomas.

Johnsson, L. G., House, W. F., & Linthicum, F. H., Jr. (1982). Otopathological findings in a patient with bilateral cochlear implants. *Annals of Otology, Rhinology, and Laryngology, 91,* 74–89.

Keidel, W. D., Kallert, S., & Korth, M. (1983). *The psychological basis of hearing.* New York: Thieme-Stratton.

Leake-Jones, P. A., & Rebscher, S. J. (1983). Cochlear pathology with chronically implanted scala tympani electrodes. *Annals of the New York Academy of Sciences, 405,* 203–223.

Liberman, A. M., Harris, H. F., Hofman, H. S., & Griffith, E. C. (1957). The discrimination of speech sounds within and across phoneme boundaries. *Journal of Experimental Research, 54,* 358–368.

Ling, D. (1976). *Speech and the hearing impaired child: Theory and practice.* Washington, DC: Alexander Graham Bell Association for the Deaf.

Luxford, W. M., & Brackmann, D. E. (1985). The history of cochlear implants. In R. F. Gray (Ed.), *Cochlear implants* (pp. 1–26). Boston: College-Hill Press.

McCandless, G. A. (1986, April 17–19). Factors which influence speech recognition in multichannel cochlear implants. Paper presented at the conference on Speech Recognition with Cochlear Implants: Issues, Progress, and Trends. New York University Medical Center, New York.

McFarland, W. (1986, March 7). The role of rehabilitation with cochlear implant patients. Presented through an ASHA teleconference, *Cochlear implants: What's happening?*

Mecklenburg, D. J. (1984, February 6–9). Results on speech tracking with the implantable hearing prosthesis. Poster presentation at the Association for Research in Otolaryngology, Dolphin Beach, FL.

Mecklenburg, D. J., & Brimacombe, J. A. (1985). An overview of the Nucleus cochlear implant program. *Seminars in Hearing, 6*(1), 41–51.

Mecklenburg, D. J., & Brimacombe, J. A. (1986, April 17–19). Descriptive data on 65 multichannel patients in relation to audiologic results. Paper presented at the conference on Speech Recognition with Cochlear Implants: Issues, Progress, and Trends. New York University Medical Center, New York.

Mecklenburg, D. J., Brimacombe, J. A., & Dowell, R. C. (1985, August 27–31). Performance profile of patients who achieve substantial open-set speech discrimination without lipreading. Paper presented at the International Cochlear Implant Symposium and Workshop, Melbourne, Australia.

Mecklenburg, D. J., & Dowell, R. C. (1986). *Training manual for the Nucleus 22-channel cochlear implant system.* Englewood, CO: Cochlear Corp.

Mecklenburg, D. J., Dowell, R. C., & De Filippo, C. (1984, August 26–30). *Speech tracking technique.* Paper presented at the XVII International Congress of Audiology, University of California, Santa Barbara, CA.

Mecklenburg, D. J., Dowell, R. C., & Jenison, V. W. (1987). Nucleus multichannel implant training manual. Englewood, CO: Cochlear Corp.

Mecklenburg, D. J., & Lee, K. J. (1986). Cochlear implants. In K. J. Lee (Ed.), *Essential otolaryngology —Head and neck surgery* (4th ed., pp. 227–238). New Hyde Park, NY: Medical Examination Publishing.

Merzenich, M. M. (1983). Coding of sound in a cochlear prostheses: Some theoretical and practical consideratons. *Annals of the New York Academy of Science, 405,* 502–508.

Michaelson, R., Merzenich, M. M., & Pettit, C. (1973). A cochlear prosthesis: Further clinical observations, preliminary results of physiological studies. *Laryngoscope, 83,* 1116.

Millar, J. B., Tong, Y. C., & Clark, G. M. (1984). Speech processing for cochlear implant prostheses. *Journal of Speech and Hearing Research, 27,* 280–296.

Moore, B. C. J. (1985). Speech coding for cochlear implants. In R. F. Gray (Ed.), *Cochlear implants* (pp. 163–179). Boston: College-Hill Press.

Norton, N. B., & Berliner, K. I. (1977). Environmental sounds: Test and training program for the hearing impaired. Paper presented at the American Speech and Hearing Association Convention, Chicago, IL.

Oller, D. K., Eilers, R. E., Vengara, K. C., & LaVoie, E. C. (1986). Tactual vocoders in a multisensory program training speech production and reception. *Volta Review, 88,* 21–36.

Osberger, M. J. (1986). Auditory training. In D. J. Mecklenburg (Ed.), Cochlear implants in children: Proceedings from a multidisciplinary colloquium. *Seminars in Hearing, 7*(4), 423–431.

Owens, E., Kessler, D. K., & Schubert, E. D. (1981). The Minimal Auditory Capabilities (MAC) battery. *Hearing Aid Journal, 34,* 9–34.

Owens, E., & Telleen, C. C. (1981). Tracking as an aural rehabilitative process. *Journal of the Academy of Rehabilitative Audiology, 14,* 259–273.

Parkin, J. (1985, September 27–29). Surgical implications. Paper presented at Current Issues in Cochlear Implantation Symposium, Park City, UT.

Parkin, J., Eddington, D., Orth, J., & Brackmann, D. (1985). Speech recognition experience with the multichannel implants. *Otolaryngology Head-Neck Surgery, 93*(5), 639–645.

Parkins, C. W., & Houde, R. A. (1982). The cochlear implant prosthesis: Theoretical and practical considerations. In D. G. Sims, G. G. Walter, & R. L. Whitehead (Eds.), *Deafness and communication — Assessment and training* (pp. 332–356). Baltimore: Williams & Wilkins.

Paterson, M. M. (1982). Integration of auditory training with speech and language for severely hearing-impaired children. In D. G. Sims, G. G. Walter, & R. L. Whitehead (Eds.), *Deafness and communication — Assessment and training* (pp. 261–270). Baltimore: Williams & Wilkins.

Patrick, J. F., Seligman, P. M., McDowell, R. C., & Blamey, P. J. (1986, April 17–19). Performance of the Nucleus speech processor in noise. Paper presented at the conference on Speech Recognition with Cochlear Implants: Issues, Progress, and Trends. New York University Medical Center, New York.

Punch, J. L., McConkey, A., Myres, W., Pope, M. L., & Miyamoto, R. T. (1985, November 22–25). Relationships among selected pre- and post-implant measures. Paper presented at Annual Convention of the American Speech-Language-Hearing Association, Washington, DC.

Raphael, L. (1986, April 17–19). Speech reception in the normal hearing. Paper presented at the conference on Speech Recognition with Cochlear Implants: Issues, Progress, and Trends. New York Medical University Center, New York.

Rebscher, S. J. (1985). Cochlear implant design and construction. In R. F. Gray (Ed.), *Cochlear implants* (pp. 74–123). Boston: College-Hill Press.

Ries, P. W. (1982). Hearing ability of persons by sociodemographic and health characteristics. *U.S. Vital Health Statistics* (Series 10, No. 140). Hyattsville, MD: U.S. Department of Health and Human Services.

Ross, M., & Calvert, D. (1984). Semantics of deafness revisited: Total communication and the use and misuse of residual hearing. *Audiology, 9,* 127–145.

Scouten, E. L. (1984). *Turning point in the education of deaf people.* Danville, IL: Interstate Printers and Publishers.

Sims, D. G. (1982). Hearing and speechreading evaluation for the deaf adult. In D. G. Sims, G. G. Walter, & R. L. Whitehead (Eds.), *Deafness and communication — Assessment and training* (pp. 141–154). Baltimore: Williams & Wilkins.

Sparks, D., Kuhl, P., Edmonds, A., & Gray, G. (1978). Investigating the MESA (multipoint electrotactile speech aid): Segmental features of speech. *Journal of the Acoustical Society of America, 63,* 246.

Staller, S. J. (1985). Cochlear implant characteristics: A review of current technology. *Seminars in Hearing, 6*(1), 23–32.

Stark, R. E., Bowman, L. A., Busse, L. A., Hasenstab, S., House, J. L., & Oller, D. K. (1986). Developmental aspects influencing implantation and rehabilitation of children. In D. Mecklenburg (Ed.), Cochlear implants in children: Proceedings from a multidisciplinary colloquium. *Seminars in Hearing, 7*(4), 371–382.

Thielmeir, M. A., Tonokawa, L. L., Petersen, B., & Eisenberg, L. S. (1985). Audiological results in children with a cochlear implant. *Ear & Hearing, 6*(3), 27S–35S.

Tong, Y. C., Blamey, P. J., Dowell, R. C., & Clark, G. M. (1983). Psychophysical studies evaluating the feasibility of a speech processing strategy for a multichannel cochlear implant. *Journal of the Acoustical Society of America, 74,* 73–80.

Tyler, R. S., Preece, J. P., & Lowder, M. W. (1983). *The Iowa cochlear implant tests.* Iowa City: University of Iowa, Department of Otolaryngology, Head and Neck Surgery.

Uttal, W. R. (1973). *The psychobiology of sensory coding.* New York: Harper & Row.

White, M. W., Merzenich, M. M., & Gardi, J. N. (1984). Multichannel cochlear implants: Channel interactions and processor design. *Archives of Otolaryngology, 110,* 493–501.

White, R. L., Roberts, L. A., Cotter, N. E., & Kwon, O. H. (1983). Thin film electrode fabrication techniques. In C. W. Parkins & S. W. Anderson (Eds.), *Cochlear prostheses: An international symposium* (pp. 183–190). New York: New York Academy of Sciences.

Wilson, B. S., & Finley, C. C. (1985). Cochlear implant. *ASHA, 27*(5), 27–35.

Wilson, B. S., & Finley, C. C. (1986). Comparison of strategies for coding speech with multichannel auditory prostheses. Paper presented at the conference on Speech Recognition with Cochlear Implants: Issues, Progress, and Trends, New York University Medical Center, New York.

9

HEARING AID ASSESSMENT AND THE AUDITORY BRAINSTEM RESPONSE

MICHAEL R. SEITZ ■

DENNIS L. KISIEL ■

Hearing aid assessment procedures in use since the 1960s have been widely criticized following the 1980 Vanderbilt Confererence. Although the Carhart procedure and its variants were subject to criticism during and after this conference, no uniform procedures have emerged to replace these comparative techniques. Methods based on audiometric parameters including loudness discomfort level (LDL), most comfortable loudness level (MCL), and threshold have all been proposed to replace speech-based procedures. Given this history of dissatisfaction, one might anticipate that clinicians would begin to explore the use of auditory evoked response techniques to assist in the selection and fitting of hearing aids, especially for individuals who are unable to respond to the more traditional hearing aid selection procedures, such as infants and people who are multiply handicapped.

Auditory evoked response techniques developed rapidly during the 1970s, following the introduction of the auditory brainstem response (ABR) procedures of Jewett and Williston (1971) and Jewett, Romano, and Williston (1970). This technique was found to be clinically useful for the measurement of the transmission of auditory information through the brainstem. The technique required no active patient participation and was not greatly affected by sedation or natural sleep as were late- and middle-component evoked potential techniques. In addition, the ABR technique is very sensitive to the mid- to high-frequency region of the cochlea (2000–4000 Hz), which is very important for the successful fitting and use of hearing aids. This region is also very important for the discrimination and identification of many of the consonants of English and contains most of the F2 and F3 formant transitions for vowels and diphthongs as well.

Thus, the ABR technique seemed appropriate to use in determining the hearing loss of hard-to-test patients and was readily adopted for testing newborns and infants.

As clinicians and researchers became more facile with the technique, some clinicians began to explore the use of ABR procedures to assist in the fitting of hearing aids, especially for the same patients who were hard to test or could not participate in more traditional hearing aid fitting procedures.

Researchers and clinicians have been attempting to utilize auditory evoked response techniques to assist in the fitting of hearing aids since the late 1960s. One of the first articles to suggest utilization of evoked response techniques in the fitting of hearing aids (Rapin & Graziani, 1967) utilized late component evoked potentials to elicit aided cortical responses from a rubella infant, who displayed a lack of response in an unaided condition. This study established that evoked responses could be derived through a hearing aid and demonstrated that evoked potential procedures might well be adapted to assist in hearing aid fitting.

The first published report that documented the use of auditory brainstem evoked responses with hearing aid users (Mokotoff & Krebs, 1976a) measured the ABRs of adult hearing aid users under three test conditions: unaided with earphones, unaided via loudspeaker, and aided via loudspeaker. In the aided condition, subjects were asked to adjust their hearing aid volume to a most comfortable listening level. This article was skeletal in detail on the exact methodology of the study, but the authors indicated that the aided ABR data compared favorably to aided behavioral data and concluded that the ABR technique had potential application in hearing aid fitting for infants who were unable to participate in normal behavioral hearing aid assessment procedures.

In the middle 1970s, a number of researchers (Cox & Metz, 1980; Mahoney, Condie, & Snyder, 1980; McPherson and Clark, 1980; Jacobson, Seitz, Mencher, & Parrott, 1981) began to experiment with the use of auditory evoked response techniques in the fitting of hearing aids. Many of the early experiments were later published or presented at national conferences and are reviewed later in this chapter. It immediately became clear to these researchers that, although the use of ABR techniques to fit hearing aids was feasible, it was also fraught with difficulties and technical problems. Since then most of the articles and presentatons that have reported on ABR and hearing aid fitting have been preliminary and descriptive in nature. Many of the early studies were not published, and thus clinicians do not have easy access to them. The early studies were also preliminary in nature and lacked the systematic controls of more rigorous investigations.

Because there are many technical difficulties associated with the use of ABR techniques to select and fit hearing aids, this chapter reviews these past studies and attempts to articulate the technical problems associated with using ABR procedures in hearing aid assessment. We hope this analysis of the technical problems and the suggestions for using ABR techniques in hearing aid assessment will assist clinicians who wish to use ABR techniques for hearing aid selection and fitting.

HISTORICAL PERSPECTIVE

The earliest published study on the use of evoked potentials and hearing aids was done by Rapin and Graziani (1967), who used the late component evoked potentials in their initial procedures. Hecox, Breuninger, and Krebs (1975) and Mokotoff and Krebs (1976) were the first to use ABRs in conjunction with hearing aids. These studies were sketchy in detail and preliminary in nature, but they did document that both brainstem and late evoked component responses could be obtained through a hearing aid from both normal and hearing-impaired subjects. These researchers also suggested that the development of appropriate evoked response procedures might be beneficial in the selection and fitting of hearing aids for hard-to-test populations.

Cox and Metz (1980) published one of the first systematic investigations on the use of auditory brainstem response techniques and hearing aid prescription. Eight adult hearing aid users with moderate-to-severe sensorineural hearing losses were paid to be subjects in this study. Three of the subjects had flat audiometric configurations, three had sloping losses, and two had precipitous losses. ABRs were obtained for both click and tone pip stimuli. The tone pips used were 1000, 2000, and 3000 Hz. Speech recognition data were also collected and compared to the ABR wave V latencies. Cox and Metz (1980) reported that hearing aid ranking by the subject's speech recognition scores generally agreed with the ABR latency rankings, with the shortest wave V latencies corrrelating with the highest speech recognition scores. They also reported that the poorest agreement occurred between the aided ABR threshold and speech recognition scores. Cox and Metz concluded that hearing aid gain adjusted to result in maximum reduction of wave V latency settings would be representative of the best gain setting for that individual. They estimated that hearing aid-ABR techniques could be 75 percent as accurate as traditional methods in the selection of hearing aids. Accuracy was related to the configuration of the hearing loss and was higher for flat and precipitous hearing losses. The authors suggested that the use of tone pip stimuli increased the accuracy of hearing aid selection. Although other investigations (Beauchaine, Gorga, Reiland, & Larson, 1986) have questioned some of the results of this early study, it still remains one of the landmark investigations in this area.

Another early study was initially reported by McPherson (1980) in an abstract and expanded later in another article (McPherson & Clark, 1983). The latter study was to assess the ABR parameters that contributed most to the selection of a hearing aid. Ten relatively young (18 to 26 years old), normal hearing subjects were used. Subjects were tested for most comfortable listening level (MCL) and loudness discomfort level (LDL) under four conditions: (1) unaided under earphones, (2) unaided in sound field, (3) unaided in sound field with a simulated conductive hearing loss of approximately 15 dB (by occluding the external auditory canal), and (4) aided sound field with an occluded external auditory canal to simulate conductive hearing loss. The effects of the simulated conductive hearing loss on the ABRs were greatest at threshold and not as severe at suprathreshold levels. McPherson and Clark concluded that the ABR wave V latency was useful in adjusting the dynamic range of the hearing aid and that compression amplification should limit wave V latency to greater than 5.3 ms, the wave V latency at which subjects reported loudness discomfort. (One needs to remember that as stimulus intensity increases, wave V latency decreases. Thus it is necessary for stimulus intensity to be limited to intensities that elicit wave V responses that exceed 5.3 ms in latency.) The authors also suggested that the hearing aid itself was the primary limiting factor in using ABR procedures for amplification selection, a point that will be addressed under technical considerations later in this chapter.

Jacobson, Seitz, Mencher, and Parrott (1981) reported a case study in which they tested a mild-to-moderate, sensorineural hearing-impaired subject under sound-field conditions using click stimuli. The hearing aid was fitted to the right ear and appropriate masking was applied to the left ear. Auditory brainstem responses were recorded under two conditions: a 50 dB HL click intensity level using three different hearing aid gain settings (40, 30, and 20 dB) and a constant hearing aid gain of 40 dB SPL and three different click intensity levels (40, 30, and 20 dB HL). The results indicated that wave V latencies changed predictably with changes in either hearing aid gain or stimulus intensity. The resultant wave V latencies for both conditions were remarkably similar at any given combination of hearing aid gain and stimulus presentation level. These data supported the clinical view that repeatable ABRs could be obtained through a hearing aid under controlled sound-field conditions when appropriate technical considerations were followed.

In 1982, Kileny presented four clinical cases in which ABR techniques were used to test hearing aid performance in children. Both click and 500 Hz tone pip stimuli were employed and compared to the aided and unaided ABRs. He concluded that ABR assessment was both feasible and clinically useful in hearing aid selection and fitting but cautioned that excessive electromagnetic artifacts caused by hearing aid receiver ringing and excessive acoustic feedback may contaminate the ABRs. These types of contamination have been documented in other ABR-hearing aid studies (Hall & Ruth, 1985; Mahoney, 1985).

Hecox (1983) reported clinical experiences with ABR techniques and hearing aids in a series of selected clinical reports on adults with a variety of hearing losses of unspecified etiology. Standard ABR procedures and click stimuli were used and differences were found in hearing aids as reflected in their individual ABRs. Some patients' response to acoustic stimuli ABRs reflected little or no benefit from amplification. Hecox described the process of amplification as an attempt to normalize the abnormal latency–intensity, input-output functions of hearing-impaired subjects. He offered the observation that patients with central nervous system disorders may not benefit from amplification as much as patients with peripheral hearing losses in terms of improved communicative abilities. This clinical viewpoint is not universally accepted, primarily because of the variety of central nervous system disorders and the lack of supporting data. The Hecox article, however, confirmed that reliable ABRs can be obtained from click stimuli for hearing-impaired subjects and that both technical and neurophysiological difficulties needed

to be explored before the usefulness of ABR-hearing aid protocols in the selection and fitting of hearing aids in the hard-to-test population can be determined.

Other researchers have taken a slightly different approach to using auditory evoked responses in the selection of hearing aids. In a series of papers, Kiessling (1982, 1983a, 1983b, 1984, 1987) described a clinical application using ABRs in hearing aid assessment. Based on earlier work by his European colleagues, Kiessling tested a number of normal hearing and hearing-impaired subjects, ranging in age from 1 to 5 years in one study and to young adults in another study. Kiessling first established normative latency-amplitude functions from which he derived a mathematical calculation for optimal hearing aid output characteristics. He did not use ABR latency data as previous researchers had but instead used ABR amplitude data, based on the assumption that ABR amplitudes reflect an individual's perception of loudness. If hearing aids are selected on the basis of ABR amplitude, then hearing aids fitted on this basis should exhibit near normal values. Utilizing unaided ABR intensity-amplitude data, a mathematical formula, and hearing aid characteristics such as average gain in dB, dynamic range, compression and type of compression, and so forth, Kiessling prescribed a hearing aid device.

Although Kiessling's method is rather complex, it is one of the few protocols that have provided a large data base on the use of ABR techniques for hearing aid selection and evaluation, especially on children. He stressed that in children hearing aid amplification needs to be introduced as early as possible, within the first year of life. As more audiometric data become available as the child matures, appropriate modifications in the hearing aid responses should be made. Kiessling proposed that the advantages of ABR assessment in hearing aid selection far outweigh the disadvantages.

Another application of evoked potentials in the fitting of hearing aids was postulated by Sanders (1983). Rather than using

ABRs, he used the slow brainstem response (SBR) or the SN_{10} response. This response is a slow negative waveform that occurs around 10 ms when tone pip stimuli with a low frequency cut-off of 30 Hz are presented. (See Hall and Ruth [1985] for a more succinct discussion of this procedure.) Sanders reported that aided SBR thresholds for hearing-impaired subjects were within 5 dB of their behavioral thresholds, thus indicating that the SBR might be useful in the selection and fitting of hearing aids. Because the number of subjects in this study was small and the effects of sedation on the SBR are not known, it may be too early to determine the effectiveness of the SBR on hearing aid assessment. This study indicates that there is still much to learn about the use of evoked potential techniques for the fitting of hearing aids.

Hall and Ruth (1985) reviewed the use of acoustic reflex and evoked response measurements in hearing aid evaluation, and their article contains a number of useful figures, tables, and graphs. They stressed the need for unaided and aided real-ear measurements of the hearing-impaired subjects rather than relying on the manufacturers' specifications of hearing aid performance. They noted that the use of electrophysiologic procedures is most appropriate for infants and difficult-to-test cases. This study clearly articulated the technical difficulties with ABR measurements. Finally, Hall and Ruth speculated on the use of late component evoked response techniques to assess some of the cognitive and linguistic functions of the young hearing-impaired persons. They concluded that use of auditory evoked responses and acoustic reflexes will assume an increasingly important role in the selection and fitting of hearing aids.

Mahoney (1985) reviewed ABR applications to hearing aid selection and fitting and commented on a number of technical problems encountered in using ABR techniques in conjunction with hearing aid selection and fitting. He recommended a test protocol for using ABR techniques in hearing aid assessments.

TECHNICAL CONSIDERATIONS

As noted previously, one of the greatest difficulties in the development of ABR techniques for hearing aid assessment is not understanding the technical considerations and complications that occur when a hearing aid is combined with electrophysiologic measurement. Rackliffe and Musiek (1983) reviewed the significant articles available at that time on the use of ABRs in hearing aid assessment. They outlined a number of problems that should be addressed in future studies. Most of these problems were technical in nature, such as the effect of the output characteristics of the hearing aid on the auditory system itself. They also questioned whether the utilization of latency–intensity measurements alone was sufficient for the selection of a specific hearing aid device or whether waveform morphology or some form of amplitude measurement or ratios should also be utilized. Rackliffe and Musiek indicated the need for stimulus presentation rate studies because stimuli can be distorted if the presentation rate is too fast for the hearing aid's electroacoustic function to handle. They also noted that present ABR-hearing aid procedures are time consuming and need to be "abridged" if they are to become clinically useful.

Other ABR problems noted included the selection of the type and polarity of the ABR stimulus, the type of transducer to be used, the optimal distance between the transducer and the hearing aid microphone, radiation artifact, the selection of appropriate electrophysiological indices (i.e., latency-intensity functions, waveform morphology, or amplitude measurements) to use for hearing aid selection, signal processing problems, earmold effects, and calibration.

Type of Transducer

As is the case with conventional ABR procedures, stimulus choice is predicated on the purpose of the evaluation. Additional determinants of stimulus types in aided

ABR procedures include the type of transducer and the electroacoustic parameters of the hearing aid. The choice of transducer includes sound-field speakers versus conventional head phones, typically placed from 2 to 8 cm from the hearing aid microphone post (nearfield or quasi nearfield). Power and efficiency characteristics allow loudspeakers to be placed a considerable distance from the hearing aid, effectively eliminating the troublesome electromagnetic artifact.

However, there is a price to be paid for using a loudspeaker to present a stimulus to a subject wearing a hearing aid (Jacobson et al., 1981; Beauchaine et al., 1986), since the distance from the speaker to the hearing aid is usually 2 to 3 ft. While temporal changes in the ABR waveform due to electromagnetic radiation are reduced, other distortions are introduced. These include excessive receiver ringing (temporal distortion) and temporal shifts in wave V latency due to speaker frequency response, resonance characteristics of the external auditory canal, and room reverberation (Jacobson et al., 1981).

An additional problem associated with using free field loudspeakers and earphones in a sound field relates to the mandatory assessment of sound pressure attenuation due to distance (Parrott, Jacobson, & Seitz, 1980; Mahoney, 1985). In the Parrott study, for example, ABRs were obtained from 30 normal hearing adults under binaural earphones and sound-field conditions. In the sound-field condition, a single speaker was placed 1 m from either ear at 0-degrees azimuth. Stimulus repetition rate was 33.3 clicks per second for both binaural earphone and sound-field conditions, and the latency-intensity functions were derived in 10 dB steps from 70 to 0 dB HL for all subjects. The results indicated that mean wave V latencies increased as intensity decreased in a similar manner for both conditions. However, when quantifying the curve functions for the sound-field and binaural earphone conditions, a steeper slope was found

for the binaural earphone condition with wave V latency being reduced by 2.85 ms over a 65 dB range compared to a wave V latency reduction of only 2.06 ms in the sound-field condition. In addition, the mean wave latency was 3.51 ms longer in the sound-field condition than in the binaural earphone condition, which was 0.60 ms longer than the calculated time of 2.91 ms for the click stimulus to travel 1 m from the speaker to each ear canal. They attributed the difference in actual wave V latency compared to the calculated wave V latency to three possibly interacting variables:

1. Differences in the frequency response characteristics between a TDH-39 earphone and the loudspeaker
2. Differences in the resonance characteristics of an occluded and unoccluded auditory canal
3. The possible effects of room reverberation, even in a sound-treated room

Although wave V latency differences existed between the two conditions, the two sets of measurements were significantly correlated and highly predictive of each other. The authors were unable to determine the individual contribution of each of the above variables to determine which, or how much, each contributed to the 0.60 ms difference from the actual to predicted wave V latency under sound-field conditions. Obviously, these variables may also contribute to changes in wave V latency under aided conditions and need to be considered in the development of any hearing aid-ABR procedure.

A standard earphone, while more readily accepted for use for ABR testing in most clinical settings, invites certain difficulties. The most common problem is establishing the distance of the loudspeaker from the hearing aid that will reduce electromagnetic radiation while providing an adequate stimulus to the ear without overdriving the hearing aid transducer.

A typical arrangement for an earphone-generated stimulus used in aided

ABR procedures was outlined by Mahoney (1985). In this procedure, a standard earphone (TDH-39) used as the transducer was placed 8 cm from the hearing aid microphone. This resulted in a 0.25 ms travel delay from the transducer earphone to the hearing aid microphone which equates to a 20 dB loss in sound pressure due to distance. This 20 dB sound pressure reduction was determined by behavioral threshold judgments, wave V latency equalization procedures, and sound pressure level comparisons between a closed 6 cc coupler and the sound-field measurements.

Hecox (1983) reported placement of an earphone 3 cm from the external auditory canal of his subjects and stated that this resulted in a 0.3 ms latency increase for wave V at that distance. In another study, McPherson and Clark (1983) placed the earphone 5 cm from the external auditory canal of their subjects and reported a 0.91 ms delay for the unaided sound-field condition and a 1.8 ms delay under the ear occluded sound-field condition. In the Jacobson and colleagues (1981) study, the loudspeaker was placed 1 m from the subjects and a 3.51 ms latency shift in the ABRs was reported. It is unclear why the shorter distances between earphone and ear canal in the McPherson and Clark (1983) and Hecox (1983) studies resulted in longer latencies than the 8 cm placement used by Mahoney (1985) in his procedure. Perhaps these differences are related to the different types of earphones used or to test room heat and sound attenuation characteristics. Whatever the reasons, the differences in wave V latency shifts reported in these studies clearly indicate that each clinic must establish an appropriate distance to use and calculate the latency shift that results if the waveform analysis is to be useful for hearing aid assessment.

Stimulus Parameters

Another important consideration is whether a stimulus input is faithfully transmitted through the hearing aid system. If the hearing aid modifies the stimulus, the resulting ABR cannot be expected to be of high quality or to accurately reflect expected latency-amplitude waveform shifts. Using a pinna-mounted earphone as a standard, researchers have already shown that a speaker, or an earphone used as a speaker, introduces both frequency and temporal distortions to the input stimulus.

Temporal Distortion

In another study, Hall and Ruth (1985) compared the temporal waveform of a 100 microsecond click transmitted through a TDH-49 earphone under three conditions:

1. Click measured directly from the earphone in a standard 6 cc coupler
2. Earphone held 2 in. from the microphone of a sound level meter
3. Earphone held 2 in. from the microphone port of a moderately powerful hearing aid attached to a 2 cc coupler of a sound level meter

Stimulus intensity was adjusted to achieve approximately equivalent peak output pressure under the three conditions.

The temporal waveform under this condition is largely predicted by the frequency response and resonance characteristics of the earphone. In this example, the result for condition 1 was one initial prominent peak followed by two or three minor oscillations covering about 0.5 ms. Condition 2 in this series resulted in a more complex waveform that reflected a phase shift of the first peak and increased oscillations extending just beyond 1.0 ms. Condition 3 resulted in an even more complex waveform with substantial receiver ringing that lasted 3.0 ms, with an additional hearing aid processing delay of 0.42 ms. This delay was significantly longer than conditions 1 and 2.

Thus, it appears that temporal distortion of a hearing aid can arise from at least three different sources. The first source, discussed previously, is caused by driving the speaker or earphone at output levels without sufficient head room (i.e., at levels producing distortion). The second source presumes that an undistorted signal is transmitted through a hearing aid with a steep acoustic peak or peaks. These peaks can become a source of ringing and distort the resultant auditory brain stem responses that are recorded. The third source that can produce temporal distortion originates from the hearing aid transducer itself. In cases where the maximum power output (SSPL90) is set too low, compared to the gain characteristics of the hearing aid, temporal ringing can result. Figure 9–1 depicts an example of ringing that resulted from an undistorted transient passed through a Unitron 1P hearing aid with a steep acoustic peak. Figure 9–2 is the companion insertion curve for the Figure 9–1 temporal display. Figure 9–2 highlights the slope of

the frequency response peaks, which are presumably the source of the temporal and ABR waveform distortions.

Temporal distortion of the phase of the input signal can result in an inversion of wave V latencies, in which wave V latencies for higher intensities are actually longer than wave V latencies for intensitites 10 to 20 dB lower. Although rarefaction versus condensation phase click stimuli generally yield similar wave V latencies for normal hearing adults, sometimes the transducer can cause changes in latency between rarefaction and condensation click stimuli. Weber, Seitz, and McCutcheon (1981) demonstrated just this phenomenon and alerted clinicians to the constant need to calibrate their earphones to ensure both that the polarity is correct and that the earphone has not developed excessive ringing or distortion, which could change the frequency characteristics of the stimulus and result in changes in ABR latency and amplitude.

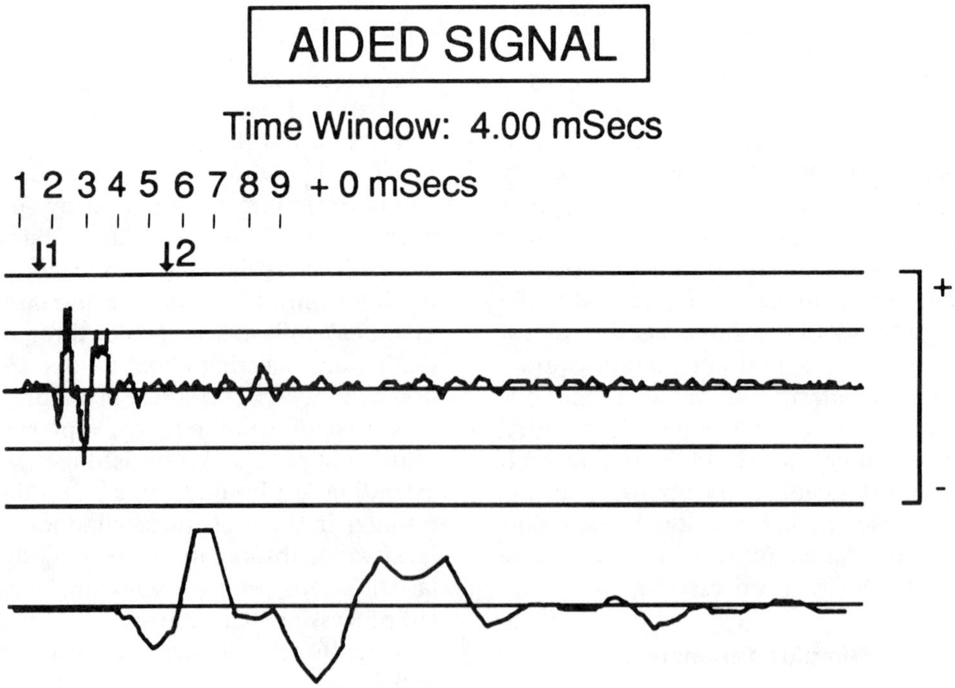

FIGURE 9–1. Temporal display of an unfiltered click waveform measured at the output of a high gain postauricular heairng aid. (See also Figure 9–2.)

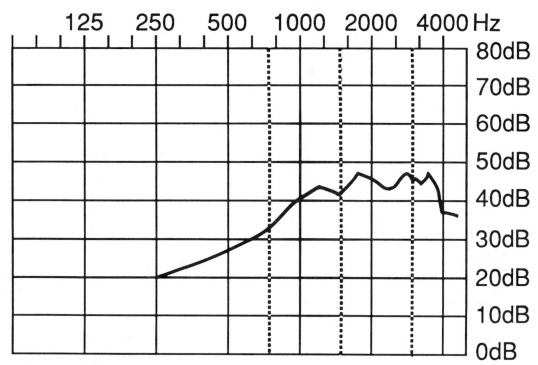

FIGURE 9–2. Insertion gain curve for the unfiltered click shown in Figure 9–1 routed through a high gain postauricular hearing aid. (See also Figure 9–1.)

Latency inversions can also occur in the ABRs of newborns and in adults with cochlear hearing losses (Coates, 1978; Stockard, Stockard, & Coen, 1983; Mahoney, 1985). Because of the possibility of latency inversion, the use of alternating monopolar clicks, measured at the eardrum plane, is often recommended for ABR-hearing aid procedures.

Latency inversion also can occur at high intensities during ABR-hearing aid testing as a result of receiver ringing. Whether this reversal is due to overdriving the earphone, hearing aid induced distortion, cochlear overload, spread of masking, or some combination of these conditions is as yet unclear. A similar phenomenon has been observed by Bobbin and Kisiel (1981) at a more peripheral level of the guinea pig auditory system.

Frequency Distortion

Frequency factors include differences in spectra generated by intensity equated clicks routed through earphones or speakers. Hall and Ruth (1985) demonstrated the types of frequecy changes that can occur in the acoustic spectra of a 100 microsecond rectangular pulse (click) delivered to a TDH-49 earphone, and Weber, Seitz, and McCutcheon (1981) have documented the types of changes in acoustic spectrum that can occur in TDH-39 earphones.

Seitz, Jacobson, and Parrott (1980), in a conference paper, reported on differences between loudspeaker- and earphone-generated click spectra. Figure 9–3 depicts the waveforms and spectra of earphone (TDH-39)- and loudspeaker-generated (Nicolet 1008) click stimuli. This figure shows

Input Intensity for all figures was 70 BNnL

Spectra readings are 0.1 to 20 KHz
on the log scale

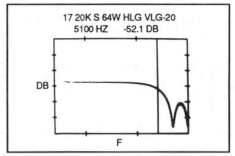

Spectrum 80 μsec of electrical click from click generator

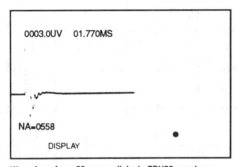

Wave form from 80 μ sec click via TDH39 earphone

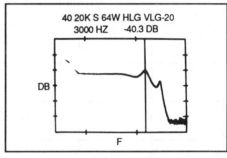

Spectrum of 80 μsec click from TDH39 earphone

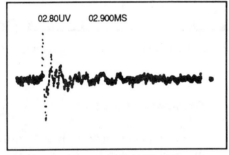

Wave form from 80 μsec click via NIC 1008 speaker

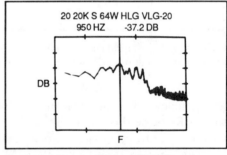

Spectrum of 80 μ sec click from NIC 1008 speaker

FIGURE 9–3. Waveforms and speaker spectra for a click generated through a TDH-39 earphone and a Nicolet 1008 loudspeaker.

the difference in loudspeaker and earphone generated click spectra. There is an additional 1 ms of ringing in the loudspeaker-generated click compared to the earphone-generated click spectra. This additional 1 ms of ringing (Figure 9–3, left) is probably due to the more dynamic movement of the speaker diaphragm, while the difference between the earphone and speaker spectra (Figure 9–3, upper and lower right) probably results from both transducer diaphragm

differences and reverberation effects of the sound-treated room.

The earphone click spectra are very clean, with major peaks occurring at 3000 and 5100 Hz, while the sound-field speaker click spectra are much broader and noisier, with the highest peak occurring much lower at 950 Hz and the last major peak occurring at 2700 Hz. In addition, the sound-field speaker generated clicks containing approximately 6 to 10 dB more high frequency energy above 4000 Hz than did the click spectrum of the earphone. These data substantiate the results of Coates and Kidder (1980), who found that clicks derived in sound-field conditions had more energy concentrated above 6000 Hz than clicks derived from earphones similar to the one used in the Seitz study. On the other hand, it is not possible to generalize from either the loudspeaker or the earphone spectra derived in the above study to other transducers. Each researcher or clinician must determine the spectra of the transducers used for stimulus presentation in ABR and hearing aid assessment techniques, whether they are loudspeakers or earphones.

It is obvious that the type of transducers used and its distance from the listener can change the energy spectra of stimuli used for ABR procedures. Add to these transducer effects changes resulting from routing click stimuli through different hearing aids and earmolds and the possible variations in ABR waveforms, latencies, and amplitudes that can occur multiply. Tonal stimuli would also be influenced by transducer type. One can predict that a 500 or 1000 Hz tone pip might be more faithfully reproduced by sound-field speakers while a 3000 Hz tone pip might benefit from earphone transducton because of the natural enhancement of the 3000 Hz region in most TDH-39 and -49 earphones. No matter what type of transducer is used, the stimulus spectrum delivered to the subject is altered by the earmold and the hearing aid. The subject's hearing loss configuration also will affect the resulting ABRs by responding differently to the resulting changes in the stimulus spectrum.

Effect of Hearing Aids on ABR Waveform

Hearing aids themselves have complex effects on the latency, amplitude, and waveform morphology of ABRs. The magnitude of these effects is so all-encompassing that the novice could easily be dissuaded from using ABR techniques in conjunction with hearing aid assessment procedures. The authors hope that such will not be the case.

One of the important measurement variables involved is the analysis of temporal delay caused by the click stimulus passing through the hearing aid. This temporal lag is specific to individual hearing aids and types (Hall & Ruth, 1985; Beauchaine et al., 1986; Kisiel & Lilly, 1986). Reports of hearing aid temporal delays range from 0.2 to 1.0 ms. Most reports of transmission delay suggest shorter delays for in-the-ear (ITE) hearing aids compared to behind-the-ear (BTE) hearing aids. Kisiel and Lilly (1986) did not observe appreciable differences when physical dimensions of hearing aid types were equalized. An obvious implication for clinicians working in this area is the need to independently assess the delay time of each hearing aid employed. Beauchaine and colleagues (1986) developed a workable procedure for this task, and use of such a procedure is recommended.

As described earlier, hearing aid performance can temporarily distort input waveforms. Temporal distortions can result from the use of hearing aid compression circuits. Early studies suggested that the total duration of unfiltered clicks was far shorter than the onset-offset time of the hearing aid compression circuits. Other studies (Hecox, 1983; Mahoney, 1985) demonstrated significant differences in latency, amplitude, and latency-intensity functions of hearing aids due to compression. Mahoney (1985) speculated that these differences may be caused by duration or interstimulus interval (ISI) changes created by the hearing aid rather than the compression circuit per se. Evidence supporting Mahoney's speculation can be found in the work of Durrant (1983) and Beattie and Boyd (1984). They demonstrated that a positive correlation exists between stimulus duration and sound pressure level. The ISI is affected in cases of temporal distortion caused by excessive receiver ringing when the end of an initial stimulus overlaps the presentation of the following stimulus. This ringing can result in distortion of the resulting waveform morphology, or even cause latency reversal. Whether these observed changes in the ABR are actually generated by this form of temporal distortion has yet to be confirmed. There is some clinical evidence to suggest that increased ISI does not affect wave V latencies above and beyond the unaided control condition for hearing aids without compression (Mahoney, 1985). More studies are needed to determine the exact effects of compression amplification and other forms of distortion on aided ABRs in hearing aid assessment procedures.

However, there is some theoretical evidence that suggests that changes in the ISI of a stimulus can affect ABR latencies or amplitudes when these stimuli are processed through a compression circuit. Gorga, Beauchaine, and Reiland (1987) demonstrated a difference in output signal amplitude under conditions of rapid change in signal level. They found a systematic relationship between the steady state and onset amplitude of a hearing aid processed click only at high stimulus repetition levels. Presumably, the offset portion of a compression circuit would never function under rapid stimulus repetition rates, thus allowing the onset and steady state portions of the click to approach equal intensity. For greater ISIs, discrepancies as large as 20 dB were reported by Braida and colleagues (1982).

Earmold Effects

Earmolds also have been suggested to influence aided ABRs. In an article reported in Hall and Ruth (1985), Swinson, Wagner, and Ruth (1984) reported on the influence of various hearing aid characteristics such as gain, tone, and volume setting, as well as earmold modifications, on acoustic click

and tone burst spectrum measured in a 2 cc coupler and real-ear probe microphone measurements on actual aided ABRs. As anticipated, the data revealed that different hearing aids uniquely shaped the acoustic waveform and spectrum in unpredictable ways. However, changes in spectral composition resulting from hearing aid settings and earmold modifications did not result necessarily in significant changes in the ABRs. This was particularly true for earmold modifications. Signal processing changes that occur with hearing aid amplification were more critical to ABR alterations than earmold configuration.

Kisiel and Seitz (1986) compared three different earmolds — a standard shell, Libby horn, and a McCrae type — on a single high gain, postauricular hearing aid with and without the presence of environmental noise. Click stimuli used in this study were delivered by a TDH-39 earphone placed 8 cm from the earmold. Preliminary results from three normal hearing subjects indicated that the three different earmolds did affect the resulting ABR latencies but these differences in wave V latencies may not be significant. For subject 1 (Table 9-1) the lowest ABR thresholds and wave V latencies were obtained with the Libby horn-normal frequency setting, while the longest wave V latencies and highest thresholds were found with the reverse Libby-low pass setting. Frequency response, however, seemed to be the primary determinant of wave V latency for subject 2 (Table 9-2).

In essence, the preliminary data indicated that earmolds and frequency response settings can affect wave V latencies to some degree, a finding that conflicts with the data derived by Swinson, Wagner, and Ruth (1984). It appears that earmolds, especially nonstandard earmolds, may have some effect on aided ABR waveforms and latencies, but the extent of these effects is not yet clear.

Most investigators agree that the technical problems that still need to be resolved center around changes in frequency

TABLE 9-1. ABR wave V latencies in ms for six frequency response-earmold combinations at 70 dBN HL for patient 1 using a Unitron E1P hearing aid in sound-field conditions.

Earmold	Frequency Response Setting of Hearing Aid	ABR Latency (in ms)
Libby	Normal	6.04
	Low-pass filter	6.88
Reverse	Normal	6.80
	Low-pass filter	6.92
Regular	Normal	6.48
	Low-pass filter	6.72

TABLE 9-2. ABR wave V latencies in ms for six frequency response-earmold combinations at 70 dBN HL for patient 2 using a Unitron E1P hearing aid in sound-field conditions.

Earmold	Frequency Response Setting of Hearing Aid	ABR Latency (in ms)
Libby	Normal	5.84
	Low-pass filter	6.72
Reverse	Normal	5.72
	Low-pass filter	6.64
Regular	Normal	5.64
	Low-pass filter	6.64

characteristics of the stimulus transducer, differences in latency shifts resulting from placing the transducer at varying distances from the hearing aid, changes in the stimulus signal resulting from the uniqueness of different design characteristics of hearing aids and types of hearing aids, and finally the presence or absence of compression circuits and their induced time delays in the hearing aids used in aided ABR procedures.

USE OF ABR MEASUREMENTS FOR HEARING AID ASSESSMENT

Investigators have compared aided and unaided ABR responses using four basic electrophysiological parameters:

1. ABR threshold and latency–intensity measurements in aided versus unaided conditions

2. Absolute wave V latency changes in aided and unaided conditions
3. Absolute wave V amplitude measures
4. Various combinations of the above three methods

Each of these approaches needs to be addressed individually.

ABR Threshold and Latency–Intensity Measurement

Researchers who used changes in ABR threshold measurements or latency-intensity (L/I) functions for their studies include Rapin and Graziani (1967), Mokotoff and Krebs (1976), Jacobson and colleagues (1981), Kileny (1982), McPherson and Clark (1983), Mahoney (1985), Hall and Ruth (1985), and Beauchaine and colleagues (1986). Some researchers attempted to correlate the aided ABR results with speech intelligibility, MCL, and LDL procedures as well.

The aided wave V threshold procedure is the simplest way to compare hearing aid function. Typically, an abbreviated L/I function is obtained in both aided and unaided conditions, and the thresholds under the two conditions are compared. The difference in dB level between the wave V latencies at threshold is determined to be the gain setting for the hearing aid. This assumption is true only if the hearing aid's amplification is similar at 1000, 2000, and 4000 Hz. If, however, the 1000 Hz response amplification is either significantly greater or less than the hearing aid's high-frequency (2000 to 4000 Hz) amplification, the ABR estimate of the ANSI gain will be either an over- or underestimate of the actual gain setting. These over- and underestimation errors also can occur in cases of low frequency amplification or extreme high frequency emphasis amplification.

In addition, Kileny (1982) and Beauchaine and colleagues (1986) stressed that auditory brainstem responses reflect only high frequency cochlear hair cell activity in the 2000 to 4000 Hz region. Normal or residual low frequency responses in hearing-impaired subjects are not reflected in the aided or unaided ABRs to click stimuli. Thus, threshold-based ABR-hearing aid assessment procedures share some of the same problems that standard pure tone thresholds have as the sole determinants of inner ear hair cell function (Pollack & Lipscomb, 1979). All "prescription" techniques, including the conventional Carhart procedures, utilize suprathreshold measures such as LDL, MCL, and speech discrimination scores to aid in the selection and fitting of an appropriate aid.

While the development of aided ABR techniques has been spurred by their potential use in fitting hearing-impaired infants and other hard-to-test persons, the use of ABR threshold data for hearing aid selection may be markedly limited. ABR

threshold procedures really address only the question: Can the patient hear something with a hearing aid that he or she cannot hear without it? If a signal is inaudible in the unaided state but evokes a potential in the aided condition, the hearing aid may be of some benefit to the patient. Evoking a brainstem response does not mean that a patient hears, but it does indicate that the auditory information is being processed along the auditory pathway. Thus, the ABR threshold procedure can identify when an auditory signal is being processed but cannot determine whether speech intelligibility will be enhanced or normal loudness function is restored.

At best, ABR threshold procedures can help determine if a hearing aid will enhance the signal processing capacity of the auditory system and which ear should be aided. The ABR threshold procedures and perhaps the newer ear canal probe tube microphone measurement techniques may be the only measures available to clinicians to estimate behavioral gain settings for hard-to-test patients.

Absolute Wave V
Latency Measurements

Other researches (Cox & Metz, 1980; Hecox, 1983; Thornton, Yardley, & Farrell, 1987) have used suprathreshold wave V latency measurements in ABR-hearing aid assessment procedures. Use of wave V latency measurements at specified suprathreshold levels can provide a basis for comparison with behavioral measurements such as speech discrimination, as Cox and Metz did in their 1980 study. However, Beauchaine and colleagues (1986) correctly pointed out that it is still unclear just how speech intelligibility is related "to the latency of onset of neural discharges in response to a click" (p. 126).

Hecox (1983) postulated that the slope of an L/I curve could reflect the presence or absence of recruitment, with sharply sloping and abbreviated L/I curves indicating recruitment. He suggested that if a clinician could normalize the L/I curve, that is, make the slope of L/I curve of a hearing-impaired subject more like the L/I slope of a normal hearing subject by manipulation of hearing aid gain or frequency, then normal loudness function would result. His assumptions, however, have been challenged by a number of other investigators (Gorga et al., 1985a, 1985b; Margolis, 1985). Margolis, for example, was not able to restore normal loudness functions for hearing-impaired listeners wearing compression amplification systems. His subjects' aided loudness functions instead reflected abnormal loudness growth typical of sensorineural hearing loss and the saturation characteristics of the hearing aids themselves.

In a more recent study, Thornton, Yardley, and Farrell (1987) developed a model which they used to predict lowest discomfort level (LDL) based on previous work with 8 normal subjects and 12 cochlear impaired patients with a mix of audiometric configurations. The authors concluded that the slope of the ABR L/I function could be used to predict loudness discomfort levels within ± 5 dB. This model was felt to be superior to those based on absolute latency or acoustic reflex thresholds. However, the sensitivity-specificity of their model for patients with mixed and conductive hearing losses is unknown. Unless the etiology and audiometric configurations of clinical patients are known, a priori estimates of loudness limiting may be in error for patients with conductive components to their hearing loss. Often, these types of hearing losses are difficult to determine in newborns and young infants.

While more study is needed to help determine just what the relationship is between suprathreshold ABR latency measurements and behavioral indicators, such as LDL, MCL, and speech discrimination, these methods offer some indication of the rate of transmission of auditory stimuli up the auditory pathway.

ABR Amplitude Measurements

ABR amplitudes are thought to be a reflection of the graded postsynaptic potentials generated by neuronal dendrites or soma, while ABR latency is thought to reflect axonal propagation up the ascending auditory pathway. Studies by physiologists such as Buchwald (1983) have supported this postulation and indicated that amplitude and latency functions reflect different physiological processes that can co-vary or independently vary. Stephens and Thornton (1976), Stockard, Stockard, and Coen (1983), and Hecox, Cone, and Blow (1981) have demonstrated that both absolute wave V amplitude and the relative wave V/I amplitude ratio (i.e., the ratio between wave V amplitude to wave I amplitude at a given intensity) may be of value in ABR diagnostic procedures.

On the other hand, Kisiel and Klodd (1982) and Rowe (1982) have demonstrated large standard deviations in absolute amplitude measures for normal young adults and older adults, so no clinical determination of "normal" amplitude variance can be made. Absolute wave V amplitudes have been observed to grow at a near linear rate but with large standard deviations for normal hearing subjects (Seitz, Morehouse, & Jacobson, 1981) and some selective groups of pathologic subjects, while non-monotonic growth rates have been observed for patients with recruitment (Hecox, 1983). In general, American researchers have been unable to demonstrate a strong correlation between loudness and ABR amplitude.

This is not the case for many European researchers. Kiessling in a series of articles (1982, 1983a, 1983b, 1984, 1987) and Stecker (1982a, 1982b) have proposed that ABR amplitudes reflect loudness perception. Evidence supporting this observation comes from the fact that widely varying gain requirements are used for similar sensitivity losses. In Kiessling's studies, gain requirements ranged from 20 dB for mild losses to 40 dB for moderate losses. These estimates were derived from electrophysiologic and psychoacoustic loudness matching experiments. A review of the varying range of gain rules based on thresholds (i.e., one-third, one-half, two-thirds) also reflects the poor correlation of loudness with ABR thresholds and indicates, as Libby (1985) noted, the need to use suprathreshold measures such as LDL or ABR amplitude measures as loudness indices.

Kiessling used projection or transformation plots to "transform" speech dynamics into the MCL range for the hearing impaired. For example, Kiessling (1982) derived gain, dynamic range, and compression type from a single projection curve. The amplitudes of wave V and the 40 and 180 dB points of the "normal speech" dynamic range were then compared with the hearing-impaired ear's identical amplitudes. The intensity levels needed to equate or normalize amplitude were then computed, and Kiessling used these figures to compute the gain and compression functions needed for the patient.

Kiessling (1983b) studied the use of this technique extensively in conjunction with more traditional hearing aid assessment techniques. He computed ABR amplitude regression curves for different threshold levels and demonstrated steeper curves for increasing hearing losses. The largest number of compression factors (50%) were in the 0.36 to 0.57 range, which exceeded the compression characteristics of 75 percent of the hearing aids then available in Germany. Gain requirements ranged from 40 to 50 dB for 62 percent of his pediatric hearing-impaired patients.

Kiessling (1987) attempted to validate his technique by comparing speech discrimination scores from adults obtained using this procedure to scores generated conventionally. Using this projection technique, he reported that he was able to successfully fit children and adults without actually recording aided ABRs. The only negative feature of Kiessling's projection procedure was the inability to predict appropriate loudness levels for specific frequencies. This limitation forced Kiessling to abandon this procedure in favor of in situ audiometry for the evoked potential procedures (Kiessling, 1987).

Initially, the technique developed by Kiessling and expanded by Stecker (1982a, 1982b) showed some promise. However, ABR amplitude and even V/I amplitude ratios have not proved as helpful in hearing aid assessments as many researchers had hoped. Obviously, more research is needed in this area before these procedures can be adapted to actual clinical settings.

Combination Approaches Using ABR Measurements

Clinicians often combine existing procedures in an effort to enhance their diagnostic accuracy. This is also true for aided ABR techniques. Some researchers have begun to use various combinations of ABR analyses in an effort to expand the usefulness of ABR procedures in hearing aid assessment.

Stecker (1982a, 1982b) was one of the first to report the use of a combination of aided ABR measurements in hearing aid assessments. He used ABR latency, threshold, and amplitude measurements to determine hearing aid frequency response and gain. He also used unaided amplitude-intensity functions, similar to those used by Kiessling (1982), to estimate compression. Stecker used 500 and 1000 Hz tone pips as well as click stimuli in his procedures. These measurements were employed to set hearing aid output at a level where further increases in hearing aid gain did not result in expected decreases in wave V latency. His study indicated that normal ABR latencies could be approximated for conductive and gradually sloping sensorineural hearing losses but not for steeply sloping sensorineural hearing losses. These steeply sloping losses often generated distorted ABR waveforms and could not approximate a normalized ABR L/I function.

Kisiel and Seitz (1986) reported use of absolute wave V latency at suprathreshold levels in combination with L/I functions and threshold measurements in their ongoing research but have not embraced the use of unaided ABR amplitude measurements in the way Stecker and Kiessling have reported.

Mahoney (1985) also used a number of ABR procedures in his measurement protocol. For example, he initiated his aided ABR procedure at 50 dB SPL (equal to approximately 70 dB on his ABR instrument). The earphone placement is 8 cm from the hearing aid microphone. If no ABR is generated at this 70 dB intensity level, the input intensity is increased in 10 dB steps. Once an ABR is generated and replicated, hearing aid gain is assessed by increasing or decreasing the volume control of the hearing aid until wave V latency stabilizes and the amplitude saturates. L/I functions are also collected at various frequency and compression settings, starting with the maximum compression setting of the hearing aid.

SUGGESTED AIDED ABR PROTOCOL

Kisiel and Seitz (1986) used a clinical aided ABR protocol similar to the one used by Mahoney (1985) and found it to be of clinical value in selecting and fitting hearing aids on very young or hard-to-test patients. The protocol is as follows.

Clinicians interested in using ABR procedures for hearing aid assessment must first establish transmission line delay due to the attenuation of sound caused by the electromechanical aspects of the hearing aid and the distance between the stimulus transducer and the hearing aid microphone. This aggregate delay is subtracted from the nominal aided wave V latency in order to arrive at a corrected ABR latency similar to standard earphone wave V latencies. Alternating clicks are recommended to reduce earphone artifact. Initial (start-

ing) intensity levels should be around 50 to 70 dB SPL. The volume control of the hearing aid is set approximately in the middle position to avoid acoustic distortion encountered in the high taper control settings. With a fixed intensity click stimulus presented to the hearing aid microphone, a L/I function is then obtained. The maximum stimulus intensity used is dictated by the following criteria:

1. Further intensity increases result in increased wave V (roll-over) latency or no change in wave V latency
2. Excessive ringing obscures the early portion of the ABR waveform
3. Morphology of the ABR waveform begins to deteriorate

The SSPL of the test hearing aid should be set conservatively (i.e., relatively low) to avoid inadvertent overstimulation with levels exceeding the person's UCL. If several hearing aids are being evaluated, the following criteria may be used to identify "superior" electroacoustic devices. Select the hearing aid

1. With the lowest or most sensitive aided ABR threshold (Note that hearing aids with high internal noise levels may have higher wave V thresholds.) (Rines, Stelmachowicz, & Gorga, 1984)
2. That approximates the "normalization" of the ABR L/I function
3. With the widest dynamic range (wave V threshold to LDL)
4. That provides the best appropriate action of the hearing aid's compression circuit (i.e., minimum distortion of the resulting waveforms)

The electrical or acoustical frequency response changes in modern analog or hybrid hearing aids will rarely affect wave V latency or amplitude. With hearing loss exceeding 75 dB, a wave V may be obtained at only one point of an L/I function or not at all (Hecox, 1983). With the present state of the art, use of the ABR in hearing aid assessment is probably more beneficial in comparing aided versus unaided conditions rather than differentiating performance of different brands of similar hearing aids.

SUMMARY AND FUTURE IMPLICATIONS

A standardized protocol for using ABRs in hearing aid assessment does not presently exist. The literature review indicates that a great deal of preliminary data has been gathered on suggested procedures and as yet unresolved technical issues. ABRs can be obtained through hearing aids with compression amplification circuits, but the amplified click stimulus output is significantly reduced in such hearing aids (Mahoney, 1985). Obviously, click-evoked ABRs can provide only information about the 2000 to 4000 Hz region. Continued exploration is needed to refine the use of freqency-specific tone pip or tone burst stimuli in notched noise or masking paradigms to determine whether such stimuli can yield better data on the presence and usefulness of residual low frequency hearing in difficult-to-test subjects. Although preliminary research has been completed on the effects of hearing aids on ABRs, these initial impressions need to be confirmed with extensive follow-up studies. For example, the effects of different stimulus repetition rates on individual hearing aids is not known, although some researchers feel that click rates around 11 per s are best. There is no consensus relative to the use of absolute amplitude or V/I amplitude ratio to determine gain settings for hearing aids. With the advent of real-ear measurement instruments, it is now possible to correlate such measures with aided ABRs. Truncated or shortened aided ABR procedures must be developed if these techniques are to be clinically useful. The present protocols cannot be completed in less than 2 hours, and many hard-to-test persons cannot tolerate the length of these procedures without sedation.

Most clinicians feel positive about the future of aided ABR techniques in the selection and fitting of hearing aid devices. There are reasons for this optimism:

- Aided ABR techniques may be the only method presently available for obtaining reliable and valid estimates for hearing aid fitting in pediatric and other hard-to-test populations.
- Behaviorally determined MCL and LCL measures have been found to be unreliable and procedure sensitive, especially for pediatric patients, while normalization of aided ABR L/I functions can indicate a hearing aid that will provide a more normal auditory pathway transmission function when the hearing aid is worn. (Project Phoenix [Hecox, 1983] is an attempt to develop a master hearing aid capable of providing electronic circuitry that would accomplish the normalization of pathologic ABRs.)
- Aided ABR procedures, like unaided ABR procedures, are not adversely affected by factors such as sedation, developmental status of the patient, or middle ear function. ABR latency, intensity, and waveform morphology are stable and repeatable. Thus, the changes that do occur in ABR waveforms reflect actual changes in auditory transmission or changes resulting from hearing aid gain, compression, or type.
- ABR parameters can be successfully correlated with a number of behavioral and audiometric findings which will be helpful in the refinement of future aided ABR techniques.
- Future utilization of frequency specific stimuli, with or without masking, will expand the applications of ABR procedures in hearing aid selection and fitting.
- Utilization of middle latency response techniques and late cortical evoked potential techniques will provide the clinician with a more accurate picture of the

hard-to-test patient's audiometric and auditory perceptual potential with a hearing aid.

■ The development of standardized procedures for use in ABR hearing aid assessments may be accomplished with the refinement of new hybrid and digital hearing aids which provide compression and amplification circuitry that can more cleanly process pure tone and click stimuli. The result of this refinement will be cleaner and more useful ABRs for hearing aid assessment and selection for hard-to-test patients.

As more clinics obtain auditory evoked response instrumentation and as the technological advancements of the last few years continue, reliable clinical protocols for the use of auditory evoked response techniques for hearing aid assessment will become a reality.

REFERENCES

Beattie, R. C., & Boyd, R. (1984). Effect of click duration on the latency of the early response. *Journal of Speech and Hearing Research, 27,* 20–75.

Beauchaine, K. A., Gorga, M. P., Reiland, J. D., & Larson, L. L. (1986). Application of ABRs to the hearing-aid selection process: Preliminary data. *Journal of Speech and Hearing Research, 29,* 12–128.

Bobbin, R., & Kisiel, D. (1981). Auditory physiology. In D. Brown & E. Daigneault (Eds.), *The pharmacology of hearing: Experimental and chemical bases.* New York: John Wiley.

Braida, L. D., Durlach, N. I., DeGennaro, S. V., Peterson, P. M., & Bustamante, D. K. (1982). Review of recent research on multiband amplitude compression for the hearing impaired. In G. A. Studebaker & F. H. Bess (Eds.), *The Vanderbilt hearing aid report: Monographs in contemporary audiology* (pp. 133–143). Upper Darby, PA.

Buchwald, J. S. (1983). Generators. In E. J. Moore (Ed.), *Basis of auditory brain-stem evoked responses.* New York: Grune & Stratton.

Coates, A. C. (1978). Human auditory nerve action potentials and brainstem evoked responses. *Archives of Otolaryngology, 104,* 709–717.

Cox, L. C., & Metz, D. A. (1980). ABER in the prescription of hearing aids. *Hearing Instruments, 31,* 12–15, 55.

Durrant, J.D. (1983). Fundamentals of sound generation. In E. J. Moore (Ed.), *Basis of auditory brain-stem evoked responses.* New York: Grune & Stratton.

Gorga, M. P., Beauchaine, K. A., & Reiland, J. K. (1987). Comparison of onset and steady-state responses of hearing aids: Implications for use of the auditory brainstem response in the selection of hearing aids. *Journal of Speech and Hearing Research, 30,* 130–136.

Gorga, M. P., Reiland, J. K., & Beauchaine, K. A. (1985). Auditory brainstem responses in a case of high-frequency conductive hearing loss. *Journal of Speech and Hearing Disorders, 50,* 346–350.

Gorga, M. P., Worthington, D. W., Reiland, J. K., Beauchaine, K. A., & Goldgar, D. E. (1985). Some comparisons between auditory brainstem response thresholds, latencies, and the pure-tone audiogram. *Ear and Hearing, 6,* 105–112.

Hall, J. W., III, & Ruth, R. A. (1985). Acoustic reflexes and auditory evoked responses in hearing aid evaluation. *Seminars in Hearing, 6*(3), 251–273.

Hecox, K. E. (1983). Role of auditory brainstem responses in the selection of hearing aids. *Ear and Hearing, 4,* 51–55.

Hecox, K. E., Breuninger, C., & Krebs, D. (1975). Brainstem evoked responses obtained from hearing-aided adults. *Journal of the Acoustical Society of America, 57,* 563.

Hecox, K. E., Cone, B., & Blow, M. E. (1981). BSAER in the diagnosis of neurological diseases. *Neurology, 31,* 832–840.

Jacobson, J., Seitz, M., Mencher, G., & Parrott, V. (1981). Auditory brainstem response: A contribution to infant assessment and management of hearing loss. In G. T. Mencher & S. E. Gerber (Eds.), *Early management of hearing loss.* New York: Grune & Stratton.

Jewett, D. L., Romano, M. N., & Williston, J. S. (1970). Human auditory evoked potentials: Possible brain stem components detected on scalp. *Science, 167,* 1517–1518.

Jewett, D. L., & Williston, J. S. (1971). Auditory evoked far fields averaged from the scalp of humans. *Brain, 94,* 681–696.

Kiessling, J. (1982). Hearing aid selection by brainstem audiometry. *Scandinavian Audiology, 11,* 269–275.

Kiessling, J. (1983a). Hirnstammaludiometrie zur objektwin Horgeratevorwahl. *Audiotechnik, 33,* 1–6.

Kiessling, J. (1983b). Clinical experience in hearing aid adjustment by means of BER amplitudes. *Archives of Otorhinolaryngology, 238*(3), 233–240.

Kiessling, J. (1984). Zur Validitat Hirnstammaudiometrischer Horgenatevorwahl [on the validity of hearing aid selection by brainstem-evoked responses audiometry]. *Laryngologie-Rhinologie-Otologie, 63,* 88–91.

Kiessling, J. (1987). Insitu Audiometry (ISA): A new frontier in hearing aid selection. *Hearing Instruments, 38*(1), 28–29.

Kileny, P. P. (1982). Auditory brainstem responses as indicators of hearing aid performance. *Annals of Otology, 91,* 61–64.

Kisiel, D. L., & Klodd, D. (1982). Short and long term test-retest reliability of ABR absolute and relative amplitudes in a normal adult population. Paper presented at the Second International Evoked Potentials Symposium, Cleveland, OH.

Kisiel, D., & Lilly D. (1986). Unpublished data.

Kisiel, D., & Seitz, M. (1986). Evoked potentials and hearing aid selection. Paper presented at the New York State Speech and Hearing Association annual convention, Kennisha, NY.

Libby, E. R. (1985). State-of-the-art of hearing aid selection procedures. *Hearing Instruments, 1,* 30.

Mahoney, T. M. (1985). Auditory brainstem response hearing aid applications. In J. T. Jacobson (Ed.), *The auditory brainstem response* (pp. 349–370). Boston: College-Hill Press.

Mahoney, T., Condie, R., & Snyder, K. (1980). Hearing aid evaluation by brainstem evoked responses: A feasibility study. Paper presented at the meeting of the American Speech-Language-Hearing Association, Detroit, MI.

Margolis, R. H. (1985). Magnitude estimation of loudness III: Performance of selected hearing aid users. *Journal of Speech and Hearing Research, 28,* 411–420.

McPherson, D. (1980). Auditory brainstem evoked responses in young hearing-impaired individuals with and without amplification. *Journal of the Acoustical Society of America, 68,* 20.

McPherson, D. L., & Clark, N. E. (1983). ABR in hearing aid utilization: Simulated deafness. *Hearing Instruments, 34,* 12–15, 66.

Mokotoff, B., & Krebs, D. (1976a). Brainstem auditory-evoked responses with amplification. Paper presented at the meeting of the Acoustical Society of America, San Diego, CA.

Mokotoff, B., & Krebs, D. (1976b). Brainstem auditory-evoked responses with amplification. *Journal of the Acoustical Society of America, 60,* S16 (Abstr.).

Parrott, V., Jacobson, J., & Seitz, M. (1980). Comparison of auditory brainstem responses under binaural earphone and sound field conditions. Paper presented at the Canadian Speech and Hearing Association Convention, Winnipeg, Canada.

Pollack, M. C., & Lipscomb, D. M. (1979). Implications of hair-pure tone discrepancies for oto-audiologic practice. *Audiology and Hearing Education, 5,* 16–36.

Rackliffe, L. M., & Musiek, F. E. (1983). An introduction to ABR in hearing aid evaluation. *Hearing Instruments, 34,* 9–10.

Rapin, I., & Graziani, L. J. (1967). Auditory-evoked responses in normal, brain damaged and deaf infants. *Neurology, 17,* 881–894.

Rines, D., Stelmachowicz, P. G., & Gorga, M. P. (1984). An alternate method for determining functional gain of hearing aids. *Journal of Speech and Hearing Research, 27,* 627–633.

Rowe, M. J. (1987). Normal variability of the BAER in young and old adults. *Electroencephalography and Clinical Neurophysiology, 44,* 459–470.

Sanders, J. W. (1983). The slow brainstem response in pure tone audiometry and hearing aid evaluation. *Hearing Instruments, 34,* 14, 16–20.

Seitz, M., Jacobson, J., & Parrott, V. (1980). Comparison of sound field and earphone derived ABRs. *ASHA, 22,* 9.

Seitz, M., Morehouse, R., & Jacobson, J. (1981). Dual hemisphere recording in brainstem evoked response and audiometry. *Biocommunication Research Reports, 3,* 1.

Stecker, M. (1982a). Objective hearing aid fitting. *Laryngology, Rhinology, and Otology, 61,* 678–682.

Stecker, M. (1982b). Objective Horgerate-Anpassung. *Laryngol Rhinol Otol* (Stuhg), 61, 678–682.

Stephens, D. S. G., & Thornton, A. R. D. (1976). Subjective and electrophysiologic tests in brain-stem lesions. *Archives of Otolaryngology, 102,* 608–613.

Stockard, J. E., Stockard, J. J., & Coen, R. W. (1983). Auditory brainstem response variability in infants. *Ear and Hearing, 4,* 11–23.

Swinson, L., Wagner, B., & Ruth, R. (1984). Effect of a hearing aid setting and earmold coupling on the waveform and spectral composition of ABR click and tone burst stimuli. Paper presented at the meeting of the Virginia Speech and Hearing Association, Norfolk, VA.

Thornton, A. R. D., Yardley, D., & Farrell, G. (1987). The objective estimation of LDL using ABER. *Scandinavian Audiology, 16,* 219–255.

Weber, B., Seitz, M., & McCutcheon, M. (1981). Quantifying click stimuli in auditory brainstem response audiometry. *Ear and Hearing, 2,* 15–19.

10

■ CLINICAL APPLICATION OF REAL-EAR PROBE TUBE MEASUREMENT

JOHN E. TECCA ■

Methods for measuring sound within the ear canal have undergone a major transformation since their introduction more than 40 years ago. Ear canal probe tube measures were essentially research tools during their first 30 years. The apparatus used to make such measurements was expensive, difficult to use, and posed some risk for clinical use due to the relatively hard-walled tubes that were used. Research conducted with early probe tube apparatus gave us much of the foundation for understanding the acoustics of the external ear (Weiner & Ross, 1946; Shaw, 1974) and the acoustics of earmolds (McDonald & Studebaker, 1970; Studebaker & Zachman, 1970).

Real-ear probe tube systems are now available for clinical applications. The measuring procedures were greatly simplified with the advent of microprocessor technology, miniature transducers, and soft probe tubes. During the last decade extensive research has been conducted on the clinical applications of real-ear measures. We have

now reached a time when audiologists can be comfortable in incorporating real-ear measures clinically.

A new procedure should have a solid rationale before it is widely adopted. The basic principles underlying the clinical use of real-ear measures follow.

The real-ear electroacoustic characteristics of amplification systems are the primary factors determining the adequacy of hearing aid fittings. It is now widely accepted that the electroacoustic characteristics of hearing aids that provide the best opportunity for optimal speech perception can be prescribed (e.g., Cox, 1983; McCandless & Lyregaard, 1983; Berger, Hagberg, & Rane, 1984; Byrne & Dillon, 1986; Libby, 1986). It is essential that methods be available to verify that the desired real-ear electroacoustic characteristics are obtained. Furthermore, the results of such measures should provide the audiologist with specific information for modifying amplification systems that are judged unacceptable. Real-ear measures are uniquely suited to meet this objective.

There is a significant interaction between ears and amplification systems due mainly to anatomical differences that occur among ears. The results of these variations is that a given hearing aid will not perform the same on different ears. These individual differences are not predicted well from standard 2 cc coupler or manikin measures (Hawkins & Haskell, 1982; Zemplenyi, Dirks, & Gilman, 1985; Mason & Popelka, 1986; Schum, 1986). Real-ear measures readily assess differences among ears. Individual differences can be measured prior to hearing aid fitting and incorporated into the prescription of choice. Real-ear measures provide the audiologist with a much better prediction of the aided performance that will be obtained.

The focus of this chapter is on clinical aspects of real-ear probe tube measures. Clinical experience and research findings are integrated in an effort to help the audiologist implement real-ear probe measures into routine clinical practice.

TEST PARAMETERS

There are presently no standards for completing real-ear measurements. Clinicians who make real-ear measures can draw on related standards, such as those applying to coupler or manikin measurements (e.g., ANSI, 1985a; ANSI, 1985b; ANSI, 1987), for guidance in determining specific test parameters. Until standards are available, each facility should make consistent use of its own "standard" procedures in order to increase the likelihood of optimizing the reliability of repeated measures. In transmitting information to other facilities, procedures should be described in sufficient detail to allow others to understand the conditions under which the real-ear measures were completed. The following sections describe some of the variables that need to be considered in selecting test parameters.

Test Environment

Audiologists are accustomed to making measures in sound-treated environments. For many procedures, maintaining very quiet conditions is essential for obtaining valid test results. A standard (ANSI, 1977) is available for permissible ambient noise levels for audiometric testing. The sound-treated room also provides an environment with a relatively short reverberation time, which can be a critical factor influencing test results. However, prefabricated sound-treated test enclosures are expensive and space consuming. It would be advantageous to many audiologists if probe tube measures could be made in nonstandard environments. There are at least two reasons that the need for a sound treated enclosure may be questioned. First, probe tube measures are generally completed at levels of at least 60 dB SPL. At these levels the signal should be sufficiently greater than ambient noise levels in most reasonably quiet rooms to avoid test artifact. Second, most test instruments incorporate circuitry to minimize the effects of extraneous sound.

Tecca (1987) compared insertion gain results obtained in a prefabricated sound-treated enclosure conforming to ANSI standards (ANSI, 1977) and a nonstandard consultation room. The two rooms are shown in schematic form in Figure 10-1. Ten adults were tested three times in each room using each of two test methods (substitution and modified comparison) and at each of two distances from the loudspeaker (1.0 and 0.5 m). This resulted in a total of 12 test conditions per subject. Test 1 and test 2 were completed sequentially within the same session without repositioning the subject or the probe apparatus. It was believed that any differences observed between these two tests could most likely be attributed to momentary environmental changes or to inaccuracies of the test instrument. Test 3 occurred on a different day, increasing the number of variables that could contribute to differences among tests.

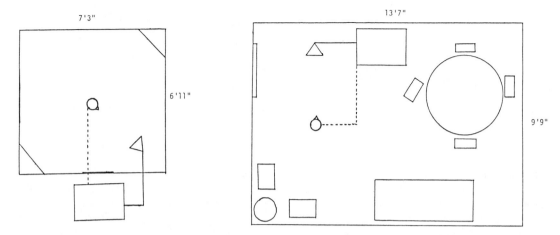

FIGURE 10-1. Schematic diagram of test arrangement used for measurement of insertion gain in a sound-treated room *(left)* and a nonstandard consultation room *(right)*. The consultation room was furnished with a round table and four chairs, credenza, a side grouping of two chairs and an end table along with the measuring equipment and patient's chair.

Mean test results indicated that very similar insertion gain results were obtained in the two rooms (Figure 10-2). Statistically significant differences were not observed between test 1 and test 2 results. Some statistically significant differences were noted in the mid- to high frequencies between test 1 and test 3. The mean differences were very small, and the statistical significance most likely occurred due to the large number of measures included in the analysis. Mean results obtained for the individual test conditions are shown in Figures 10-3 and 10-4. Again, it can be seen that very similar results were obtained across conditions.

The most important measure for clinical applications is probably the standard deviation of the difference between test 1 and test 3. These results are shown in Table 10-1. Standard deviations are slightly larger for the insertion gain measures completed in the nonstandard room. The mean intrasubject standard deviation from 500 to 4000 Hz was 2.92 dB in the sound-treated room and 3.41 dB in the nonstandard room. Thus, the mean difference of the standard deviations was on the order of 0.5 dB. Overall, the results indicate that valid insertion

gain results can be obtained outside of the prefabricated sound treated enclosure.

Specific environments can affect the validity of the results, therefore it is prudent for the audiologist to measure ambient levels in the proposed test room prior to initiating insertion gain measures to determine if there is a sufficient difference between ambient levels and signal levels to avoid contamination. Additionally, it is desirable to compare insertion gain results obtained for several subjects in the pro-

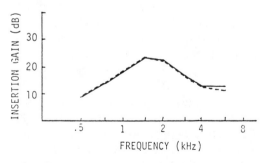

FIGURE 10-2. Mean insertion gain for 10 subjects in each test room. Data were averaged across all conditions. *Dashed line* = sound treated room; *solid line* = nonstandard consultation room.

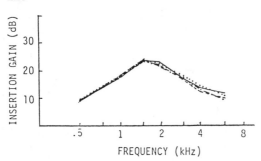

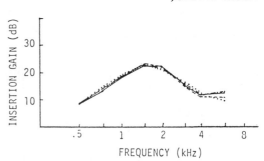

FIGURE 10–3. Mean insertion gain obtained at a distance of 1 m from loudspeaker for 10 subjects under four conditions. *Solid line* = nonstandard consultation room, modified comparison method; *dashed line* = sound treated room, modified comparison method; *dotted line* = nonstandard consultation room, substitution method; *dots and dashes* = sound treated room, substitution method.

FIGURE 10–4. Mean insertion gain obtained at a distance of 0.5 m from loudspeaker for 10 subjects under four conditions. *Solid line* = nonstandard consultation room, modified comparison method; *dashed line* = sound treated room, modified comparison method; *dotted line* = nonstandard consultation room, substitution method; *dots and dashes* = sound treated room, substitution method.

posed test room with those obtained in a sound-treated room prior to initiating clinical measures.

Test Signal

Standard measures of hearing aid performance are made using pure tone signals in very quiet enclosures that have high sound absorption. It has been demonstrated that reliable insertion gain results can be made with discrete frequency test signals in audiometric test rooms (Tecca, Woodford, & Kee, 1987). However, a discrete frequency signal is at risk for interaction with the test environment in reverberant rooms. It is desirable to use an alternative signal whenever possible. Available options include warble tones, narrow band noise, speech spectrum noise, composite noise, and clicks. The choice depends on the options available with the specific test instrument. Signal processor-type hearing aids present a special problem, which is discussed later in this chapter. They should be evaluated using a broadband signal in order to accurately measure the effect of the processor.

Distance from Sound Source

Traditionally real-ear probe tube and manikin measures made in research applications have placed the loudspeaker 1 m from the subject. Much of the research was conducted in anechoic test chambers. In clinical work, testing is conducted in reverberant test rooms, either standard audiometric test enclosures or nonstandard test rooms. In such environments there is a greater opportunity for interaction between the sound emanating directly from the loudspeaker and reflected sound. It is desirable to minimize this possible source of contamination of test results. A review of the clinical probe tube literature reveals that distances ranging from 20 cm to 1.5 m have been recommended. Testing at closer distances with small loudspeakers creates the risk of entering the near field. When this occurs, small changes in distance, such as those attributable to head movements, may translate into relatively large measurement errors.

Tecca (1987) was interested in knowing the effect of distance from sound source on insertion gain test results. He compared the

TABLE 10-1. Standard deviations for the differences between insertion gain measured on test 1 and test 3 for eight conditions in study 1. Also included is the data from study 2, which was conducted under actual clinical conditions using the modified comparison method in the nonstandard consultation room at a distance of 1 m from the loudspeaker. Study 2 data were obtained from 11 consecutive patients.

| Conditions | | | Frequency (Hz) | | | | | | | |
Type of room	Method	Distance (in m)	500	750	1000	1500	2000	3000	4000	6000
STUDY 1										
Nonstandard	Substitution	1	3.87	3.56	2.76	2.39	1.87	1.70	2.69	5.31
Sound treated	Substitution	1	3.92	4.25	3.61	1.85	1.71	1.96	2.46	3.71
Nonstandard	Modified comparison	1	4.85	4.14	3.47	3.38	2.64	2.49	2.90	7.47
Sound treated	Modified comparison	1	4.62	3.57	3.56	1.71	2.20	1.48	3.33	5.52
Nonstandard	Substitution	0.5	4.60	4.89	3.18	1.65	1.64	2.42	3.05	7.32
Sound treated	Substitution	0.5	3.41	3.67	3.59	2.30	2.91	1.64	2.59	3.59
Nonstandard	Modified comparison	0.5	4.55	4.24	3.53	2.36	2.62	2.62	2.73	5.85
Sound treated	Modified comparison	0.5	3.62	3.62	3.21	1.87	1.35	1.89	1.85	5.55
STUDY 2										
Nonstandard	Modified comparison	1	1.37	3.42	3.45	3.82	3.98	3.82	3.00	8.34

results obtained at two distances, 1.0 and 0.5 m, in two environments, an audiometric test room and a nonstandard consultation room. Other details of this study were discussed previously under the section heading test environment. The results revealed essentially no differences between the two distances in either room (Figures 10–3 and 10–4; Table 10–1). At the outset of this study, a 20 cm distance was also included in the experimental design. This distance was eliminated after a pilot study indicated it was unpleasant for subjects at the 0-degree azimuth that was being utilized.

Clinical experience has shown that patients feel more comfortable with the loudspeaker placed at a distance of 1 m, at least when 0-degree azimuth is used. When this information is considered along with the above data and the recommendation of re-

lated standards, it seems appropriate to routinely use a 1 m distance. Exceptions to this guideline may include the use of azimuths other than 0 degrees.

Azimuth

Most prior research has made use of 0-degree azimuth. It is relatively easy to locate a patient at this azimuth by instructing the patient to look directly at a focal point in the center of the loudspeaker cone. Killion and Revit (1987) reported that reduced variability of repeated measures is obtained when the loudspeaker is placed 45 degrees to the side and at 45 degrees elevation (Figure 10–5). They found that this placement reduced the average within the subject test-retest standard deviation up to 1 dB rela-

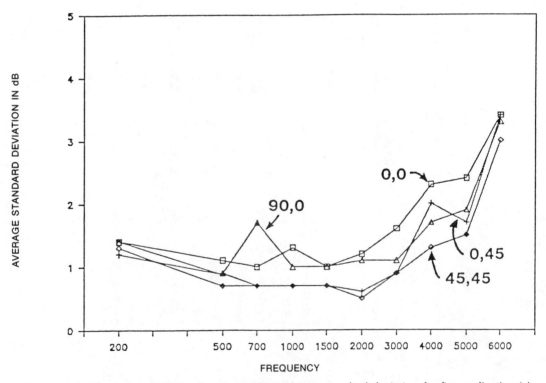

FIGURE 10–5. Test-retest variability (average within-subjects standard deviation for five replications) in insertion gain for four loudspeaker locations. From M. C. Killion and L. J. Revit. Insertion gain repeatibility versus loudspeaker location: You want me to put my loudspeaker WHERE? *Ear and Hearing, 8*(5, Suppl.), pp. 68–73. Copyright 1987 Williams & Wilkins. Reprinted with permission.

tive to 0-degree azimuth. Although the effect of this placement is desirable, Killion and Revit did not provide instructions for how the 45-degree elevation is to be achieved in the clinical setting. At the present time, none of the manufacturers of probe equipment offer a speaker stand to allow the clinician to easily achieve this azimuth. Additionally, use of this azimuth requires repositioning the patient or loudspeaker between measures on the two ears.

Another azimuth likely to be chosen for clinical measures is 90 degrees in the horizontal plane. Placement of a loudspeaker at this angle is achieved with relative ease. The Killion and Revit (1987) data showed this azimuth to have slightly better test-retest variability than 0-degree azimuth. However, such an orientation may interact with directional microphones and compromise results. The patient or loudspeaker also has to be reoriented between measures on the two ears.

Use of a 0-degree azimuth has some pragmatic advantages for routine clinical applications. However, the audiologist may wish to use alternative orientation in order to achieve slightly improved repeatability of measure; and it is necessary to use orientations other than 0 degrees for special applications, such as measuring directional microphone effects, head shadow effects, or effects of CROS-type amplification systems.

Probe Tube Insertion Depth

Placement of the probe tube in the external auditory canal is one of the sources of greatest variability in making real-ear measures. Two guidelines should be followed in determining probe tube insertion depth. First, the insertion depth should not be great enough to permit the probe tube to touch the tympanic membrane. Results comparable to those obtained at the tympanic membrane can be obtained at a point 6 to 8 mm away from its surface (Dirks & Kin-

caid, 1987). This placement greatly reduces the risks of causing the patient discomfort or injury. The effect of distance from the tympanic membrane on the SPL measured is shown in Figure 10–6. Second, the insertion depth should be at least 4 to 5 mm beyond the lateral tip of the earmold (Burchard & Sachs, 1977). This placement moves the tip of the probe tube out of the transitional sound field and reduces the likelihood of test artifact.

The probe tube insertion depth chosen for clinical applications is dependent on the

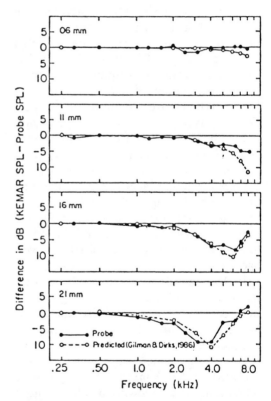

FIGURE 10–6. Differences in dB between KEMAR eardrum and probe measured SPL with the tip of the probe located at several distances from an ear simulator microphone mounted in a KEMAR manikin. Predicted results calculated from data presented in Dirks and Kincaid's Figure 2 are shown for comparison. From D. D. Dirks and G. E. Kincaid. Basic acoustic considerations of ear canal probe measurements. *Ear and Hearing, 8*(5, Suppl.), 60–67. Copyright 1987 Williams & Wilkins. Reprinted with permission.

particular test being conducted. If the audiologist wishes to obtain precise measures of ear canal sound pressure levels (SPLs), the tip of the probe tube should be within 6 to 8 mm of the surface of the eardrum (Dirks & Kincaid, 1987). For example, this placement is highly desirable if the audiologist is interested in determining real ear SSPL-90. If the audiologist is interested only in relative measures, such as those obtained in measuring insertion gain, then any distance beyond the transitional sound field is acceptable. Some of the more sophisticated probe systems now provide a mechanism for determining rather precisely the distance of the probe tube tip from the tympanic membrane. Sullivan (1988) has also described a method for manually calculating distance from the tympanic membrane.

Consideration of ear canal anatomy helps put the above distances into perspective. The average adult ear canal is 24 mm in length. The average earmold tip extends 10 mm into the ear canal (Cox, 1979). Adding the minimum 5 mm to the length of the average earmold places the tip of the tube at a depth of 15 mm. This is 9 mm away from the tympanic membrane. It follows then that extending the tip of the probe tube about 7 mm beyond the tip of the average earmold achieves the goal of accurately reflecting SPLs at the eardrum with minimal risk of actually touching its surface. Alternatively, audiologists may wish to mark their probe tubes so that they are routinely inserted 16 to 18 mm into the ear canal. This placement will usually result in a placement 6 to 8 mm from the tympanic membrane while allowing a safety margin for variability in ear canal length.

Regardless of the insertion depth chosen by the clinician, it is critical that the same distance be maintained throughout testing with the same patient. Significant movement of the tube between aided and unaided measures can result in large errors (Hawkins & Mueller, 1986). Although movements of several millimeters between measures may produce minimal error, there is an interaction between distance from the

tympanic membrane and error associated with tube movement (Dirks & Kincaid, 1987). Variability is smallest when the probe tube is close to the tympanic membrane.

Head Restraint

Head restraint is usually used in research applications of probe tube measures. Some form of head restraint is desirable as it helps ensure that the distance and azimuth relative to the loudspeaker will be maintained throughout the test. Killion and Revit (1987) demonstrated that variability associated with different loudspeaker azimuths is due to small head movements. Head restraint should be expected to reduce the likelihood of error. Clinically, it is often difficult to use head restraint, even the passive restraint provided through the use of a headrest. Some patients are simply unable to position themselves against a headrest. Also, headrests do not always have adequate adjustment to bring them to the patient's desired position.

Tecca (1987) used a headrest to control subject position in his study evaluating the effects of test room, test method, and distance from the sound source on insertion gain test results. In a follow-up study using the same test parameters with a group of consecutive clinic patients, a headrest was not used. Although the effect of the headrest was not directly evaluated in Tecca's (1987) study, examination of the results does provide some insight regarding its effect. The mean intrasubject test-retest standard deviation was 3.41 in the first study and 3.23 in the second study (Table 10–1). It seems reasonable to conclude that when care is taken to instruct the patient to sit still and to look at a focal point during the testing that eliminating a headrest is acceptable.

Signal Level

Various signal levels have been suggested for completing insertion gain measures. There are three considerations in selecting a test level:

1. The test level should be great enough to avoid contamination by ambient noise levels. Ambient levels should be measured with a sound level meter prior to initiating probe tube measures. Most current probe systems make use of tracking filters or a method of Fourier analysis so that extracting the signal from background noise is now much less of a problem than it was with earlier test systems.
2. The test level should not be so great as to send the hearing aid into saturation or to activate its compressor circuitry. If compression is activated, the results will obviously be erroneous, showing less amplification than the system is capable of delivering at the chosen volume setting. If it is suspected that the hearing aid has been overdriven, the measure should be repeated with a lower input level. The results from the two tests should show parallel frequency response curves separated by a distance equal to the difference in dB of the two input levels.
3. The test level should not be so great as to cause discomfort to the patient.

Levels of 60 to 70 dB SPL are routinely acceptable. The 70 dB SPL level is used in most cases. This level generally exceeds ambient levels even in nonstandard rooms, usually does not send linear hearing aids into saturation, and rarely causes the patient discomfort. Lower levels are most frequently required to avoid saturation of high power hearing aids and with compression hearing aids. Higher levels are usually required to measure the saturation sound pressure level (SSPL) of a hearing aid.

TEST METHOD

The audiologist can either use a one- or two-microphone measurement system. In its most basic sense this choice is between using a substitution method, which incorporates one microphone, and a modified comparison method, which incorporates two microphones for making real-ear measures (Preves & Sullivan, 1987). The substitution method compares the SPL measured at the calibration point, which is the point where the center of the subject's head will be located, and the SPL measured in the ear canal. This method allows measurement of all head and body diffraction effects on the test signal along with the effects introduced by the ear and hearing aid. The modified comparison method uses a control or reference microphone to monitor sound level at some point near the ear. This microphone provides real-time correction in signal level for variations due to equipment, ambient conditions, or patient movement. The test microphone is located in the patient's ear canal as it is in the substitution method.

The substitution method is clearly a more "pure" measurement method. However, it requires more careful placement of the patient relative to the calibration point, and greater care must be taken to maintain the patient's position during the test. Tecca (1987) compared the insertion gain results obtained using the substitution and modified comparison methods in an audiometric test room and a nonstandard consultation room. Results were essentially the same for both methods (Figures 10–2, 10–3, 10–4, Table 10–1). Tecca concluded that, in general, clinical use of the modified comparison method is advantageous because it affords greater control of patient and ambient factors during testing.

There are specific cases in which a control microphone cannot be used. The most common case encountered clinically is the measurement of insertion gain at different azimuths with CROS-type amplification systems. A control microphone located near the test ear will negate azimuth effects. Consequently, a substitution method should be used. This allows for a remarkable display of head shadow effects and the elimination of these effects when a hearing aid microphone is located on the nontest ear.

TEST PROTOCOL

The clinician has many factors to consider in deciding on a specific test protocol for routine use in making real-ear measures. Many of these factors were discussed in the section on test parameters. Under ideal circumstances, testing is completed in a sound-treated room using a broad band test signal. A substitution method is used. The probe tube is positioned within a few millimeters of the tympanic membrane, and some form of head restraint is used. A pair of loudspeakers are oriented 45 degrees to each side at 45 degrees elevation. Unfortunately, in the clinical world, the audiologist does not always operate under ideal circumstances. Decisions often must be made between the ideal and the practical, with careful consideration given to the increased variability that may result from the compromise. The following test protocol has been found to be effective for routine clinical applications. The variability associated with this protocol under actual clinical conditions is shown in Table 10–1 as the results for study 2.

1. Otoscopic examination of the ears should always be completed before placing a probe tube in the ear canal. This examination is essential to determine whether a condition is present that might contraindicate probe tube measures. It also helps the clinician formulate an estimate of canal length and shape, which facilitates placement of the probe tube.
2. The patient is situated 1 m from the loudspeaker using an azimuth of 0 degrees.
3. The probe tube is marked so that its tip will protrude about 7 mm beyond the lateral end of the earmold or in-the-ear (ITE) hearing aid. The length of the earmold or hearing aid canal is measured and a reference point on the ear is identified for positioning the mark on the probe tube. This usually is easily accomplished by placing the earmold or hearing aid in the ear and noting a point that aligns with its lateral-most edge. A point near the intertragal notch usually works well. The earmold or hearing aid is removed, and the probe tube is placed along its inferior surface so that the tip of the tube extends about 7 mm beyond its medial tip. A mark is made on the tube at the point where it aligns with the earmold's lateral-most point. The mark is adjusted to allow for differences in the lateral point on the earmold and the reference point on the ear.
4. The probe tube is inserted into the ear canal. The tube may be anchored in place.
5. The patient is instructed to look directly ahead at a focal point in the center of the loudspeaker and told not to move or talk until the sound stops.
6. Wearer frequency response is measured (Preves, 1987a). This response is also called ear canal resonance, external ear resonance, or external ear effect.
7. The earmold or hearing aid is placed on top of the probe tube. Alternately, the tube may be removed from the ear canal and reinserted through a hole specially drilled through the earmold to accept the probe tube. The tube may also be inserted through the vent tube. The clinician must be aware, however, that placing the tube through a medium-to-small vent effectively reduces the diameter of the vent with consequent alterations in low-frequency response. Placing the tube alongside the earmold introduces a slit vent. This generally does not introduce a significant acoustic effect in a vented earmold but is likely to reduce amplification measured below about 500 Hz in an unvented amplification system (Pedersen, 1982).
8. Insertion gain is determined. The instrumentation may do this automatically and plot an insertion gain curve, or gain may be determined at discrete frequencies by moving the cursor and using a command to subtract the difference between the wearer frequency response and in situ gain frequency response curves.

9. The obtained insertion gain values are compared to desired target values.
10. The hearing aid or earmold is modified as needed to better approximate target values.
11. Aided measures and comparisons are repeated to verify outcomes.

RELATIONSHIP OF INSERTION GAIN TO OTHER MEASURES

Insertion Gain Compared to Functional Gain

There is a natural tendency to compare various measures of hearing aid performance. These comparisons provide the audiologist with a cross check of the validity of test results. The relationships among measures can also be used to determine the validity of the procedure. Intuitively, insertion gain and functional gain are different methods for measuring the same aspect of hearing aid performance. Insertion gain determines the difference in SPL developed at a given point in the auditory canal for unaided and aided conditions. Functional gain determines the difference in sound-field thresholds for unaided and aided conditions, which are presumably due to changes in ear canal SPL. Yet, if a clinician compares the results of the two procedures on a given patient, it is likely that large differences will be observed.

Harford (1981) reported preliminary results comparing functional and insertion gain for a group of 17 hearing-impaired subjects. His results indicated that on the average results obtained with the two measures were similar but large variability was observed. Further studies examining this question were not immediately forthcoming. Audiologists were left to their own devices to determine whether insertion gain measures were acceptable for clinical use. Subsequently, several studies dealing with this issue were published (Zemplenyi, Dirks, & Gilman, 1985; Mason & Popelka, 1986; Dillon & Murray, 1987; Tecca & Woodford, 1987).

Each of these studies indicated that insertion gain and functional gain were essentially equivalent measures. Dillon and Murray's (1987) study was unique because it compared several behavioral and electroacoustic methods. They determined the average of several methods to provide an estimate of "true gain," then compared the results obtained with the individual methods to this estimate of "true gain." They noted very similar performance among methods but particularly for the methods of functional and insertion gain judged to be of the highest accuracy (Figure 10-7).

Tecca and Woodford (1987) also found that functional and insertion gain methods

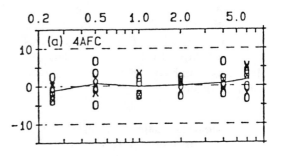

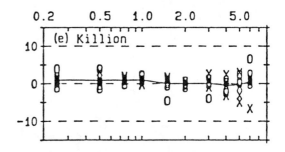

FIGURE 10-7. Group mean and individual subject median gain determined by the 4AFC functional and the Killion probe microphone techniques relative to "true" gain. Positive values indicate that the measured gain was greater than the calculated "true" gain. From H. Dillon and N. Murray. Accuracy of twelve methods for estimating the real ear gain for hearing aids. *Ear and Hearing, 8,* 2–11. Copyright 1987 Williams & Wilkins. Reprinted with permission.

provided equivalent results on the average. However, they noted that in individual cases substantial differences in results were often observed between the two methods. They noted that very few cases agreed within ± 5 dB at all frequencies. Most cases agreed within ± 10 dB at all frequencies, but it was not uncommon to find differences in excess of 10 dB for at least some frequencies. They concluded that differences of at least ± 10 to ± 14 dB (± 2 SD) must be allowed to make certain that real differences were present when functional gain and insertion gain test results were compared in individual cases. These results were in good agreement with the results of Killion (1982), which were based on theoretical variables. The differences that were observed in individual cases were most likely attributable to the combined error associated with the measurement variables of both procedures. Tecca and Woodford recommended that clinicians avoid comparing the two measures clinically.

Real-Ear Gain Compared to Coupler Gain

It is now widely accepted that measures of 2 cc coupler gain do not provide an accurate representation of real-ear gain. This finding has been demonstrated through comparisons of real-ear gain to coupler gain (Pascoe, 1975; Hawkins & Haskell, 1982; Hawkins & Schum, 1984; Zemplenyi, Dirks, & Gilman, 1985; Mason & Popelka, 1986). In reviewing the results of the various studies reported, the most striking difference occurs in the region of the primary external ear resonance where real-ear gain is consistently observed to be less than coupler gain (Figure 10–8). Reasonably good agreement is generally observed between real-ear gain and coupler gain in the lower frequencies when an occluding earmold is used.

REPEATABILITY OF INSERTION GAIN MEASURES

The repeatability of any test should be determined prior to its clinical use. It is important to define which aspect of test repeatability is of interest to the clinician. For example, it may be anticipated that the variability obtained within a test session will be less than the variability obtained between test sessions. Numerous factors can contribute to test variability, including the

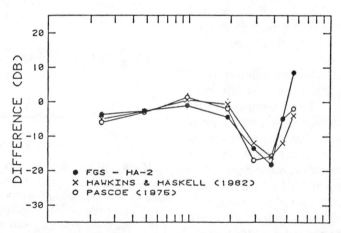

FIGURE 10–8. Mean difference in dB between functional gain and HA-2 coupler gain from Zemplenyi, Dirks, and Gilman, 1985 (●), Hawkins and Haskell, 1982 (X) and Pascoe, 1975 (O). From J. Zemplenyi, D. Dirks, and S. Gilman. Probe-determined hearing-aid gain compared to functional and coupler gains. *Journal of Speech and Hearing Research, 28*, 394–404. Copyright 1985 American Speech-Language-Hearing Association. Reprinted with permission.

variability inherent to the test system, variability of the environment, subject variables such as changes in distance and azimuth to the loudspeaker, time between test and retest, and examiner variables. The following is a summary of some of the major factors to be considered and the variability associated with them.

Immediate Test-Retest

Immediate test-retest variability refers to differences found between measures that are completed sequentially within the same session without removing the earmold. Test-retest variability is attributed to environmental changes, patient movement, and the stability of the measuring equipment. Tecca (1987) found no significant differences between sequential tests completed using two different test rooms (prefabricated sound-treated room and nonstandard consultation room), two different test methods (substitution and modified comparison) and two different distances from the loudspeaker (1 and 0.5 m). The modal difference observed was 0 dB and the range of differences did not exceed 2 dB. The application of this data is in assessing the effect of changes in hearing aid controls made without removing the earmold. For example, an audiologist may want to adjust a low frequency potentiometer while the patient listens and then verify the changes in insertion gain. Immediate test-retest differences in excess of 2 dB should be considered significant.

Short-Term Test-Retest

Short-term test-retest variability refers to differences found between measures that are completed sequentially within the same session with the earmold removed between tests. The variability found is due to all of the factors described for immediate test-retest variability plus the variability associated with earmold placement. Ringdahl and Leijon (1984) and Tecca and colleagues

(1987) have reported test-retest data under these conditions. In general, intrasubject test-retest standard deviations were on the order of 1.5 to 2.5 dB. The application of this data is in assessing the effect of earmold alterations. For example, an audiologist may wish to decrease insertion gain in the low frequencies through vent modification and then to verify the results. Differences in excess of 3 to 5 dB (2 SD) are considered significant.

Long-Term Test-Retest

Long-term test-retest variability refers to differences found between measures completed during two different sessions. This variability is due to all of the factors described for immediate and short-term test-retest variability plus the additional variability associated with a prolonged time between sessions. Data on long-term test-retest has been provided by Tecca and colleagues (1987) and Tecca (1987). In general, test-retest standard deviations have been on the order of 3.0 to 3.5 dB. The application of this data is in assessing an individual's performance with an amplification system over time. For example, an audiologist may want to compare insertion gain measured at the time of hearing aid fitting with that obtained later, such as at an annual recheck or at a time when the patient returns to the office complaining that the hearing aid is not functioning properly. Differences in excess of 6 to 7 dB (2 SD) are considered significant.

ADVANTAGES AND LIMITATIONS OF PROBE TUBE MEASURES

Like other clinical procedures, probe tube measures have both advantages and limitations. In this section several of these factors are briefly described. Limitations that require detailed explanation are covered more thoroughly elsewhere in this chapter. The following is a list of advantages of probe tube measures, based on direct clinical experience and reports of others (Hawkins & Mueller, 1986).

1. Probe tube measures offer an objective electroacoustic method for assessing the real-ear performance of amplification systems.
2. When carefully administered, probe tube measures have very good reliability on repeated testing.
3. Probe tube measures provide a means of rapidly obtaining accurate results when assessing the performance of amplification systems on difficult-to-test populations, such as young children and developmentally delayed adults.
4. Probe tube measures obtain information across the entire frequency range of interest, not only at octave or 0.5 octave intervals.
5. Probe tube measures are not influenced by the slope of audiometric threshold curve. Spurious results may be obtained with sound-field behavioral measures that use warble tone or narrow band stimuli due to an interaction of signal bandwidth and a sharply sloping hearing loss.
6. Probe tube measures are not contaminated by internal hearing aid noise or modest amounts of room noise, which can be a problem with behavioral sound-field threshold testing with patients who have hearing levels better than about 30 dB HTL (Rines, Stelmachowicz, & Gorga, 1984).
7. Probe tube measures allow easy assessment of amplification on the poorer ear of individuals with unilateral or asymmetrical hearing losses, eliminating the need for occluding or masking the better ear as in functional gain measures.
8. Probe tube measures do not require the use of audiometric test rooms to obtain valid results.
9. Probe tube measures are more time efficient than behavioral methods when multiple conditions are being assessed.
10. Probe tube measures allow direct measurement of wearer frequency response so that it can be incorporated in a hearing aid prescription.
11. Probe tube measures provide an accurate method for determining whether overamplification is occurring.
12. Probe tube measures can detect the effect of minimal hearing aid tone adjustments and earmold modifications.

Although this is an impressive list of the advantages of probe tube measures, it is important to be aware of the limitations of the procedure. Probe tube measures are not a panacea and, at times, their use can cause frustration. The following is a list of limitations that have been encountered clinically.

1. Probe tube measures are contraindicated when a significant accumulation of cerumen is present in the ear canal. Even moderate amounts of cerumen can make proper placement of the probe tube difficult. Due to the tiny internal diameter of the probe tube, even a very small amount of cerumen can block its opening. Repeated attempts to place a probe tube in such cases can be exasperating.
2. Placement of a probe tube in narrow and unusually curved ear canals can be difficult and time consuming. Accurate placement requires patience and experience.
3. Placement of a probe tube between the earmold and the ear canal wall introduces a slit vent, which may significantly alter low-frequency results when occluding earmolds or small vents are used (Pedersen, 1982).
4. Probe tube induced venting may allow acoustic feedback to occur before the desired volume setting is reached.
5. Changes in probe tube insertion depth can cause large differences in test results. Great care must be taken to ensure that the location of the probe tube is not disturbed.
6. Passive cooperation of the patient is required. Inserting a probe tube into the ear canal of an active infant can be difficult at best.

7. In some cases of profound hearing loss, unaided thresholds may be vibrotactile. Insertion gain results may be misleading in such cases, suggesting greater audibility of aided signals than actually occurs (Stelmachowicz & Lewis, 1988).
8. Probe tube measures do not measure hearing. They are of little value without valid hearing test results.

APPLICATIONS OF PROBE TUBE MEASURES

There are two primary applications of probe tube measures: prediction and verification. As a predictor, probe tube measures are used in conjunction with behavioral test results to select a specific set of electroacoustic characteristics for a given patient's hearing aid. This set of characteristics would be predicted to match the desired hearing aid prescription. As a verifier, probe tube measures are used to determine if an amplification system conforms to the prescription. There are many specific applications of probe tube measures. Some of the more

important applications are detailed in the following sections.

Wearer Frequency Response

Perhaps the most fundamental and important probe tube measure is wearer frequency response. This measure is also commonly referred to as the field-to-drum transfer function, the external ear resonance, the ear canal resonance, or the external ear effect. This measure determines the natural amplification afforded by the external ear in relation to an external reference point. An example of the average wearer frequency response is shown in Figure 10–9. This response is more accurately called the manikin frequency response because it was obtained from the KEMAR manikin. It is representative of the average adult wearer frequency response. Little resonance usually occurs below 1000 to 1500 Hz with a rapidly rising resonance above 1500 Hz. The resonance peak typically occurs in the vicinity of 2500 to 3000 Hz and on the average occurs at 2700 Hz.

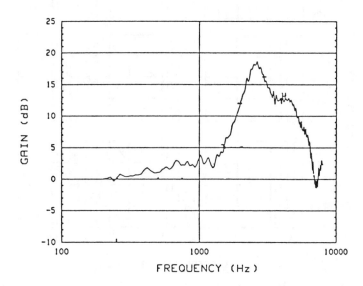

FIGURE 10–9. The "free field" response of the unaided simulated ear. From E. D. Burnett and L. B. Beck. A correction for conventing 2 cm³ coupler responses to insertion responses for custom in-the-ear nondirectional hearing aids. *Ear and Hearing, 7,* 257–265. Copyright 1987 Williams & Wilkins. Reprinted with permission.

The peak amplitude of the KEMAR primary resonance is 17 dB. There is considerable variability among individuals in the frequency location of the primary resonance, the overall shape of the resonance, and the magnitude of this resonance peak.

There is evidence that wearer frequency response is age dependent due to changes in size of the external ear. Kruger (1987) presented data that demonstrated a systematic decrease in the primary external ear resonance frequency from about 6000 Hz for the newborn to adult values of about 2700 Hz by age 2 years (Figure 10–10). The implication is that if an infant is fitted with an amplification system on the basis of median adult external ear characteristics, more than expected real-ear gain may be ob-

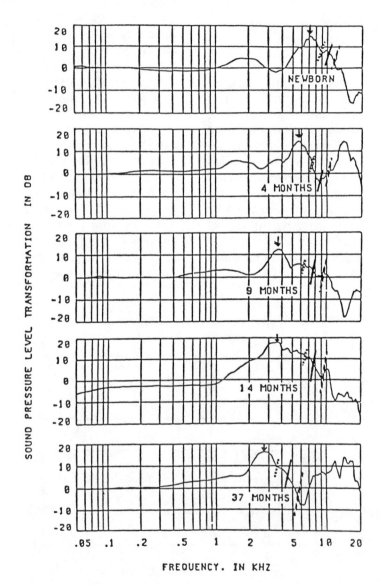

FIGURE 10–10. Diffuse field to ear canal sound pressure level transformation for a newborn, and 4-, 9-, 14- and 37-month-old children. The estimated upper frequency is indicated for an accuracy of ±3 dB *(dotted line),* ±5 dB *(solid line),* and ±10 dB *(dashed line).*

tained in the 2000 to 3000 Hz region, while less amplification may be obtained in the higher frequencies. Furthermore, the pattern of insertion gain may be expected to systematically change during the first 2 years of life as the infant grows. Kruger (1987) suggests that adjustable compensation for these changes should be provided in hearing aids. Such changes present a real challenge to the audiologist. Most hearing aids do not provide adequate frequency adjustment in the high frequency range. The choices for the audiologist are to alter earmold plumbing or to change hearing aids. The audiologist must also consider the pragmatic problems of expense, obtaining adequate patient follow-up, and not disrupting the intervention process. This is certainly not to say that changes should not be made. It simply indicates that in some cases having more information actually complicates case management.

It is also important to be aware that there may be considerable differences in the wearer frequency response for right and left ears of the same individual, adult or child. These differences are usually attributable to small anatomical variations. They may cause the same hearing aid to behave differently on the two ears of the same individual. For these reasons, in prescribing hearing aid characteristics, it is important to give careful consideration to the specific wearer's frequency response rather than using an average such as the manikin frequency response.

Insertion Loss

Inserting a hearing aid or earmold into the ear disrupts its natural resonance properties. The extent of this disruption is termed insertion loss. Before an individual realizes any functional amplification, a hearing aid must replace what it takes away. Insertion loss is approximately equivalent to the inverse of the wearer frequency response. However, the specific amount of insertion loss also depends on the location of the hearing aid microphone (Madafarri, 1978) and, perhaps to a lesser degree, on the extent of occlusion of the ear. The SPL developed at the input to the hearing aid microphone is influenced by its location. Greater input levels at the hearing aid microphone effectively offset a portion of the insertion loss. Input SPLs are lowest for behind-the-ear (BTE) hearing aids, greater for the ITE hearing aids, and greatest for the in-the-canal (ITC) hearing aids. The differences occur because instruments with microphones located in the concha benefit from the boost in SPL contributed by the concha's resonance effects. Although differences in microphone input SPL's are typically small, they may approximate 5 dB at some frequencies. Theoretically, if the microphone could be located within the ear canal, there would be no insertion loss. The important clinical conclusion of this information is that BTE hearing aids require more gain than ITE hearing aids to develop the same insertion gain. Similarly, ITE hearing aids require more gain than ITC hearing aids (Sullivan, 1989).

Measuring insertion loss is a simple matter. Initially, the wearer frequency response is measured in the usual manner. The probe microphone is then removed from the ear canal and a hearing aid of the desired type is carefully fitted. The probe microphone is located at the same point as the hearing aid's microphone. A frequency response curve is then generated. Subtracting this frequency response curve from the wearer frequency response curve gives the insertion loss. Note that this method does not account for any sound that is transmitted through an unoccluded ear canal or vent. This factor may be significant for the low frequencies, but its contribution is likely to be negligible in the mid- to high frequencies due to the typical emphasis of amplification in these regions. Other measurement schemes may be developed to account for the amount of external ear occlusion.

Using Wearer Frequency Response and Insertion Loss to Specify Hearing Aid Frequency Response

Wearer frequency response and insertion loss may be measured at the time that a hearing aid is recommended so that their effects may be incorporated into the prescription. These measures can be made for any type of hearing aid, but it is most helpful with custom hearing aids. It is possible to test a patient with a BTE hearing aid before a final recommendation is made. This test allows the audiologist to be very confident of the way that the recommmended hearing aid will perform at the time of fitting. However, patients with custom ITE or ITC hearing aids cannot be tested with these instruments until the time of fitting.

Many audiologists rely on the manufacturers to select the desired ITE hearing aid characteristics for a patient. While this is effective in some cases, there is great variation among manufacturers or within the same manufacturer in selecting amplification characteristics for identical audiometric characteristics. The results obtained depend on the prescriptive techniques used by the manufacturer, or perhaps solely on the skill of a designated manufacturer's employee, to select the appropriate response matrix. Of additional concern is the fact the specific patient's external ear characteristics are not accounted for in the selection process. If such a method is used, it is hoped the audiologist is familiar with and in agreement with the selection method used by the manufacturer.

Wearer frequency response or insertion loss can be incorporated with audiometric test results to prescribe the desired electroacoustic characteristics of hearing aids. Such an approach allows a closer approximation of the characteristics desired than is obtained through the use of average wearer frequency response data. The desired result, of course, is to avoid extensive modifications at the time of hearing aid fitting and to reduce the frequency with which hearing aids must be returned to the manufacturer for exchange or circuit modification, which is costly and time consuming for both the fitter and the manufacturer. More significantly, such actions may undermine the patient-audiologist relationship and delay the aural rehabilitation process.

Probably the most accurate method for integrating wearer frequency response and insertion loss to the hearing aid prescription involves making real-ear and coupler measurements. The following method is similar to one recommended by Skinner, Pascoe, Miller, and Popelka (1982). Insertion gain measures are made with a reasonably appropriate BTE hearing aid. Ideally, the patient's own custom earmold is used. The insertion gain measured is compared to the insertion gain prescribed. The differences between the two insertion gain curves are determined. These difference values serve as a set of correction factors. The 2 cc coupler response of the hearing aid is then measured with all controls held constant. The correction factors are subsequently added to the measured coupler response to determine the desired coupler response. Manufacturer specifications can be consulted to identify BTE instruments that have the desired frequency-gain characteristics. If an ITE or ITC instrument is ordered, additional correction factors can be added to account for differences between these instruments and BTE instruments (Mason & Popelka, 1986). The desired coupler response can then be ordered from the manufacturer.

A computational method also may be used by incorporating the 2 cc coupler to real-ear correction factors described by Burnett and Beck (1987). Initially, the wearer frequency response of the patient must be measured. This response is compared to the "free field" response of the unaided manikin. A set of correction factors is computed as the difference between the patient's wearer and the manikin frequency response.

The insertion gain desired is determined using the formula of the audiologist's choice. The insertion gain is then converted to 2 cc coupler gain by using the correction factors provided by Burnett and Beck (1987). Finally, the difference between the patient's wearer and the manikin frequency responses is applied to account for the differences between the characteristics of the patient and the manikin. The result is 2 cc coupler frequency response characteristics that should produce the prescribed insertion gain for the patient. A similar method was recently described by Mueller (1989).

This method is most accurate for non-directional fully occluding ITE hearing aids as this type of instrument was used by Burnett and Beck (1987) in their research. However, this qualification does not present a serious limitation for clinical applications. Most ITE hearing aids do not incorporate a directional microphone. Venting primarily effects low frequency response. The audiologist may request additional low frequency gain when a vented instrument will be used. Correction factors also may be used, such as those described by Lybarger (1985). Since vent diameter is relatively easy to vary, the instrument can be fine-tuned at the time of the fitting. It should be noted that data indicating the predictive error associated with this procedure are not presently available.

A second computational method is easier to use, although it is probably not as precise as the method just described. Initially, the prescribed 2 cc coupler response is determined from the desired formula. The measured insertion loss for the patient is added to the coupler response, thereby increasing the amount of coupler gain requested. It is assumed that the prescriptive method used did not include average ear effects in its derivation of coupler gain. The derived coupler results are then sent to the manufacturer as the desired frequency-gain characteristic to be used in preparation of the hearing aid.

Measurement of Insertion Gain

Perhaps the most frequent application of probe tube technology is for the mea-surement of insertion gain. Recall that insertion gain is the difference in the SPL developed at a specific point in the ear canal with and without a hearing aid. This measure is believed to provide the best estimate of the modification the hearing aid makes on environmental sounds and speech. In most cases, determination of insertion gain is a straightforward procedure, although there are a number of cases that require modifications to the procedures described previously in this chapter in order to obtain valid results.

Mild-to-Moderate Gain
Linear Hearing Aids

The majority of hearing-impaired individuals are fitted with mild-to-moderate gain, linear hearing aids with SSPLs between 100 to 115 dB. For these cases, the test protocol described earlier in this chapter usually provides valid measures of insertion gain.

Low SSPL–High Gain
Linear Hearing Aids

The audiologist must remain cognizant of the relationship between input level, gain, and hearing aid saturation in measuring insertion gain. Use of too high an input level can drive the hearing aid into saturation, which is particularly easy to do with hearing aids that have low SSPL or high gain. Insertion gain results obtained under such conditions will be inaccurately low. Saturation may occur within a narrow frequency range or across a wide range of frequencies. In the latter case, saturation should be readily apparent in the relative flatness of the response curve. If the saturation is restricted to a narrow frequency range, it may not be readily apparent from examination of the response curve (Figure 10–11). The audiologist can minimize the likelihood of this problem by attending to the manufacturer's specifications of the hearing aid's 2 cc coupler gain and SSPL-90. With this information, a reasonable in-

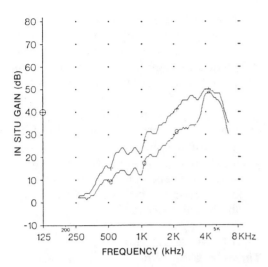

FIGURE 10–11. Example of a hearing aid driven into saturation within a narrow frequency region due to the input level.

ference can be made about whether the routine input level will drive the hearing aid into saturation. A reduced input level should be used any time it is believed that the standard level will drive the hearing aid into saturation. One method of determining whether the hearing aid is saturated is to obtain results with two different input levels, such as 60 and 70 dB SPL. The resulting response curves should be parallel and separated by 10 dB. At any point where the curve obtained with the 70 dB input is not 9 to 10 dB greater than the curve obtained with the 60 dB input, saturation has occurred.

Some probe tube systems are capable of rapidly generating input-output functions at a specific test frequency for a hearing aid. An input-output function allows determination of the exact level at which the hearing aid was driven into saturation. It must be remembered that a hearing aid may function linearly at one frequency and be in saturation at another. This factor suggests that the test frequency must be chosen judiciously or multiple test frequencies should be used.

As a final caution in this section, the audiologist must be certain that the input level chosen to avoid saturation is not too low. It is possible for the test signal to be contaminated by ambient noise levels.

Directional Hearing Aids

The azimuth of the loudspeaker in relation to the hearing aid wearer's head is a significant variable when testing directional hearing aids. Routinely, a 0-degree azimuth should be used to measure the maximum insertion gain of the hearing aid for a given volume control setting. Changing the loudspeaker azimuth should produce decreases in insertion gain if the hearing aid's directional microphone is working properly.

There may be cases when the audiologist wants to measure the real-ear directional effects of a hearing aid. In this case, insertion gain curves can be generated at several azimuths. To most accurately accomplish the measurement of directional effects, a substitution method should be used. Methods that use an active control microphone correct for differences in SPL at the reference point due to changes in the orientation of the head to the loudspeaker. This factor may introduce measurement artifact, but the effect should be small if comparisons are made between 0- and 180-degree azimuth.

CROS-type Hearing Aids

As for directional hearing aids, loudspeaker azimuth is an important variable in measuring insertion gain for CROS-type hearing aids. At least two types of insertion gain measures are important for CROS hearing aids. The first is a measure of insertion gain at 0-degree azimuth, which allows determination of the appropriateness of the pattern of amplification. This measure is particularly important when there is concern about overamplifying an ear with relatively normal hearing. In this case, the measurement procedures used are the same procedures used for mild-to-moderate gain linear hearing aids.

The second insertion gain curve is obtained with a 270-degree azimuth. At this azimuth, the loudspeaker is oriented directly at the more impaired ear where the CROS microphone is located. The probe tube, obviously, must remain in the opposite ear where the CROS receiver is located. This measure indicates the effectiveness of the CROS system in picking up sound in the most adverse orientation.

Ideally these measures should be made with the instrumentation set to display aided and unaided results so that the results will show azimuth effects separately for aided and unaided conditions rather than displaying only the derived insertion gain curve for each condition (Figure 10–12). The benefit of displaying the results in this manner is that the head shadow effects are more clearly observed. This information is especially valuable for the unaided comparison of 0- and 270-degree azimuths. Showing the hearing aid wearer this result is an effective way of explaining why communication difficulty is experienced due to head shadow and how the hearing aid helps overcome this problem.

It is critical that a substitution method be used for these measures. The use of an active control microphone offsets head shadow effects by maintaining a constant signal level alongside the better hearing ear in which the probe tube is located. An exception to this condition exists if the test instrument permits separation of the control microphone from the probe apparatus. In this case, the control microphone is relocated for different azimuths.

Compression Hearing Aids

Care must be taken in selecting the input levels for measuring the insertion gain of compression hearing aids. The input level should be low enough so that the hearing aid is not driven into compression. Use of higher levels causes erroneously low insertion gain to be measured. Specific measurement procedures are the same as those discussed in the section on low SSPL–high

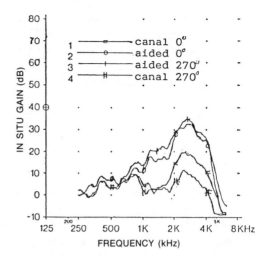

FIGURE 10–12. Example of in situ gain results obtained with a CROS-type hearing aid. Head shadow effects are readily apparent in the unaided measures. The similarity of aided results in the 0-degree and 270-degree orientation are also shown.

gain linear hearing aids. If the audiologist wishes, an input-output function also can be determined. This function shows the effect of the compressor as signal level is varied.

Signal Processor-Type Hearing Aids

The term signal processor-type hearing aids is used to describe a class of hearing aids whose output is varied according to the input. It differs from traditional compression amplification in that it does not simply reduce gain across the frequency range when its threshold of activation is exceeded. Most commonly, this type of hearing aid reduces low frequency amplification in response to increasing levels of background noise. However, modification of different portions of the frequency spectrum also can be accomplished by certain signal processor-type hearing aids.

Accurate measurement of the performance of this type of hearing aid requires the use of a complex test signal (Heide, 1987). Insertion gain may be measured at several input levels in order to obtain a composite of the effect of the signal processor. This measure gives the audiologist valuable information for making inferences regarding the effect of the processor in environments with different levels of background noise. It is also helpful in readjusting the processor on follow-up visits in response to patient complaints.

Measuring the performance of signal processor-type hearing aids with pure tone or relatively narrow band signals produces an exaggerated low frequency response (Heide, 1987). Many current insertion gain systems do not offer a complex test signal as an option. If tonal or narrow test stimuli must be used, the input level should be below the activation threshold of the processor, which will result in a measure that reflects the performance of the instrument in its unactivated mode.

Probe-induced Feedback

There are cases where placing a probe tube between the hearing aid or earmold and the ear canal wall induces acoustic feedback. This response occurs because the presence of the probe tube creates a slit vent. In most cases the effect of the slit vent is negligible because a comparatively large vent is used in the earmold. The effect of the slit vent is most frequently significant when a high gain hearing aid is used or when the preferred volume setting is at a point where the hearing aid is already very near oscillation. Testing the hearing aid while it is in oscillation produces erroneous insertion gain results. Several methods can be used to avoid this problem.

A small hole can be drilled through the earmold to serve as a passage for the probe tube. If the problem is anticipated, the probe tube hole can be requested of the laboratory when the earmold is ordered. The probe tube is plugged after testing is completed. The particular problem of this approach is that there often is not sufficient room within the ear canal to accomodate the probe tube hole.

Alternatively, the probe tube can be inserted through an existing vent rather than passing it along the canal wall. This approach generally eliminates the feedback problem because it not only eliminates the slit vent but also effectively reduces the vent diameter. The problem with this approach is that it alters the low frequency response compared to the response obtained without the probe tube in the vent hole. The magnitude of the effect depends on the relationship between the size of the vent and the outside diameter of the probe tube. For a very large vent, the presence of the tube may not significantly alter the results because it does not comprise a significant reduction in effective vent diameter. For a small vent, the presence of the tube may reduce the effective vent diameter so significantly that the results are similar to those obtained for an occluding earmold.

A third method uses a combination of real-ear and coupler methods. If the presence of the tube causes acoustic feedback at the desired hearing aid volume control setting, the hearing aid should be removed from the ear without disturbing the volume setting. The hearing aid then is placed on the appropriate 2 cc coupler and its frequency response is measured. The gain of the hearing aid then is reduced to a point that allows measurement of insertion gain without feedback. A second frequency response curve is obtained on the coupler. The difference between the two frequency curves is determined. It is most convenient if the test system does this computation automatically. The derived values serve as a set of correction factors for the insertion gain results. The hearing aid is returned to the user's ear, again being careful not to disturb the volume setting. The insertion gain is determined and the correction factors derived from the coupler measures are added to the measured insertion gain. The result is the insertion gain that would have been derived at the higher volume setting. The only apparent disadvantage to this approach is that it requires several extra minutes to complete. A similar method described by Sullivan (1988) for inferring real-ear SSPL90 can also be used for this application. Sullivan's method is described in the next section.

Saturation Sound Pressure Level

Real-ear hearing aid SSPL can be measured with relative ease using probe tube instrumentation. Two different methods have been described in the literature: a direct method in which SSPL is measured from the ear canal of the patient while the hearing aid is worn (Hawkins, 1987a) and an indirect method in which real-ear SSPL is inferred from a combination of real-ear and coupler measures (Sullivan, 1987). Hawkins (1987a) also noted that it is possible to predict real-ear SSPL by applying average 2 cc to real-ear difference values. However, since this method relies on average data, it is likely to be significantly different from true SSPL values whenever the patient does not have average external ear characteristics.

The real-ear method described by Hawkins (1987a) is analogous to standard coupler methods for measuring SSPL90. He recommends that the hearing aid be set to its full-on volume position, or the highest volume position possible without acoustic feedback, while it is on the ear with the probe tube in place. A 90 dB SPL signal is then introduced to the field and an in situ response curve is generated. After evaluating the adequacy of the results, the hearing aid output control can be readjusted, if needed, and the measure repeated.

Sullivan (1987) recommended that the indirect method of inferring real ear SSPL-90 be used. He noted that there is some risk of causing emotional and acoustic trauma to the patient due to the high output levels developed in the ear canal. There also should be concern for avoiding loudness discomfort for the tester or other observers in the test room. If the audiologist has carefully attended to previously determined loudness discomfort levels for the patient and these values were considered in select-

ing the limiting levels of the hearing aid, the risks are rather small. However, unless there is no alternative, a procedure that provides maximum protection to the patient and minimizes the risk of litigation for the audiologist is desirable.

The procedure described by Sullivan (1987) is easily accomplished through the use of routine coupler and real-ear in situ measures. The audiologist should first determine the coupler SSPL90 of the hearing aid. The hearing aid is then adjusted to either the reference test position or, preferably, to the wearer's preferred volume setting. A coupler frequency response curve is then generated. Next, the hearing aid is placed on the patient's ear with the probe tube in place without altering the volume setting. An in situ frequency response curve is then obtained.

The inferred real-ear SSPL90 is derived through simple addition and subtraction. The difference between the coupler and real-ear frequency response curve is determined. This set of difference values is the patient's own coupler to real-ear transfer function for the specific hearing aid–earmold under test. The transfer function is then applied to the coupler SSPL90 in order to determine the real-ear SSPL90.

The approach described by Sullivan (1987) appears to meet the test of a method that provides reasonable estimates of real-ear SSPL90 with minimal risk to the patient. However, there is an element of face validity to the direct measurement of real-ear SSPL90 that will probably continue to be attractive. If real-ear SSPL90 measures are made, a conservative approach should be considered. If a hearing aid with adjustable SSPL is being used, the control should be set to a point that would unquestionably keep the hearing aid output below the wearer's loudness discomfort level in the presence of a 90 dB SPL input. A series of real-ear SSPL90 measures then can be made with increasingly higher hearing aid output settings. The final measurement is made at the point where the patient first indicated that the loudness had become uncomfortable. For hearing aids without an adjustable output level, the signal level should be gradually increased from an initial level that clearly keeps the output below the wearer's loudness discomfort level to the point where the patient first indicated that the loudness had become uncomfortable.

Verifying the Effect of Modifications

Real-ear measures provide a rapid and accurate means of verifying the effect of hearing aid or earmold modifications (Figure 10–13). As modifications are made, sequential insertion gain measures can be made in order to determine whether the desired goal has been reached. It is often surprising, if not frustrating, to find that a specific modification did not produce the expected real-ear result.

Speech Intelligibility Prediction

There has been interest in applying speech intelligibility predictors to the evaluation of amplification systems (Pavlovic, 1984; Humes et al., 1986; Pavlovic, Studebaker, & Sherbecoe, 1986; Humes, Boney, &

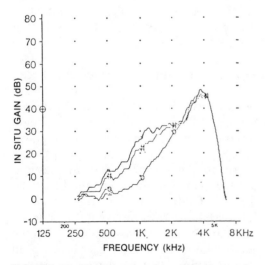

FIGURE 10–13. Example of in situ gain results obtained with several different settings of a hearing aid tone control.

Loven, 1987; Pavlovic, 1988). Both the articulation index and the speech transmission index have been evaluated as methods for predicting the benefits of amplification for speech intelligibility without actually performing speech recognition tests. Such methods perform a series of calculations to determine the amount of spectral information available to an individual for understanding speech. Although the results of these measures do not necessarily provide a precise prediction of speech recognition ability, they do provide an accurate means of determining the proportion of the speech spectrum available to the hearing aid wearer under various conditions. It is assumed that the condition that transmits the greatest proportion of the speech spectrum affords the highest speech intelligibility (Pavlovic, 1988).

Speech intelligibility predictors may be valuable to the audiologist in comparing hearing aids or various settings of the same instrument. The use of speech intelligibility predictors enables the audiologist to reduce the measured frequency response information to a single number, greatly simplifying the analysis. These predictors should help audiologists determine whether differences observed among amplification conditions are significant. However, input from the patient regarding perceived sound quality and intelligibility should not be overlooked.

Insertion gain measures are used to determine the amount of amplification of the speech spectrum that occurs with various amplification systems. The insertion gain values measured at specific frequencies are inserted into complex formulae. Computer software is available to facilitate computations (Humes, 1988; Popelka, 1988). However, a recently proposed articulation index method has simplified the computations to the point that it can be quickly calculated using addition and subtraction (Pavlovic, 1988).

Assistive Listening Devices

The application of real-ear probe tube measures is not limited to hearing aids.

Real-ear measures also provide a powerful method for measuring the amplification characteristics of assistive listening devices. The output of essentially any audio system can be measured with a probe tube system.

Hawkins (1987b) described a method for measuring the real-ear performance of FM systems. The approach is similar to the procedure described previously for measuring the performance of standard hearing aids. The major difference is that an 80 dB SPL test signal is used. The choice of input level is based on earlier work of Hawkins and Schum (1985), which showed that the typical level of speech at the input to an FM microphone is 80 to 84 dB SPL rather than the typical 60 to 65 dB SPL input level to a hearing aid microphone. The difference in input level is due to the closer proximity of the speaker's mouth to the FM microphone than to the hearing aid microphone.

There are two reasons why using the higher input level for measuring the performance of FM systems is important. First, the goal of real-ear measures is to determine whether the output levels in the ear canal approximate target values. Output level is determined primarily by the addition of the input level and the gain of the amplification system. By definition then, 20 dB less gain is required to develop the same output level with an 80 dB than with a 60 dB SPL input level, assuming system linearity. If this premise is ignored, the consequence may be to prescribe excessive gain from the FM system.

The second reason for using the higher input level relates to the saturation of the FM system. It is important to be certain that the amplification system will not be in saturation during typical use. Measuring the performance of the FM system with an input typical of that encountered in actual use conditions helps to determine if the system is being overdriven by the desired volume settings. If a 60 dB SPL input signal is used and excessive gain is prescribed, the system may be routinely driven into saturation when used.

Hawkin's (1987b) method is schematized in Figure 10–14. A modified comparison method is used to control the signal level near the test ear. Often the in situ gain of the patient's own hearing aid is mea-

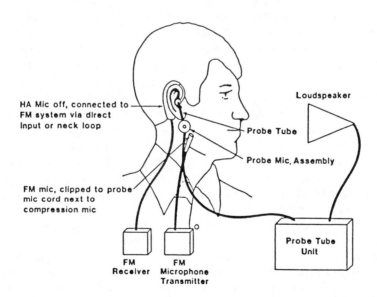

FIGURE 10–14. Arrangement to measure the real-ear response of an FM system attached to a hearing aid with an ear canal probe tube measurement device. From D. B. Hawkins. Assessment of FM systems with an ear canal probe tube microphone system. *Ear and Hearing, 8,* 301–303. Copyright 1987 Williams & Wilkins. Reprinted with permission.

sured first, using a 60 dB SPL input level if possible. The outputs measured with the personal hearing aid serve as target values for the output of the FM system. This method assumes that the patient is wearing an "optimal" hearing aid and that the same output levels are desired for both the hearing aid and FM system (Hawkins & Schum, 1985). The patient then is fitted with the FM system. Any method of coupling the FM system to the ear can be used (e.g., button receiver, direct audio input, neck loop, silhouette). If the patient's personal hearing aid is to be used in the coupling, to minimize variability associated with disturbing the placement of the probe tube, it should not be removed from the ear.

The FM microphone should be placed close to the control microphone to maintain a flat frequency spectrum at its input. A tie-clip FM microphone may be clipped to the probe assembly. Larger microphones may be held in place with a microphone stand and laboratory clamp.

The FM volume control should be adjusted to the preferred setting. This adjustment can be accomplished either by having the patient adjust the volume to a comfortable setting while listening to conversation or by the audiologist adjusting the volume until the same level is developed in the ear canal as with the hearing aid for a specific frequency. An 80 dB SPL input signal centered at 1000 Hz is used for this adjustment.

Finally, the in situ output of the FM system is measured with an 80 dB SPL test signal. The measured levels then are compared to the levels obtained with the personal hearing aid. It is convenient to make comparisons if hearing aid and FM measures can be displayed on the same graph. Adjustments can be made to the FM controls or the earmold, if a button receiver is used, until the hearing aid and FM curves are aligned as closely as possible. A sample of results obtained with this measurement method is shown in Figure 10–15.

An alternative measurement approach is placing the FM microphone within 6 to

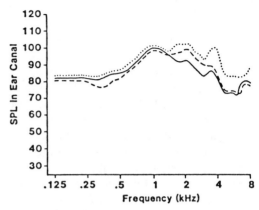

FIGURE 10–15. Output sound pressure levels in the ear canal for three measurement conditions utilizing the technique shown in Figure 10–14. The *dotted line* is the output of the hearing aid alone. The *dashed line* is the output with the hearing aid coupled to an FM system via a neck loop. The *solid line* represents a connection via direct input. The FM receiver volume control wheel was adjusted such that the output at 1000 Hz was the same as with the hearing aid alone.

10 in. of the loudspeaker. This closer proximity decreases the SPL developed in the test room while maintaining the desired signal level at the FM microphone. Lower levels in the test room are less annoying to the tester and any observers. This approach requires that the control microphone be detachable from the probe assembly. Alternatively, a substitution method could be used, eliminating the control microphone. However, use of the substitution method requires greater care to maintain a constant frequency response at the input to the FM microphone at different locations in the test space. Most likely, the system would have to be recalibrated at the closer location.

The same procedures used for FM systems can be used with other assistive listening devices. It is common to find that assistive listening devices that do not use a custom earmold produce less real-ear gain prior to feedback than the maximum gain reported by the manufacturer. Measurements with a probe system define the effective range of user volume. It is unlikely that routine real-ear measures are cost justified in fitting inexpensive assistive listening devices. However, it is worthwhile to evaluate such devices on several ears in order to develop in-house real-ear specifications.

Real-Ear Measures in Patient Counseling

There is a compelling attraction for many patients to focus on the computer screen during real-ear measures. There are times when it is difficult to keep the patient oriented properly at the test location because of efforts to observe the computer screen; therefore, it is desirable to position the patient so that the screen can be watched throughout measurements. This decreases variability due to patient movement and also opens the door to many patient questions about the test procedure. Without providing detailed technical explanations of real-ear measurement procedures, the patient can be given an overview of the purpose of the procedure and a description of the results, and the patient can actually observe changes produced by a hearing aid as they occur. This practice has proved very useful in explaining the goals of amplification and describing why a particular hearing aid is effective or another in not. The patient usually feels more involved in the process, and has heightened confidence in the expertise of the audiologist. This situation greatly facilitates informational counseling and results in a better educated consumer.

PURCHASING A PROBE TUBE SYSTEM

Purchasing a probe tube system is a major decision. There are now many systems available to choose from. Systems vary widely in their measuring capabilities, features, and costs. Preves (1987b) provided a detailed review of many commercially available systems. The primary consideration should be the intended purpose of the system. Does the audiologist want to use the system exclusively for real-ear measures? Does the audiologist want to be able to make real-ear and coupler measures? Does the audiologist also want to be able to measure hearing with the system? Does the audiologist want a system that will provide general computing capabilities for office management functions? The answers to these questions greatly narrow the range of choices. The audiologist then can take a detailed look at the specific features of each appropriate system. Perhaps, arrangements can be made with an equipment distributor to use the system chosen for a brief time to obtain some hands-on experience. This step can be time consuming, but only through the actual use of a system can its quirks be revealed. Because these systems are expensive, it seems worth the added effort. Table 10–2 provides a list of desirable features for probe tube systems.

CONCLUSION

There is little doubt that real-ear measures of hearing aid performance are an extremely valuable clinical and research tool. Computerized probe tube measures provide audiologists the opportunity to be more precise than ever before in specifying hearing aid performance. This chapter described a number of applications of probe tube measures. However, as Hawkins (1988) suggested, real-ear measurements are still in their infancy and the future likely will reveal new and interesting ways to use them.

The ultimate goal of the audiologist in fitting amplification must be improved speech perception. It is important to understand that probe tube measures do not provide a direct measure of this goal. The results of electroacoustic measures allow audiologists to make inferences about speech perception, that is, they provide information that can be integrated with audiometric tests to determine audibility of the speech spectrum. Jerger (1987) provided

TABLE 10–2. Summary of some of the desirable features to be considered in selecting a probe microphone system. Features desired for applications other than real-ear measures, such as coupler measurers or general computing, are not included.

- Menu driven command structure
- Video terminal
- Many test frequencies
- Frequency range is under operator control
- Input levels 50–90 dB SPL
- Input levels can be changed without losing data
- Choice of several test stimuli, including a broad band signal and tape recorded speech
- Allows different means of sound field equalization (e.g., substitution method or modified comparison method)
- Reference microphone can be moved with respect to probe microphone
- Includes circuitry to minimize effects of ambient noise
- Measures in situ and insertion gain
- Sufficient memory to store and display several response curves
- Any two response curves can be subtracted
- Response curves can be averaged
- Difference curves or average curves can be displayed and printed
- Unwanted test results can be easily erased
- Capable of displaying target insertion gain values from different formulae
- System can be inexpensively upgraded with software changes
- Printer is fast

Much of the information included in this table was abstracted from Preves (1987b).

perspective on this matter. He reminded us that spectral audibility does not ensure that the information is useful to a disordered auditory system: "The notion that speech-based measures have been discredited and will now be replaced by 'objective' measures of frequency response in the real ear may reflect an overly simplistic view of the complexity of auditory disorder" (p. 51). There is value in the clinical assessment of speech recognition ability with amplification systems. The audiologist should be challenged to determine which speech recognition measures are most effective and when to apply them. Real-ear probe tube measures and speech recognition measures are complementary and not at odds with one another.

It is also important to remember that probe tube systems do not measure hearing. Probe tube measures are of little value without valid hearing test results. Audiometric threshold test results serve as the basis for making inferences about changes in audibility of sound created by specific amplification systems. Measures of insertion gain alone do not provide a means for determining changes in the audibility of sound.

The audiologist must also be very concerned with providing the patient with an amplification system that provides a pleasing sound quality. Many hours of clinical time are spent in adjusting amplification systems to enhance sound quality based on patient complaints. Real-ear measures provide a means to objectively identify the source of these complaints. Unfortunately, the results obtained often do not provide the desired explanation. Audiologists may be tempted to tell the patient: Objective test results do not identify a problem so you will have to adjust to it. Certainly, there may be times when this is appropriate, but in general, the audiologist should not be bound by the technology and should seek solutions for unsatisfactory sound quality. Again, the use of real-ear measures and reliance on subjective impressions are not at odds with one another. They offer different input, both of value. The patient's feelings should never be forgotten.

In summary, real-ear measures are an invaluable tool in clinical practice. They provide the audiologist with a practical means of routinely answering complex clinical questions. They should be integrated as a part of the total armamentarium of the audiologist.

ACKNOWLEDGMENTS

I would like to thank Jane Phillips for collecting portions of the data presented in this chapter and Cindy Beachler for helpful review comments on an earlier draft of this work.

REFERENCES

ANSI. (S3.1-1977). *American National Standard criteria for permissible ambient noise during audiometric testing.* New York: American National Standards Institute.

ANSI. (S3.36-1985a). *American National Standard for a manikin for simulated in situ air borne acoustic measurements.* New York: American National Standards Institute.

ANSI. (S3.35-1985b). *American National Standard methods of measurement of hearing aids under simulated in situ working conditions.* New York: American National Standards Institute.

ANSI. (S3.22-1987). *American National Standard specification of hearing aid characteristics.* New York: American National Standards Institute.

Berger, K. W., Hagberg, E. N., & Rane, R. L. (1984). *Prescription of hearing aids: Rationale, procedures, and results* (4th ed.). Kent, OH: Herald Publishing House.

Burkhard, M. D., & Sachs, R. M. (1975). Anthropometric manikin for acoustic research. *Journal of the Acoustic Society of America, 58,* 214–222.

Burnett, E. D., & Beck, L. B. (1987). A correction for converting 2 cm³ coupler responses to insertion responses for custom in-the-ear nondirectional hearing aids. *Ear and Hearing, 8*(5, Suppl.), 89–94.

Byrne, D., & Dillion, H. (1986). The National Acoustic Laboratories' (NAL) new procedure for selecting the gain and frequency response of a hearing aid. *Ear and Hearing, 7,* 257–265.

Cox, R. M. (1979). Acoustic aspects of hearing aid-ear canal coupling systems. *Monographs in Contemporary Audiology.* Minneapolis, MN: Maico Hearing Instruments.

Cox, R. M. (1983). Using ULCL measures to find frequency/gain and SSPL90. *Hearing Instruments, 34*(7), 17–21, 39.

Dillon, H., & Murray, N. (1987). Accuracy of twelve methods for estimating the real ear gain of hearing aids. *Ear and Hearing, 8,* 2–11.

Dirks, D. D., & Kincaid, G. E. (1987). Basic acoustic considerations of ear canal probe measurements. *Ear and Hearing, 8*(5, Suppl.), 60–67.

Harford, E. R. (1981). A new clinical technique for verification of hearing aid response. *Archives of Otolaryngology, 107,* 461–468.

Hawkins, D. B. (1987a). Clinical ear canal probe tube measurements. *Ear and Hearing, 8*(5, Suppl.), 74–81.

Hawkins, D. B. (1987b). Assessment of FM systems with an ear canal probe tube microphone system. *Ear and Hearing, 8,* 301–303.

Hawkins, D. B. (1988). Some opinions concerning real ear probe tube measurements. *Hearing Instruments, 39*(7), 28, 50.

Hawkins, D. B., & Haskell, G. B. (1982). A comparison of functional gain and 2 cc coupler gain. *Journal of Speech and Hearing Disorders, 47,* 71–76.

Hawkins, D. B., & Mueller, H. G. (1986). Some variables affecting the accuracy of probe tube microphone measurements. *Hearing Instruments, 37*(1), 8–12, 49.

Hawkins, D. B., & Schum, D. J. (1984). Relationships among various measures of hearing aid gain. *Journal of Speech and Hearing Disorders, 49,* 94–97.

Heide, J. (1987). Testing electroacoustic performance of ASP and nonlinear hearing aids. *Hearing Journal, 41*(4), 33–35.

Humes, L. E. (1988). And the winner is . . . *Hearing Instruments, 39*(7), 24–26.

Humes, L. E., Boney, S., & Loven, F. (1987). Further validation of the Speech Transmission Index (STI). *Journal of Speech and Hearing Research, 30,* 403–410.

Humes, L. E., Dirks, D. D., Bell, T. S., Ahlstrom, C., & Kincaid, G. E. (1986). Application of the Articulation Index and the Speech Transmission Index to the recognition of speech by normal-hearing and hearing-impaired listeners. *Journal of Speech and Hearing Research, 29,* 447–461.

Jerger, J. (1987). On the evaluation of hearing aid performance. *ASHA, 29,* 49–51.

Killion, M. C. (1982). Individual insertion gain estimates: A comparison of methods. Paper presented at the American Speech-Language-Hearing Association Convention, Toronto, Canada.

Killion, M. C., & Revit, L. J. (1987). Insertion gain repeatability versus loudspeaker location: You want me to put my loudspeaker WHERE? *Ear and Hearing, 8*(5, Suppl.), 68–73.

Kruger, B. (1987). An update on the external ear resonance in infants and young children, *Ear and Hearing, 8,* 333–336.

Libby, E. R. (1986). The 1/3–2/3 insertion gain hearing aid selection guide. *Hearing Instruments, 37*(3), 27–28.

Lybarger, S. F. (1985). Earmolds. In J. Katz (Ed.), *Handbook of clinical audiology* (3rd ed.). Baltimore: Williams & Wilkins.

Madafarri, P. L. (1974). Pressure response around the ear. *Journal of the Acoustical Society of America, 56,* S3(A).

Mason, D., & Popelka, G. R. (1986). Comparison of hearing-aid gain using functional, coupler, and probe-tube measurements. *Journal of Speech and Hearing Research, 29,* 218–226.

McCandless, G. A., & Lyregaard, P. E. (1983). Prescription of gain/output (POGO) for hearing aids. *Hearing Instruments, 34*(1), 16–21.

McDonald, F. D., & Studebaker, G. A. (1970). Earmold alteration effects as measured in the human auditory meatus. *Journal of the Acoustical Society of America, 48,* 1366–1372.

Mueller, H. G. (1989). Individualizing the order of custom hearing instruments. *Hearing Instruments, 40*(2), 18–22.

Pascoe, D. P. (1975). Frequency responses of hearing aids and their effects on the speech perception of hearing-impaired subjects. *Annals of Otology, Rhinology and Laryngology, 84*(Suppl. 23), 1–40.

Pavlovic, C. V. (1984). Use of the Articulation Index for assessing residual auditory function in listeners with sensorineural hearing impairment. *Journal of the Acoustical Society of America, 75,* 1253–1258.

Pavlovic, C. V. (1988). Articulation Index predictions of speech intelligibility in hearing aid selection. *ASHA, 30,* 63–65.

Pavlovic, C. V., Studebaker, G. A., & Sherbecoe, R. L. (1986). An Articulation Index based procedure for predicting the speech recognition performance of hearing-impaired individuals. *Journal of the Acoustical Society of America, 80,* 50–57.

Pedersen, B. (1982). Probe placement for sound pressure measurements in the aided ear. *Scandinavian Audiology, 11,* 281–283.

Popelka, G. R. (1988). The CID method: Phase IV. *Hearing Instruments, 39*(7), 15–18.

Preves, D. A. (1987a). Some issues in utilizing probe tube microphone systems. *Ear and Hearing, 8*(5, Suppl.), 82–88.

Preves, D. A. (1987b). A comparison of probe microphone systems. *Audecibel, 36*(3), 10–19.

Preves, D. A., & Sullivan, R. F. (1987). Methods of sound field equalization for real ear measurements with probe microphones. *Hearing Instruments, 38*(1), 16–20.

Rines, D., Stelmachowicz, P. G., & Gorga, M. P. (1984). An alternate method for determining functional gain of hearing aids. *Journal of Speech and Hearing Research, 27,* 627–633.

Ringdahl, A., & Leijon, A. (1984). The reliability of insertion gain measurements using probe microphones in the ear canal. *Scandinavian Audiology, 13,* 173–178.

Schum, D. J. (1986). Inter-subject variability effects on coupler to real ear correction curves. *Hearing Instruments, 37*(3), 25–26.

Shaw, E. A. G. (1974). Transformation of sound pressure level from the free field to the eardrum in the horizontal plane. *Journal of the Acoustic Society of America, 56,* 1848–1861.

Skinner, M. W., Pascoe, D. P., Miller, J. D., & Popelka, G. R. (1982). Measurements to determine the optimal placement of speech energy within the listeners auditory area: A basis for selecting amplification characteristics. In G. A. Studebaker & F. H. Bess (Eds.), *The Vanderbilt hearing aid report: Monographs in contemporary audiology.* Upper Darby, PA.

Stelmachowicz, P. G., & Lewis, D. E. (1988). Some theoretical considerations concerning the relationship between functional gain and insertion gain. *Journal of Speech and Hearing Research, 31,* 491–496.

Studebaker, G. A., & Zachman, T. A. (1970). Investigation of the acoustics of earmold vents. *Journal of the Acoustical Society of America, 47,* 1107–1114.

Sullivan, R. F. (1987). Aided SSPL90 response in the real ear: A safe estimate. *Hearing Instruments, 38,* 36.

Sullivan, R. F. (1988). Probe tube microphone placement near the tympanic membrane. *Hearing Instruments, 39*(7), 43–44, 60.

Sullivan, R. F. (1989). Custom canal and concha hearing instruments: A real ear comparison. *Hearing Instruments, 40*(4), 23–29, 60.

Tecca, J. E. (1987). Insertion gain measures in nonstandard rooms. Presentation at the American Speech-Language-Hearing Association Convention, New Orleans, LA.

Tecca, J. E., & Woodford, C. M. (1987). A comparison of functional gain and insertion gain in clinical practice. *Hearing Journal, 40*(6), 23–27.

Tecca, J. E., Woodford, C. M., & Kee, D. K. (1987). Variability of insertion-gain measurements. *Hearing Journal, 40*(2), 18–20.

Wiener, F. M., & Ross, O. H. (1946). The pressure distribution in the auditory canal in a progressive sound field. *Journal of the Acoustical Society of America, 18,* 401–408.

Zemplenyi, J., Dirks, D., & Gilman, S. (1985). Probe-determined hearing-aid gain compared to functional and coupler gains. *Journal of Speech and Hearing Research, 28,* 394–404.

■ CLINICAL APPLICATION OF SOUND-FIELD AUDIOMETRY

ROBERT E. SANDLIN ■

Procedures used in the selection and fitting of hearing aid devices have ranged from rather ubiquitous statements of "Try it, you'll like it" to the careful application of sophisticated formulae to determine the desired electroacoustic performance characteristics of the recommended hearing aid. Although no one method has gained universal acceptance, measurements obtained in a calibrated sound field offer advantages not evident in other procedures used to arrive at an informed decision relative to the selection of the appropriate hearing instrument.

Sound field assessment was introduced as a clinical procedure in the late 1930s at the University of Wisconsin's Speech and Hearing Center under the direction of Dr. Robert West (West, Ansberry, & Carr, 1957). During World War II, sound-field testing for determining hearing loss was commonplace in rehabilitation centers treating returning veterans who had hearing impairment as a result of their war experiences.

The guiding principle that dictated the early use of sound-field assessment procedures was to gain information about the patient's response to selected acoustic stimuli with and without the hearing aid in place. Although hearing aid selection criteria differed from one center to the next, the general assumption was that the instrument that yielded the most advantageous performance, when compared with unaided responses, was the instrument of choice. Uses of sound-field testing as a valuable and reliable tool were reported by Carhart (1946), Ross and Duffy (1961), Duffy (1967), Victoreen (1973), Duffy (1978), Goldberg (1981), Zelnick (1982), and others who sought ways to improve professionals' ability to establish the electroacoustic responses needed for specific hearing impairment levels.

Sound-field audiometry has been employed as a clinical test for decades and has established utility in the evaluation, selection, and verification of hearing aid devices. It is a significant part of the clinical armamentarium used in the evaluation process. According to Preves (1984, p. 16), "The highest level of realism attainable is that of sound field audiometry — i.e., the amount by which the hearing aid changes the patient's hearing threshold levels, it is also a behavioral measure that includes the final decision making process of each hearing aid wearer as to whether a sound is heard or not heard."

Periodically, every audiologist or hearing aid dispenser is forced to review his or her clinical practices in light of technical and procedural contributions to the hearing aid evaluation process. Nowhere is this more apparent than in selecting the hearing aid of choice and verifying its performance when worn by the hearing-impaired recipient.

There are major concerns to be resolved in selecting and fitting hearing aid devices. Primary among these concerns is the performance of the hearing aid when fitted to the user of the device and measured in a sound field. There is no comparable procedure for obtaining a number of psychoacoustic data that are essential for proper instrument selection. Another clinical matter that needs resolution, of course, is verification that the instrument(s) selected yields results consistent with the amplification needs of the patient based on criteria established by the fitter of the device. The primary advantage of sound-field testing is that unaided and aided psychoacoustic measurements are made in the same physical environment and under the same test conditions, wherein the only significant variable is the hearing aid itself. This fact, in and of itself, is a compelling reason for including sound-field measurement in the evaluation process.

It is unwise to assume that hearing aid measurements determined by coupler response, for example, are equivalent to psychoacoustic data obtained in a sound field under conditions of actual use (i.e., when the hearing instrument is fitted to the pa-

tient). The primary assumption of any hearing aid evaluation strategy is that the data obtained provide sufficient reliability and validity to permit the audiologist or the dispenser to select the appropriate hearing aid system for the individual under test.

It is important for the audiologist or the dispenser to realize that the hearing evaluation process is, or can be, a suitable method for obtaining psychoacoustic data that contribute to the use and acceptance of hearing aid amplification, that such data reflect the patient's response to a number of selected acoustic stimuli, and that these responses are invaluable in determining the specific electroacoustic characteristics that contribute to maximum utilization of hearing aid devices. Further, subsequent testing in a sound field, following a period of hearing aid use, may indicate the necessity for modification of the hearing aid response, as well as the magnitude of such changes.

This chapter reviews some of the advantages to be gained from the use of sound-field audiometry in hearing aid evaluation that cannot be obtained in other ways. In sound-field testing the test environment must be controlled to permit measurement of selected psychoacoustic performances that can delineate one hearing aid's performance from another.

There is no general consensus among professionals who select and fit hearing aids regarding the auditory processes that need to be measured to yield information to clearly describe the magnitude of the hearing deficit. Even if there were general agreement regarding the battery of clinical tests to be used, there is no agreement regarding the electroacoustic characteristics needed to best compensate for the hearing loss. Given this lack of consensus, each audiologist or dispenser develops his or her own hearing aid selection and fitting philosophy to meet whatever measurement criteria are employed to determine a successful fitting. The problem is, of course, that, given an identical hearing loss, a number of different electroacoustic responses may be recommended to compensate for the impairment, depending on the selection and fitting biases of the individual making the decision. In other words, given a specific hearing disorder of sufficient magnitude to warrant the use of hearing aid amplification, the instrument of choice may not necessarily be the device that provides maximum utility but rather the device that reflects the fitter's bias. Fitting practices that include measurements of unaided and aided responses are important. Sound-field analysis is one of the assessment methods that can be employed in the selection and decision-making process.

Sound field audiometry can be applied to any hearing aid fitting formula that relies on specific psychoacoustic data and not solely on patient acceptance of hearing aid amplification. Sound-field measurement is an excellent tool for verifying whether the actual aided responses approach the predicted target responses consistent with the fitter's bias and acceptance criteria.

INSTRUMENTAL VERSUS FUNCTIONAL MEASUREMENTS

There is considerable interest in the recent contributions of computer-assisted probe microphone measurement to hearing aid assessment. From a rather simplistic viewpoint, probe microphone measurement is an objective instrumental assessment. Sound-field audiometry is related directly to a functional procedure which is best defined as an unaided measurement in a controlled acoustic field in which the patient is the responder to a number of acoustic stimuli.

Reports vary greatly relative to the magnitude of test-retest error when using functional measures in a calibrated sound field. From an instrumental perspective, even granting that a correction factor, whether for 2 cc or other coupler volumes, gives reasonable assessment of functional responses, the coupler measurement is representative only of a fraction of the tests employed in

accumulating sufficient information about the unaided and aided hearing status of the person under test. Lybarger (1978) observed that a standard 2 cc coupler fails to achieve appropriate loading of the microphone relative to impedance, volume, and diffraction and yields output responses that vary significantly from functional measures. The argument should not be whether sound-field audiometry is better than or equivalent to instrumental measurements but whether sound-field audiometry provides essential bits of unaided and aided information that cannot be achieved by other means.

For example, relative to real-ear measurement, there is a rather close correspondence (Zemplenyi, Dirks, & Gilman, 1985; Hawkins & Mueller, 1986; Mason & Popelka, 1986; Hawkins, Montgomery, & Prosek, 1987) between functional and insertion gain measurement, and it is commonly agreed that insertion gain could be used to express acoustic gain. However, coupler gain versus either functional or insertion gain fails to offer a clinically acceptable method of assessing gain function. Sound-field audiometry is something more than the assessment of functional gain relative to threshold changes. Threshold measurements are important and constitute a significant part of the unaided and aided evaluation. However, other psychoacoustic or psychophysical measurements can be accomplished best in a sound-controlled environment. Such measures include unaided and aided assessment of:

- Preferred listening level
- Uncomfortable listening level
- Speech discrimination function
- Binaurality
- Speech in noise
- Dynamic range
- Roll over phenomena
- Central processing disorder
- Speech reception threshold
- Difference limen for frequency and intensity
- Loudness growth

One of the major tasks facing the clinician is to arrive at an informed decision about the functional utility of a given hearing aid device. To this end, it is important that the person using the amplification device participate in the decision-making process. Most users of hearing aid devices adjust the gain of their hearing aids until a most comfortable, or preferred, listening level is achieved. Ideally, the amount of functional gain measured in a sound field, when compared to insertion gain, yields an average difference of 1 dB when compared across frequencies. With the exception of 6000 Hz, the actual variations are well within the range reported for functional gain measurements. Additionally, it is well established that 2 cc coupler measurements of hearing aid output do not adequately reflect real-ear gain. Real-ear gain can be defined best as the difference between the aided and unaided threshold sensitivity. Pascoe (1975) labeled this difference as functional gain. There is adequate defense for using either probe-tube assessment or functional measures in assessing unaided and aided responses to acoustic stimuli. Certainly, one of them is necessary to obtain an accurate measurement (Mason & Popelka, 1986).

If one computes differences between functional and coupler gain, a correction factor (arithmetic correction) could be developed to permit real-ear gain to be based on coupler measurements (Hawkins & Schum, 1984). However, the utility and applicability of selected measures are of concern. When utilizing an average correction factor to approximate a coupler measurement, an error of as much as 15 dB can be generated in the estimation of real-ear gain, due in part to variations in ear canal size.

It is not appropriate to take average correction factor data and apply them to individual subjects due to known variations in ear canal size and shape and in the compliance of the tympanic membrane itself (Gilman, Dirks, & Stern, 1981; De-Jonge, 1983). Add to the possible sources of error the variations in earmold configuration (Lybarger, 1978; Killion, 1987) as well

as threshold variances to test stimuli (Byrne & Dillon, 1981), and the magnitude of the problem becomes evident. Without question, instrumental analysis of hearing aid devices yields useful information in a clinical setting. However, data obtained with a standard 2 cc coupler fall short of providing the clinical information necessary to make the most appropriate decision relative to hearing aid selection.

There is not a one-to-one correspondence between coupler and functional gain measurements. There is a closer correspondence between insertion gain (IG) and functional gain (FG) than between coupler gain (CG) and FG. The data suggest that IG and FG best approximate real-ear gain. IG is the method of choice in gathering objective information about the spectral distribution of the acoustic signal at the eardrum. The evidence is too compelling to conclude otherwise. However, since a hearing aid evaluation is, or can be, something more than the determination of threshold sensitivity change, sound-field assessment to evaluate unaided and aided responses to a number of acoustic stimuli can serve an important function.

There is little to be gained by presenting protracted defenses of the relative merits of IG, CG, or FG. Simply stated, IG yields reliable and repeatable measurements relative to acoustic pressures at or near the eardrum. Such data are most useful. Additionally, CG provides reliable and repeatable measurements of the electroacoustic performances of hearing instruments. Probe microphone measurement for the selection and fitting of hearing aid devices offers a useful technique for assessing hearing aid amplification and contributes to a more informed and meaningful selection process.

Limitations of sound-field measurement related to functional gain assessment compared to real-ear insertion gain (probe microphone) were reviewed by Byrne, Dillon, and Dillon (1987). They include (1) aided thresholds for hearing losses of 40 dB HTL or less may reflect the internal noise of the hearing aid and result in an underestimation of functional gain; and (2) for the severely hearing impaired, unaided thresholds may not be measurable because of testing equipment limitations. They postulated that, compared to functional gain measurements, insertion gain assessment protocols were more accurate, applicable virtually to all cases, and quick and easy to apply.

Probe microphone measurements provide more objective data relative to the frequency-intensity characteristics of the input signal when measured at or near the eardrum. There is no question regarding the ability of a given probe microphone system to show characteristic changes in the output signal of a hearing aid when the input intensity is changed or specific internal frequency shaping circuits are modified. The application of probe microphone assemblies and their subsequent value in specifying certain electroacoustic characteristics related to formula applications has gained general acceptance. The formula employed calculates the recommended gain function of the instrument at selected frequencies.

In sound-field analysis, the concern is with the psychoacoustic assessment of the human auditory system. What is the person under test responding to and can the acoustic stimuli to which the person is responding be used to select the appropriate hearing aid? Here is the crux of the problem: Without measuring certain psychoacoustic functions, can hearing aid devices that provide optimal output responses to an impaired auditory system be fitted?

Jerger (personal correspondance, 1987) presented some provocative thoughts by suggesting that

Although systems for the measurement of real ear gain of hearing aids represent a significant technologic advance over analogous closed coupler measurements in quantifying the frequency response of a hearing aid system, it is important to remember that successful fitting of a hearing aid involves much more than the determination of the optimal frequency re-

sponse. The audiologist must answer the following questions:

1. Is the use of any hearing aid appropriate?
2. What is the best arrangement and configuration of the hearing aid system (e.g., BTE, ITE, canal aid; monaural vs. binaural; CROS, BICROS, etc.)?
3. Does the patient perform adequately with the recommended aid in the sense of understanding speech in realistic environments?
4. Is there a better solution than a hearing aid (i.e., assistive listening device)?

To answer these questions, a thoughtful and responsible audiologist must necessarily incorporate into the evaluative system measures that go far beyond the real ear frequency response. They will typically involve some measure of the patient's ability to understand real speech in a realistic environment. They may involve quality judgments, paired comparison, adaptive measures of signal-to-noise ratio, or more traditional speech audiometric measures. Whatever their nature, however, they will broaden the evaluative spectrum beyond the narrow confines of frequency responses.

The following measures are recommended. For phases of the evaluation process that require assessment of instrument performance, probe microphone results are less variable than sound-field measures and have direct clinical utility in instrument fitting and selection processes. Sound-field measurements lend themselves to gathering essential psychoacoustic measurements in the determination of the electroacoustic needs of the patient and serve as a valuable tool in hearing aid selection strategies.

TESTING ENVIRONMENTS AND PATIENT CONSIDERATIONS

Most audiologists and dispensers do not need to be reminded that applied clinical procedures must interface with appropriate test environments and other matters related to subject placement and response protocols. Even though this chapter is concerned with the clinical aspects of sound-field audiometry, a brief discussion of procedural matters is in order.

Attending to matters related to the validity and repeatability of sound-field measurements is the essence of good clinical practice. For an analysis of some of the technical aspects of sound-field measurement, the reader is referred to Volume I of this handbook (Chap. 5).

Reliable sound-field measurements require that specific test conditions be maintained. Necessary controls include:

- Establishing permissible ambient noise levels in the sound field
- Seating the patient away from reflective surfaces during test sequences
- Placement of calibrated speakers in the field
- Selection of acoustic stimuli to be employed in the assessment process
- Patient-speaker distance
- Control of head movement within the field during testing

Control of the parameters listed is of significant value and deserves discussion.

Ambient Noise

In general an ambient noise level at or below 45 dBA has a minimal effect on achievement of data sufficiently reliable to adequately compare hearing aids and their acoustic performances when worn by the individual. It is possible that some interference with organic threshold assessment is present at these levels (Macrae & Frazer, 1980; Zemplenyi, Dirks, & Gilman, 1985). However, unless one can afford to construct sound treated rooms that eliminate all ambient noise, the clinician must contend with some possible error in threshold assessment, regardless of magnitude.

Figure 11-1 shows averaged hearing threshold sensitivity for normal hearing persons to pure tone stimuli in a sound field having a 45 dBA ambient noise level. All threshold values are expressed in sound

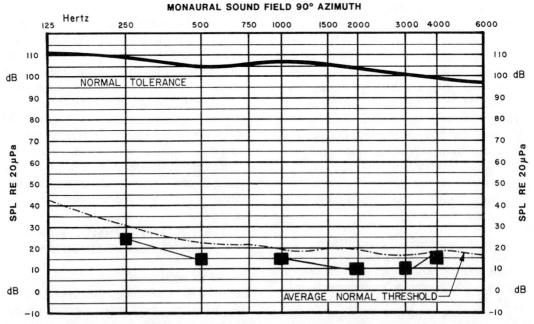

FIGURE 11-1. Average threshold sensitivity of normal hearing subjects to selected pure tone stimuli measured in a 45 dBA ambient environment with the speaker at 90-degree azimuth and approximately 9 in. from the subject's ear. Reprinted with permission of Dyn-Aura Engineering Laboratories.

pressure level (SPL). Threshold measures are well within the normal hearing range. All measurements were made with the sound source at 90-degree azimuth, with the sound field speaker placed approximately 9 in. from the subject's ear. The sound field was measured using a calibrated Type 2 sound level meter placed where the subject's head would be positioned during test. It is unlikely that values exceeding these threshold levels would be obtained in the aided mode. However, aided values approximating normal threshold sensitivity would be advantageous to the user of the hearing aid.

Macrae (1982) has suggested that

> The purpose of aided vs. unaided sound field threshold testing is to obtain an estimate of the real ear insertion gain of the hearing aid. The accuracy of the estimate depends, among other things, on the validity of the aided threshold. Invalid aided thresholds are caused by masking produced either by the internal noise output from the hearing aid or by ambient testroom noise amplified by the aid or by a combination of both. (p. 48)

Therefore, to check the validity of the obtained thresholds, Macrae and Page (1980) and Macrae and Frazer (1980) suggested that as the gain of the aid is varied the tester observes whether the aided threshold levels are altered as a function of gain changes. They suggested further that the equivalent input noise of the hearing aid under test can be measured and then correction values can be applied to achieve an estimate of the levels at which the aided thresholds are no longer valid. In general, however, "... invalid aided threshold levels improve when the gain of the hearing aid is increased and worsen when it is reduced (because the internal noise output of the hearing aid does not increase at the same rate as the gain when the volume is turned up" (Macrae, 1982, p. 48). Although these procedures have clinical utility, the reader

is cautioned to fully understand the procedures involved in arriving at realistic estimates of the possible effects of equivalent noise by reading in its entirety the 1982 article by Macrae.

Relative to the presence of ambient test room noise, Macrae (1982) suggested that, when evaluating an individual with near normal thresholds at some frequencies, the permissible ambient level should be controlled so that it has no masking effect on unaided thresholds obtained in a sound field that would correspond to a hearing threshold level (HTL) of 0 dB at frequencies where the sound-field thresholds are normal. If the ambient noise is not controlled and subsequently produces invalid results, then the real-ear insertion gain is underestimated as a result of the invalid, aided threshold measurements. If the audiologist or the dispenser suspects that invalid measures are being reflected in the sound-field test results, an examination of the effects of the ambient noise level or the equivalent noise level of the hearing aid is recommended.

Speaker-to-Ear Distance

There is no clinically contraindicated reason why a calibrated sound-field speaker cannot be placed 9 in. from the patient's ear during the evaluation process, and there is no reported measurement artifact that would obviate this ear-to-speaker distance. The effect of the near field can be reduced by using a loudspeaker with the smallest diameter speaker diaphragm necessary to produce an acceptable, low distortion output that is well within the frequency range of clinical interest. It should be understood, however, that a small diameter speaker diaphragm may not produce the output pressures needed for higher output signal levels if the speaker-subject difference approaches 1 m or greater.

The reverberant field effect can be significantly reduced by avoiding reflecting surfaces in close proximity to the person being tested (D'Antonio, 1986; Preves & Sullivan, 1987). One of the obvious advantages of placing speakers 9 in. from the subject's head is that standing waves are significantly reduced, permitting pure tone stimuli to be employed without the usual measurement errors that occur as speaker-subject distances are increased. Certainly, there is a much more direct correspondence with the standard acoustic reference for auditory assessment, that is, pure tone measurements are a traditional part of the clinical evaluation of the auditory system. The use of a pure tone signal in the hearing aid evaluation process provides a direct comparison with the more conventional measures of auditory performance. Another significant advantage is that the undistorted output of the speaker system is potentially less than for speaker systems that are placed 1 m or more from the subject. This statement is not an indictment of

the more conventional protocol of placing the subject 1 m from the speaker with the sound source at 0-degree azimuth when signals other than pure tones are employed. It suggests only that a 9 in. ear-to-speaker distance with the sound source at 90-degree azimuth provides certain benefits in the evaluation process. Chief among them is the use of a pure tone signal in selecting the electroacoustic performance to best compensate for the patient's acoustic deficit.

Figure 11-2 shows the orientation of the subject in a sound field relative to speakers placed at 90-degree azimuth. Reflections from the patient's head, or reflections from the speaker enclosure or projector, do not constitute a measurement error of sufficient magnitude to reduce its utility in achieving reliable measurement of unaided or aided responses. Positioning of the subject relative to reflective surfaces within the test room is critical. Acoustic

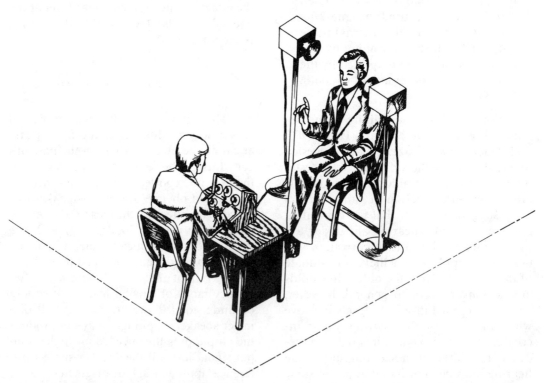

FIGURE 11-2. Orientation of the subject in a sound field relative to speaker placement at 90-degree azimuth. (Courtesy of Hyman Goldberg.)

analysis of the sound room using a calibrated sound level meter can determine possible signal distortion as a function of reflected sound energy. Further, controlling sound levels in the confined field, or space where the subject's head will be during testing, is important relative to reducing standing waves and their subsequent interference with a constant level test stimulus at the ear. In order to eliminate unwanted intensity changes in the test stimulus, which are present in an acoustically uncontrolled sound field, sound energy must be concentrated at the place of measurement. The rationale here is that errors due to standing waves are significantly reduced due to the attentuated level of reflected test signals.

Pure Tone Stimuli

Various acoustic stimuli have been employed in the sound field during the hearing aid evaluation process. Each stimulus (warble tone, narrow band, damped wave train, and AM/FM modulated signals) has its value and limitation. In the main, each type of stimulus has been employed to reduce problems associated with standing waves. Although pure tone signals are logical choices and have the highest correspondence with the way in which the auditory system is traditionally assessed, standing waves can constitute a significant problem when tests are conducted in a more conventional arrangement where the subject-speaker distance is 1 m or greater. This is not meant to suggest that test room design cannot reduce significant standing wave interference but rather that the test chamber construction and configuration do not permit accurate pure tone assessment when the subject-speaker distance is set at 1 m (D'Antonio, 1986).

Moving the sound field speaker closer to the head of the subject under test reduces measurement error due to standing waves. Further, the speaker design, plus reduced speaker-subject distance, contributes to reduction in measurement error when pure tones are the stimuli of choice.

Woodward and Tecca (1985) suggest that, "If use of pure tones in a sound field yield reliable measures of auditory sensitivity, the application of these stimuli in assessment of functional gain for various modes of amplification may prove more accurate than alternative stimuli. When a hearing aid is introduced, the potential for client response to components of frequencies other than the normal test frequency or any alternative stimuli may be affected not only by the slope of an individual audiogram, but also by the frequency response of the hearing aid and the interaction of these two variables" (p. 22).

Subsequent to their observation, Woodward and Tecca conducted a study to determine the efficiency of pure tone assessment in a sound field. They concluded that pure tone assessment is a "feasible option" for the examiner if careful attention is given to the proper positioning of the subject in a calibrated sound field. These conclusions assume, of course, that head position does not vary appreciably and that sound levels at the position of the subject's head are known. The clinical utilization of pure tone stimuli is encouraged as part of the evaluation process if test room conditions can be met, although there is no doubt that the accuracy of the data obtained can be influenced negatively by the test environment, test stimuli, and test procedure.

SPEECH DISCRIMINATION ASSESSMENT

Without qualification, the single most compelling reason for hearing aid use is to improve the hearing-impaired individual's ability to understand speech. While there is considerable disagreement among investigators regarding the speech stimulus of choice in the evaluation process, there is no disagreement that improved speech discrimination ability is the desired goal. The issue is whether clinical measures of discrimination function using standardized monosyllabic words have value in the selection and fitting of hearing aids. Reliance on the traditional CID W-22 word lists to delineate discrimination superiority among hearing aids is suspect. The reader is referred to Konkle and Molloy (Chap. 7) regarding a speech-based hearing aid evaluation to better understand the validity and reliability of speech-based testing in the hearing aid evaluation and selection process.

Regardless of the speech materials used to aid in the selection of the hearing aid device, such aided performance measurements can be made only in a controlled sound-field environment. If they are to be valid measures of aided performance, the acoustic environment in which discrimination scores are obtained should be monitored. Unusually high ambient noise levels will be reflected negatively in the discrimination score and will reduce the significance of speech discrimination tests in the decision-making process. This is especially relevant when comparing several hearing aids and selecting from among them the one that is the most propitious based on discrimination score differences. From a practical standpoint, almost any routine audiometric procedure or discrimination task can be carried out in a sound-field environment. The primary task remains that of selecting clinical test procedures that separate the appropriate hearing aid from the inappropriate, or the best from the adequate.

The underlying value of sound-field testing is that it provides a stable acoustic environment in which unaided responses can be compared to aided responses, regardless of the number of hearing aids evaluated. If speech discrimination differences among hearing aids are of major concern, regardless of the speech stimulus used, then sound-field assessment is a means by which the differences can be assessed realistically.

Understanding Speech in Noise

Every audiologist or dispenser is familiar with the problem that hearing-impaired individuals have in understanding the intended message (speech) in the presence of a background noise sufficient to interfere with the discrimination process. One of the major reasons for hearing instrument rejection is the inability to achieve adequate performance in various ambient noise backgrounds.

The ability to determine speech discrimination function in changing noise backgrounds is an important clinical procedure in the adequate management of the hearing-impaired patient. Many hearing aid devices that reduce the effects of background noise and maintain a favorable signal to noise ratio are available. Through sound-field aided measurements, the actual performance of a patient in a given noise-filled environment can be evaluated. Instrumental analysis of specific automated noise suppression circuitry defines only the electroacoustic performance of the hearing aid, not the psychoacoustic realities.

As mentioned previously, one of the more common complaints of hearing-impaired persons is not understanding speech in the presence of noise. The inability to function adequately in noise is not always eliminated or even significantly reduced by hearing aid use. There is, however, a clinical procedure that may assist the clinician in measuring the extent of signal detection and word recognition of the hearing-impaired individual in a noisy environment (Goldberg, 1981). With the patient seated in a sound-field environment, the hearing aid is adjusted to achieve a preferred listening level (PLL) (see Vol. I, Chap. 2). A speech-shaped noise is presented through a calibrated sound-field speaker at 70 dB SPL. A 3000 Hz pure tone signal at 70 dB SPL is presented to the patient. By reducing the intensity of the 3000 Hz pure tone signal in 5 dB steps while holding the speech noise constant, the *signal in noise* (SIN) can be determined. Essentially, the question is: How far down into the noise can the 3000 Hz signal go before it is no longer detected by the person under test? For normal hearing subjects, a 3000 Hz signal can be attenuated approximately 30 dB before it is no longer detected in a constant level speech-shaped noise. For a 1000 Hz signal in an identical environment, the average attenuation is 15 dB.

The implications of these tests are readily apparent. For patients who approximate normal SIN function in the aided condition, the audiologist or the dispenser can predict much less difficulty for speech discrimination tasks in noise than would be experienced by individuals who perform more poorly on this particular test in an identical noise environment.

It should be noted here that audiometric configuration and aided thresholds for the frequency range evaluated are not the only factors influencing the detection of pure tone or complex signals in noise. The pathologic status of the auditory system may also influence the ability to detect a signal in noise, regardless of the specific hearing aid selected or its level of electro-acoustic sophistication.

BINAURAL HEARING AND AIDED BINAURALITY

Binaural hearing is important and provides processing of information that is not possible monaurally. A method of achieving aided binaurality in the sound field can be extremely useful to the user of amplifying devices. The following procedures are suggested in setting the gain control of the hearing aids to achieve binaurality within the limitations of the hearing aid and the magnitude of the auditory deficit.

The patient is positioned with the head oriented properly and at an equal distance between two sound-field speakers. The speakers are at 90-degree azimuth and 9 in.

from the ear. A speech-shaped noise is introduced at 65 dB SPL. The patient is instructed to adjust the volume control of each hearing aid until midline balancing of the speech-shaped noise is achieved, that is, the speech-shaped noise appears to be in the center of the head. Although the procedure is straightforward, clinicians are cautioned to be aware that patients tend to move the head laterally in an attempt to achieve midline balancing rather than adjusting the gain control of the individual hearing aid. Usually, a simple instruction is sufficient to avoid this error. Head restraint can be utilized but should not be necessary when testing adults able to follow simple instructions.

Some clinicians prefer to employ pure tone stimuli in achieving aided binaurality, since more frequency specific information can be advantageous. Utilizing essentially the same procedure employed in achieving midline balancing for a speech-shaped noise, the frequencies most commonly used are 500, 1000, 2000, 3000, and 4000 Hz. The greater the degree of binaurality that can be achieved, regardless of the test stimulus employed, the more efficiently the patient can utilize the hearing aid amplification system. The hearing health professional is urged to consider using sound-field testing procedures in establishing binaurality when hearing instruments are used for bilateral impairment.

In some instances, due to other factors that control the loudness growth of an applied signal, it is recommended that loudness matching in establishing binaurality be assessed for input signals from 50 to 80 dB in increments of 5 dB. In instances where significant disparity exists, improved binaurality may be achieved by instrument modification or, in some cases, by selecting different hearing aid devices whose electroacoustic performances are more appropriate to the task at hand.

It is not always possible to achieve true binaurality at all input intensities due to pathological conditions of the auditory system or performance limitations imposed by the hearing aid device.

HEARING AID EVALUATION FORMULAE

The myriad formulae and clinical procedures recommended for use in the hearing aid selection process are somewhat overwhelming (Lybarger, 1944; Berger, 1976; Byrne & Tonnison, 1976; Shapiro, 1976; Berger, Hagberg, & Rane, 1977; Lybarger, 1978; Harford, 1981; Libby, 1982; McCandless & Lyregaard, 1983; Duffy & Zelnick, 1985; Libby, 1985; Byrne & Dillon, 1981; Libby, 1986; Westermann & Libby, 1988). Each formula is purported to provide the desired hearing aid output response characteristics needed by the patient to maximize speech understanding; yet theoretically, the required electroacoustic performance determined by one formula may differ substantially from the performance characteristics determined by another. Nonetheless, continued refinement of hearing aid evaluation formulae is to be encouraged. As more precise measurements of function are developed and as more appropriate hearing aid circuitry is designed to compensate for the hearing deficit, acoustically impaired persons are better served in the selection of hearing aids.

In essence, the controversy over methods of assessment and verification is a healthy one. Whether one favors probe microphone assessment or sound-field assessment in formula application, objective evidence of performance is being sought. Therefore, the question should not be "Is one better than the other?" but rather "What does each provide that lends itself to realistic measurement?"

Many of the formula approaches to hearing aid evaluation lend themselves to sound-field assessment to verify whether predicted gain functions are achieved when the hearing aid is fitted. In some formulae approaches, no attempt is made to establish the permissible maximum power output (SSPL90) of the hearing aid device based on uncomfortable loudness level (ULL) measures. While general consensus is not forthcoming from those involved in the hearing aid selection process, ULL measurements are critical to the selection process. Failure to control the maximum power output (SSPL90) of the instrument can lead to less than adequate hearing aid use, or even to rejection of the device. Sound-field evaluation of the patient's tolerance level to specific acoustic energies is tantamount to appropriate hearing instrument selection. The tolerance level obtained is directly translatable to the required SSPL-90 of the hearing aid device. However, the determination of ULL can be influenced by the instructions given to the patient. The best instruction is one that reflects the SSPL90 of the selected instrument and does not violate loudness sensitivity.

LOUDNESS FUNCTION

One of the most perplexing problems facing the audiologist or the dispenser is selecting the amplification system that best meets the patient's need regarding a loudness function that is mediated, in part, by the presenting pathology. The question is whether the selected hearing aid amplifies too much or too little, based on loudness growth generated by a given input signal. The ability to assess loudness function, or an approximation of it, results in the selection of hearing aid devices that achieve maximum utility. Loudness growth is closely coupled to the patient's dynamic range. It is generally accepted that the width of the dynamic range is often frequency specific. In other words, the dynamic range is greater, or wider, for the low frequency range than it is for the high frequency range for many individuals with impaired auditory function. Even a cursory examination of this fact suggests that sound-field assessment of differential dynamic range function provides invaluable data in determining the recommended electroacoustic performance of the hearing aid.

Figure 11–3 illustrates differential dynamic range function. Certainly, the patient's loudness function cannot be assessed by procedures other than psychoacoustic measures. Intensity is a physical quantity. It lends itself to measurement of the *size of the acoustic event* giving rise to hearing sensation. However, the psychological consequence of loudness is more closely related to the *quantity of the acoustic sensation.* In the fitting of hearing aid devices, loudness sensation plays a vital role in the selection of an appropriate amplification system.

Sound-field audiometry presents a viable method of accomplishing unaided and aided assessment of loudness function. Its importance to the instrument selection process is to be encouraged in the evaluation process.

CASE STUDIES

It is generally conceded by professionals who select and fit hearing aid devices that at least three basic functions should be assessed: threshold sensitivity, PLL, and ULL. The reasoning is simply that threshold sensitivity gives the hearing health professional a reference point from which to predict the patient's ability to detect acoustic stimuli. The PLL in the aided mode should, if possible, permit the patient to hear comfortably all of the critical elements of speech to achieve maximum discrimination. The SSPL90 of the aid should be set at a level slightly below the patient's ULL, thereby eliminating the necessity for constant adjustment of the hearing aid volume control in changing acoustic environments. The emphasis given to these three measurements is not meant to imply that other sound-field tests pale by comparison. It suggests only that, if the out-

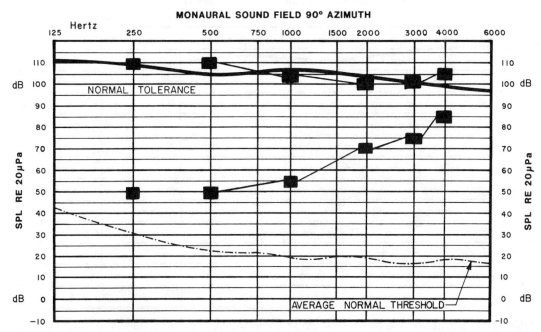

FIGURE 11-3. Differential dynamic range (area between closed squares) as a function of frequency for a hearing-impaired listener. Note the reduced dynamic range for frequencies above 1000 Hz.

put response of the hearing aid meets the requirements of threshold, PLL, and ULL, the probablity of patient success with amplification is enhanced greatly.

Notwithstanding the possible limitations imposed by discrete frequency measurements, the following theoretical case studies suggest some of the advantages of sound-field evaluation. The reader should keep in mind that the case studies given here are hypothetical. However, they do approximate the responses of hearing-impaired individuals seen for a hearing aid evaluation and the selection and fitting of a hearing aid.

In Figure 11–4 unaided threshold responses suggest a hearing impairment that is significantly more pronounced in the high frequency range. The aided threshold data indicate only a minimal acoustic gain when the hearing aid was adjusted to the patient's MCL using a speech input of approximately 65 dB SPL. When analyzing the aided data, some clinical observations

are evident. The average acoustic gain for frequencies above 1000 Hz approximates 15 dB. Although this gain provides some improvement in high frequency sensitivity, it falls short of providing high frequency information adequate to discriminate clearly among several consonant sounds.

However, assuming that the hypothetical individual shown in Figure 11–4 was fitted with a linear amplifier, if threshold sensitivity is improved by increasing the use gain of the hearing aid, then the MCL, which was set previously by the user of the device, is exceeded. Subsequently, if such volume control adjustments are made, the user frequently will adjust the volume setting to again obtain the desired MCL to reduce negative reaction to inputs that exceed acceptable listening levels. In this case, two things need to be considered to achieve optimal use: modification of the frequency response to permit significantly improved threshold sensitivity without violation of MCL or ULL values or selection of a differ-

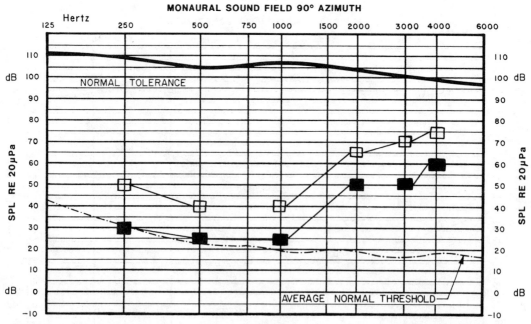

FIGURE 11–4. Unaided and aided threshold values indicating that high frequency sensitivity is inadequate for maximum discrimination of acoustic events. Open squares indicate unaided sensitivity and closed squares indicate aided function when the hearing aid is adjusted to the patient's MCL.

ent hearing aid that has the capacity to improve threshold sensitivity while maintaining acceptable MCL and ULL function.

The functional gain values shown in Figure 11-5 indicate that the electroacoustic response of hearing aid A imposes limitations on signal perception and discrimination of high frequency sounds. Not only can some consonant confusion be predicted by reason of limited acoustic gain above 1000 Hz but the distance at which certain acoustic inputs can be detected can be computed fairly accurately. The better the improvement in threshold sensitivity, the more effectively an impaired auditory system can perceive acoustic signals at specific distances. Consider, for example, a person who can *just* detect a speech signal in the unaided mode at a distance of 10 ft. Now, assume that a hearing aid is fitted and adjusted to improve that person's threshold sensitivity by 10 dB. This means that the

same signal can now be detected at three times the initial distance, or 30 ft, that is, the person could move back to a distance of 30 ft and still perceive the speech signal. However, if the hearing aid can improve the threshold sensitivity by 20 dB, as suggested by hearing aid B, then the same speech signal can be detected at 10 times the distance or 100 ft. Now, the same individual could move 100 ft from the signal source and perceive its presence.

Notice the change in functional gain values at 2000 Hz for the discrete sound-field audiogram shown in Figure 11-5. Hearing aid A provided a threshold improvement of 10 dB, or a three-fold increase in threshold sensitivity, with subsequent improvement in signal detection. While this offers a substantial improvement in signal detection, it falls short of what could be provided by a hearing aid device with a different electroacoustic per-

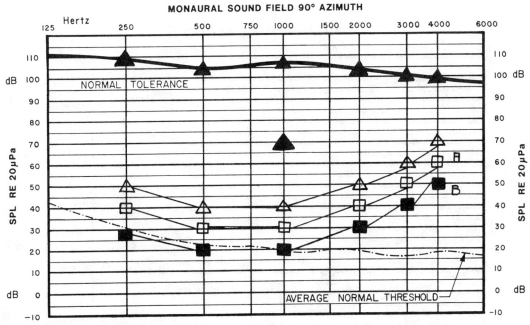

FIGURE 11-5. The sound-field audiogram shown suggests aided changes in threshold sensitivity and resulting improvement in distance hearing without violation of MCL or ULL. Unaided values are indicated by the open triangles. The open squares are response values for hearing aid A and the closed squares are response values for hearing aid B. The closed triangles are representative of aided MCL and ULL values.

formance. For example, hearing aid B improved threshold sensitivity at 2000 Hz by 20 dB, thus improving signal detection ability at that frequency tenfold compared to the unaided state.

This kind of aided analysis provides useful information to the clinician in judging whether the instrument selected provides what is deemed to be an adequate instrument for the hearing impairment present. Such analyses have immediate application in the decision-making process. This is especially true given currently available hearing aid instrumentation that permits modification of output responses in a number of ways (i.e., gain, slope, MPO, frequency range, etc.). Sound-field audiometry, therefore, provides an acceptable method of plotting several psychoacoustic responses from which decisions can be made as any specific electroacoustic parameter is altered.

Obviously, functional gain measures provide something more than assessment of signal detection at specified distances. They can determine, for example, whether the gain provided exceeds desired optimum levels.

Consider the audiometric data displayed on the sound-field audiogram shown in Figure 11–6. Of particular interest are the threshold responses shown at 250, 500, and 1000 Hz. It is apparent that if too much acoustic gain is presented at these frequencies, the patient will change the volume control setting to eliminate overamplification of the lower frequencies. Subsequently, there will be a reduction of high frequency sensitivity, which reduces the use value of the amplified high frequency range. The patient now finds himself between "a rock and a hard place." He or she must accept excessive or unwanted low frequency amplification to perceive and more efficiently use high frequency information for better speech understanding or reduce low frequency amplification to maintain an acceptable MCL and lose

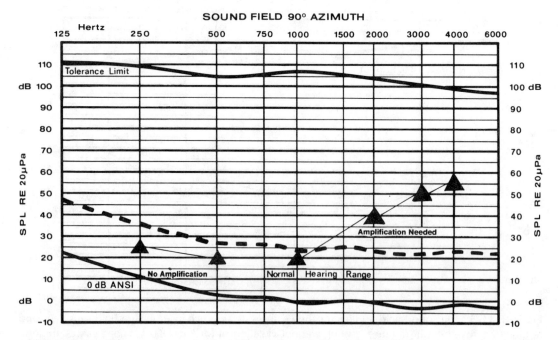

FIGURE 11–6. The unaided thresholds shown indicate normal hearing between 250 and 1000 Hz. There is a significant loss of hearing above 1000 Hz requiring amplification for optimal discrimination function. Amplification of the lower frequency range may interfere significantly with MCL function and speech discrimination ability.

high frequency information. Obviously, if excessive gain is present in the frequency range between 250 and 1000 Hz, the upward spread of masking may interfere with discrimination function.

There is a reasonable alternative which can be exercised. The low frequency response of the selected hearing aid can be changed by circuit modification or by appropriate venting of the earmold. Sound-field analysis can also provide a reliable and permanent record of the effect of circuit or venting alterations by obtaining psychoacoustic responses associated with those changes to determine acceptability.

Acoustic gain is not the only value that can be analyzed by sound-field audiometric procedures. Let us consider, in a limited way, the usefulness of sound-field audiometry in assessing speech discrimination function. Speech discrimination scores have limited value in predicting either the integrity of the auditory system or the function-

al efficiency of the hearing aid. However, sound-field measurement can provide a general assessment of speech performance. For example, consider the information in the hypothetical sound-field audiogram shown in Figure 11–7. In the unaided mode, monosyllabic words presented at 65 dB SPL yielded a discrimination score of 46 percent. Hearing aid A increased the discrimination score to 70 percent. Hearing aid B, which provides sufficient gain to permit identification of all speech sounds, improved the score to 84 percent. The conclusion drawn is simply that as more of the critical elements of the speech spectrum are perceived, the probability of correct identification of the intended message increases.

It is interesting that, had instrument B been fitted to the impaired ear in the first place, improved discrimination function would have been predicted by virtue of the speech spectrum now perceived by the user of the device. The actual score itself is, in

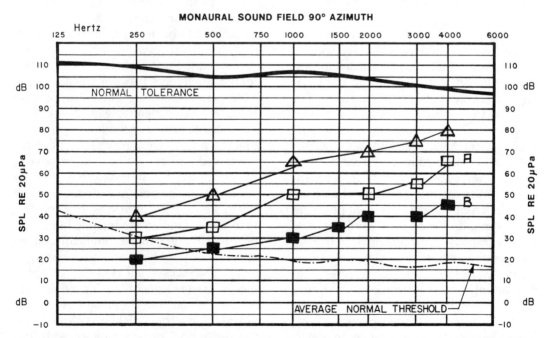

FIGURE 11–7. Speech discrimination scores as a function of change in threshold sensitivity. The speech input signal is 65 dB in the unaided and aided mode. In the aided mode, the instrument is adjusted to the preferred listening level. The open triangles represent the unaided thresholds. The open squares represent threshold values for hearing aid A and the closed squares represent threshold values for hearing aid B. The discrimination scores are 52, 70, and 86 percent, respectively.

part, a function of the auditory system's integrity and is not predicated solely on the hearing aid's ability to reinstate perception of the speech spectrum.

Sound-field analysis provides the audiologist or the dispenser with clinical evidence that the speech spectrum is audible and that the hearing aid under test yields a discrimination function either equal to or better than that achieved in the unaided mode when the speech signal is at a comfortable listening level.

The example given in Figure 11–7 suggests that as the aided response improves perception of the speech spectrum discrimination improves. However, the discrimination score obtained using hearing aid B does not reflect amplification use over time. Some improvement in speech discrimination performance would be expected as the user of the device adjusts to acoustic information not heard for some time.

INTER-OCTAVE ASSESSMENT

One of the limitations of discrete sound-field audiometry is that interoctave information, which may be needed to provide frequency data essential to the hearing aid selection process, is missing. For example, in threshold assessment and functional gain measurements, simply measuring 500, 1000, 2000, 3000, and 4000 Hz does not provide an ongoing assessment of the patient's response sensitivity to frequencies between octaves. Computer-assisted probe microphone measurement produces a fairly rapid display of a continous frequency response. This information in both the unaided and aided modes is very useful in determining whether there are significant interoctave aberrations that would reduce the utility of the hearing aid or encourage its rejection. Probe microphone measurements are appropriate in determining the adequacy of the hearing instrument selected.

PATIENT COUNSELING

One of the most useful tasks performed by the audiologist or hearing aid dispenser is offering realistic and pertinent information about the use of hearing aid amplification systems. It is one thing to assess the function of the auditory system and arrive at desired electroacoustic parameters to be reflected in the hearing aid of choice. It is, however, quite a different matter to explain the performance of the hearing aid and its probable advantages to the user of the device. To those who work with the hearing impaired, it is apparent that many persons who have hearing losses are reasonable candidates for hearing aids but are reluctant to accept hearing aid amplification because they are uncertain of the advantages to be gained. New hearing aid candidates, who experience hearing aid amplification for the first time, may mistrust the audiologist or the dispenser who recommends specific instruments. In such instances, the individual should be presented with tangible and demonstrable evidence that the hearing aid to be used performs at predictable and useful levels.

Sound-field test results that indicate significant changes between aided and unaided performance are often instrumental in helping the patient to gain insight into the probable benefit of the hearing aid. For example, if there are appreciable differences in unaided and aided threshold responses, the patient can be counseled that not only will he or she be able to hear more of the speech signal, thus improving the probability of understanding the intended message, but also will experience a significant change in the ability to hear and understand at greater distances. Such counseling cannot only reduce the fears of hearing aid use, but can also demonstrate the advantages of amplification in a sound field and clearly indicate differences in performance with and without the hearing aid, as related to improved intelligibility and distance hearing.

Other useful procedures to improve patients' acceptance of hearing aid amplification through effective counseling practices include demonstration of binaural versus monaural hearing aid use, formal speech discrimination tests, and speech understanding in noise. Obviously, it is the magnitude of the differences in performance between the unaided and the aided state that makes the advantages to be gained by hearing aid use clear to the patient.

Although, on the surface, it may sound like a negative approach to effective counseling, sound-field audiometry can also be used to demonstrate the limitations of hearing aid amplification. For example, there are types of hearing impairment and information processing deficits that make it impossible for the hearing aid to provide significant changes in a patient's ability to discriminate speech at a level thought possible by the recipient of the hearing aid. Although such limited capacity does not rule out the use of amplification, it is important for the patient to understand the limitations imposed without rejecting the hearing aid itself. If various listening or performance tasks are carried out in a sound field, the individual is better able to assess the reduced ability to function and, at the same time, appreciate the value of hearing information not available to him or her without the hearing aid. In essence, the task is to provide the patient with straightforward information about the limitations of the device but at the same time let the person know that a hearing aid is still useful and provides awareness of acoustic stimuli not possible without the hearing aid amplification system.

Sound-field audiometry is also a valuable asset in effective counseling in follow-up care of the patient. Patients' complaints can frequenctly be identified and remedied by judicious use of selected audiometric procedures. For example, if a person frequently experiences loudness discomfort, sound-field analysis may indicate that discomfort is apparent when the output signal of the instrument is only slightly above the person's MCL. Therefore, the SSPL90 should be reassessed and the permissible output should be controlled to fall within the LDL of the individual using the hearing aid device.

In reality, almost any complaint that the person has regarding hearing aid use can be assessed through sound-field procedures. Consider, for example, the following patient complaints, which can be identified and resolved through sound-field procedures: insufficient gain at selected frequencies, speech understanding in noise, excessive gain at one or more frequencies, quality judgment of hearing aid performance, and other factors that may arise from time to time.

Above all else, hearing aid use depends on the patient's acceptance of the device that was recommended. Although the audiologist or the dispenser may employ the latest in technological advances and the most current evaluation procedure, the person's reaction to amplified sound must be managed in such a manner as to encourage acceptance and continued use of the hearing aid. Sound-field testing is often an effective tool in determining the nature of the patient's complaint and the modification of the hearing aid response needed to reduce or resolve the magnitude of the complaint.

Deborah Law (personal communication, 1988) suggested that in most instances when individuals with mild or ski slope hearing losses are fitted with hearing aids they are unaware of marked improvement in speech discrimination function in acoustically stable and quiet environmental situations. As a patient management strategy, she places the person in a sound field and presents phonetically balanced, monosyllabic words in a background of speech-weighted noise at various S/N ratios, while holding the speech output constant. She reasons that for many patients who have mild or ski slope losses, discrimination for the CID W-22 monosyllabic words is often equal in the unaided and aided mode in a quiet listening environment. To demonstrate to the patient that the hearing aid is of significant value, aided and unaided assessment is conducted with the competing noise (speech noise) at a set S/N ratio. As an alternative practice, she also tests the patient in a sound-field environment in which the noise remains constant and the signal strength is varied. The aided discrimination scores should reflect, in part, the value of the hearing aid when S/N ratios are changed.

The value of these procedures is to reinforce the use of amplification, based on demonstrable evidence that the individual's ability to perform is enhanced by hearing aid use. Law has found that, if these procedures are conducted at the time of the initial fitting of the device, fewer problems are encountered and a much more positive attitude about amplification is established.

Goldberg (1981) suggested that patient management can be enhanced by explaining that "the finished sound field audiogram which contains an unaided and aided readout is one of the best means of representing the contribution of the hearing aid and, at the same time, indicating a person's improved hearing as it relates to normal hearing. If the person who is fitted is a hearing aid user, an aided measurement (in a sound field) utilizing his current hearing aid versus a newly fitted aid will indicate the degree of improvement provided by the new aid when related to the old aid" (p. 186).

Any psychoacoustic assessment employed in the decision-making process for determining the appropriate hearing aid should have meaning to the current user of hearing aid amplification or to the individual who is contemplating its use. Obviously, one of the important aspects of any hearing aid's performance is related to the discrimination of acoustic events (i.e., speech and other informational hearing signals) in

a variety of listening environments. The more objective data presented to the patient relative to the contributions of the hearing aid, the easier it is to provide the necessary follow-up care, including modification of output response when indicated by patient performance. Employing the advantages of sound-field assessment relative to psychoacoustic measurements can make patient management more effective.

The role of the hearing health professional includes hearing assessment, instrument selection, and patient management. These roles are not mutually exclusive tasks but must co-exist if the individual is to be well served in a manner that is not misleading, either in the expectation of what the hearing aid device can provide or in the ability of the person to process information, regardless of its level of amplification. Sound-field testing is an excellent means of demonstrating the realities of hearing aid use. Coupled with other patient management strategies, it can provide the audiologist or the dispenser and the patient with valuable information with which to make intelligent decisions about hearing aid amplification systems and their acceptance.

SUMMARY

Sound-field audiometry is a useful tool in the evaluation, selection, fitting, and verification processes of hearing aid use. It provides a method of assessing unaided and aided responses to specific acoustic stimuli in a controlled acoustic environment in which the measures obtained reflect the contributions of the hearing aid when compared with unaided responses to identical stimuli in an identical acoustic field.

Sound-field analysis does not imply that other measurement protocols are not pertinent to the decision-making processes in the selection of hearing aid devices. Without question they are. The recent contributions of probe microphone assessment have been most beneficial in analyzing the spectral distributions of the signal at the patient's eardrum in the aided and unaided mode.

In the final analysis, the individual patient's response to selected acoustic stimuli in a controlled environment is important in determining the appropriateness of the hearing aid device with which the person has been fitted.

REFERENCES

Berger, K. (1976). Prescription of hearing aids: A rationale. *Journal of the American Audiology Society, 2,* 71–78.

Berger, K., Hagberg, E., & Rane, E. (1977). *Prescription of hearing aids: Rationale, procedures and results.* Kent, OH: Herald Publishing House.

Byrne, D., & Dillon, H. (1981). Comparative reliability of warble tone thresholds under earphones and in a sound field. *Australian Journal of Audiology, 3,* 12–13.

Byrne, D., Dillon, A., & Dillon, H. (1987). The National Acoustics Laboratories (NAL) new procedures for selecting the gain and frequency response of a hearing aid. *Ear and Hearing, 7,* 257–265.

Byrne, D., & Tonnison, W. (1976). Selecting the gain of hearing aids for persons with sensorineural hearing impairments. *Scandinavian Audiology, 5,* 51–59.

Carhart, R. (1946). The selection of hearing aids. *Archives of Otolaryngology, 44,* 1–18.

D'Antonio, P. (1986, Sept.–Oct.). Control room design incorporating RFZ, LFD and RPG diffusions. *dB,* 47–55.

DeJonge, R. (1983). Computer similarity of hearing aid frequency response. *The Hearing Journal, 36,* 27–31.

Duffy, J. K. (1967). Audio-visual speech audiometry and a new audio-visual speech perception index. *Maico Audiological Library Services, 5*(9), 1–3.

Duffy, J. K. (1978). Sound field audiometry and hearing aid advancement. *Hearing Instruments, 29*(2), 6–12.

Duffy, J. K., & Zelnick, E. (1985). A critique of past and current hearing aid assessment procedures. *Audecibel, 34,* 10–23.

Gilman, S., Dirks, D. D., & Stern, R. (1981). The effects of occluded ear impedance on the eardrum SPL produced by hearing aids. *Journal of the Acoustical Society of America, 70,* 370–386.

Goldberg, H. (1981, Fall). Sound field audiometric measurements. *Audecibel,* 183–186.

Harford, E. R. (1981). A new clinical technique for verification of hearing aid response. *Archives of Otolaryngology, 8,* 462.

Hawkins, D. B., & Montgomery, A. A., & Prosek, B. E. (1987). Examination of two issues concerning functional gain measurements. *Journal of Speech and Hearing Disorders, 52,* 56–63.

Hawkins, D. B., & Mueller, H. G. (1986). Some variables of testing the accuracy of probe tube microphone measurement. *Hearing Instruments, 1,* 8.

Hawkins, D. B., & Schum, D. J. (1984). Relationships among various measures of hearing aid gain. *Journal of Speech and Hearing Disorders, 49,* 94–97.

Jerger, J. (1987). Personal correspondence.

Killion, M. C. (1987). Earmold options for wideband hearing band hearing aids. *Journal of Speech and Hearing Disorders, 46,* 10–20.

Law, D. (1988, December 10). Personal correspondence.

Libby, E. R. (1982). In search of transparent insertion gain hearing aid responses. In G. Studebaker & F. Bess (Eds.), *The Vanderbilt hearing aid report: Monographs in contemporary audiology.* Upper Darby, PA.

Libby, E. R. (1985). State of the art of hearing aid selection procedures. *Hearing Instruments, 1,* 30.

Libby, E. R. (1986). The 1/3–2/3 insertion gain hearing aid selection guide. *Hearing Instruments, 3,* 27–28.

Lybarger, S. F. (1944). Patent application S.N. 543, 278, July 3, 1944, as reported in Lybarger, S. F. (1944). Selective amplification — A review and evaluation. *Journal of the American Audiology Society, 3*(6), 259–260.

Lybarger, S. F. (1978). Earmolds. In J. Katz (Ed.), *Handbook of clinical audiology* (2nd ed., pp. 508–523). Baltimore: Williams & Wilkins.

Macrae, J. H. (1982). The validity of aided thresholds. *Australian Journal of Audiology, 4*(2), 48–54.

Macrae, J., & Frazer, G. (1980). An investigation of variables affecting aided thresholds. *Australian Journal of Audiology, 2,* 56–62.

Macrae, J. H., & Page, S. (1980). A procedure for checking the validity of aided thresholds. *NAL Informal Report* (No. 69). Sydney, Australia: National Acoustics Laboratories.

McCandless, G. A., & Lyregaard, P. E. (1983). Prescription of gain output (POGO) for hearing aids. *Hearing Instruments, 1,* 16–21.

Mason, D., & Popelka, G. (1986). Comparison of hearing aid gain using functional, coupler, and probe-tube measurements. *Journal of Speech and Hearing Research, 29,* 218–226.

Pascoe, D. P. (1975). Frequency responses of hearing aids and their effect on the speech perception of hearing impaired subjects. *Laryngology, 84*(Suppl. 23, No. 5, Part 2), 5–40.

Preves, D. (1984, July). Levels of realism in hearing aid measurement techniques. *The Hearing Journal, 37,* 13–19.

Preves, D., & Sullivan, A. F. (1987). Sound field equalization for real ear measurements with probe microphones. *Hearing Instruments, 1,* 21.

Ross, M., & Duffy, J. (1961). Report on sound field audiometry. Paper presented at the American Speech and Hearing Convention, Chicago, IL.

Shapiro, I. (1976) Hearing aid fitting by prescription. *Audiology, 15,* 163–173.

Victoreen, J. (1973). *Hearing enhancement.* Springfield, IL: Charles C. Thomas.

West, R., Ansberry, M., & Carr, A. (1957). *The rehabilitation of speech* (3rd ed.) New York: Harper.

Westermann, S., & Libby, E. R. (1988). Real ear measurements and their implications. In R. E. Sandlin (Ed.), *Handbook of hearing aid amplification. I. Theoretical and technical considerations.* Boston: College-Hill Press.

Woodward, C. M., & Tecca, J. E. (1985). The use of pure tone stimuli in a sound field. *Hearing Journal, 38,* 21–27.

Zemplenyi, J., Dirks, D., & Gilman, S. (1985). Probe-determined hearing aid gain compared to functional and coupler gains. *Journal of Speech and Hearing Research, 28,* 394–403.

Zelnick, E. (1982). Selecting frequency response. *Hearing Aid Journal, 35*(3), 31.

■ Author Index

Abrams, S., 89
Adkins, W. V., 153
Abberton, E., 182
Adler, A., 24
Ahlstrom, C., 248
Alencewicz, C. M., 190
Alpiner, J. G., 144, 156, 158, 159
American National Standard Institute (ANSI), 167, 175, 226
Anderson, C. V., 155
Ansberry, M., 157
Antonelli, A., 89, 90
Arnst, D., 50, 90
Ashley, J., 148
Atchley, R. C., 142
Atherly, G. R., 158
Atkinson, A., 22, 24, 25

Bagwell, C. L., 90
Banfai, P., 182, 183
Baran, J. A., 88, 89
Barber, B., 92, 93
Barford, J., 156, 160
Barker, R. G., 4
Barley, M., 197
Baver, B., 33
Baxter, J. H., 160
Beasley, D. S., 89, 90
Beattie, J. A., 149
Beattie, R., 171, 213
Beauchaine, K. A., 205, 208, 213, 214, 215, 216, 217
Beck, E., 170
Beck, L., 35, 36, 37, 239, 242, 243
Becker, G., 148
Becker, M., 173
Beckmann, N. J., 52, 94

Bell, T., 175, 248
Bender, D., 31
Benitez, J., 88
Bentler, R. A., 125
Berger, K. W., 92, 94, 157, 169, 172, 225, 268
Bergman, M., 90, 135
Bergstrom, L., 114
Berkowitz, A., 94, 147
Berlin, C. I., 89
Berliner, K. I., 192
Bess, F. H., 90, 124, 125, 126, 167, 169, 170
Bienvenue, G., 153
Bilger, J. H., 89
Bilger, R. C., 153, 171
Binnie, C. A., 125
Birk-Nielsen, H., 158
Birren, J. E., 142
Blackington, B., 154, 155
Blamey, P. J., 180, 185
Blood, G. W., 149
Blood, I. M., 149
Blow, M. E., 217
Blumfield, V., 90
Bobbin, R., 211
Bocca, E., 89
Bolton, B., 4
Boney, S., 248
Boorsma, A., 168
Boothroyd, A., 192
Bosatra, A., 90
Botwinick, J., 151
Bowlby, J., 5, 7
Bowmeester, J., 153
Boyd, R., 213
Brackmann, D. E., 179, 182
Braida, L. D., 170, 214
Bratt, G., 170

■ SUBJECT INDEX